The Good Samaritan Nurse in a Secular Age

Teresa Lynch

This book is published by
Grosvenor House Publishing Ltd
Link House
140 The Broadway, Tolworth, Surrey, KT6 7HT.
www.grosvenorhousepublishing.co.uk

A CIP record for this book
is available from the British Library

ISBN 978-1-80381-295-3
eBook ISBN 978-1-80381-619-7

I am sincerely grateful for the invaluable support during the writing of this book to:

Dr John Duddington, editor of *Law and Justice: The Christian Law Review* and secretary of the Medical Ethics Alliance, for his patient, kind and constructive support and encouragement.

Mr David Galloway, past President of the Royal College of Physicians and Surgeons of Glasgow, for his generous time and useful questions.

I would like to thank the nursing and medical contributors who wrote the foreword:

Mary Farnan, secretary of the UK Association of Catholic Nurses, England and Wales.

Professor Patrick Pullicino, retired Professor of Neurology and also for his helpful comments on the manuscript.

With thanks also to the following who read and offered comments on the manuscript:

Dr Gosia Brykczynska, executive committee member of the UK Association of Catholic Nurses, England and Wales and President of the European Region of the International Catholic Committee of Nurses and Medico-Social Assistants (CICIAMS).

Dr Tony Cole, retired paediatrician and Chair of the Medical Ethics Alliance.

Dr Majid Katme, past President of the Islamic Medical Association in the UK. Leader of the Pro-life, Pro-family Muslim campaign in the UK/UN.

I dedicate this book to the memory of my devoted parents,
my mother, a good listener and great artist and my father,
a true physician advocate for all his patients.

In tribute to all the patients, good nurses, doctors, care support
workers, students, and other members of the multidisciplinary
teams that I have met throughout my career.

With thanks to my family and friends for
all their support and encouragement.

Contents

Acronyms used and their meanings

The following acronyms are used throughout this book.

Acronym	Meaning
AMA	American Medical Association
ACP	American College of Physicians
APG	All Party Group
APPG	All-Party Parliamentary Group
BMA	British Medical Association
CANH	Clinically-assisted nutrition and hydration
CDS	Continuous deep sedation
CEO	Chief Executive Officer
CHI	Commission for Health Improvement
CPR	Cardiopulmonary resuscitation
CPS	Crown Prosecution Service
CQC	Care Quality Commission
CQUIN	Commission for Quality and Innovation
DCD	Donation after circulatory death
DBD	Donation after brain death
DH	Department of Health
DID	Dignity in Dying
DNACPR	Do not attempt cardiopulmonary resuscitation
ECHR	European Court of Human Rights
EMA	European Medicines Agency
EPA	Enduring power of attorney
FATE	Friends at the End
FDA	Food and Drug Administration
GMC	General Medical Council

Acronym	Meaning
GSF	Gold Standard Framework
GSFCH	The Gold Standard Framework in Care Homes Programme
HNA	Holistic needs assessment
HSE	Health and Safety Executive
IEAs	Immediate and essential actions
IDD	Imminent death organ donation
IMCA	Independent Mental Capacity Advocate
i/v	Intravenous (into a vein)
JFK	John F. Kennedy
LCP	Liverpool Care Pathway
LPA	Lasting power of attorney
MAiD	Medical Assistance in Dying
MCA	Mental Capacity Act
MCS	Minimally conscious state
NCPC	The National Council for Palliative Care
NHS	National Health Service
NICE	National Institute for Health and Care Excellence
NMC	Nursing and Midwifery Council
PALS	Patient Advice and Liaison Service
PEG	Percutaneous endoscopic gastrostomy
PHSO	Parliamentary and Health Services Ombudsman
PICC	Peripherally inserted central catheter
PVS	Persistent vegetative state
RCN	Royal College of Nursing
RCOG	Royal College of Obstetricians and Gynaecologists
RCP	Royal College of Physicians
RCUK	Resuscitation Council UK

Acronym	Meaning
ReSPECT	Recommended Summary Plan for Emergency Care and Treatment
RN	Registered nurse
RIG	Radiologically inserted gastrostomy
s/c	Subcutaneous (under the skin)
SPUC	Society for the Protection of Unborn Children
UDDA	Uniform Determination of Death Act (USA)
UKCC	United Kingdom Central Council for nursing, midwifery and health visiting (replaced by the NMC)
UN	United Nations
WHO	World Health Organisation
WMA	World Medical Association

Foreword

A nursing perspective

St Augustine in his teachings describes an *Exitus* and *Reditus*, that we come from God and eventually return to God, and tells us that life is our journey through that process – a journey which is often tortuous and trialled with various forms of adversity that can affect our physical, mental and spiritual well-being. While the Church provides rites of passage through the sacraments to help us on that journey, we are intrinsically interdependent, so we all depend on the vocations and skills of trained professionals and carers such as doctors and nurses and other key workers that support those professions, many of whom have selflessly put their own lives at risk to ensure the care and well-being of so many others during the COVID-19 pandemic. Sadly, some have lost their own lives in the process.

The pandemic raised many ethical concerns where stretched resources and lack of equipment led to decisions being made as to whose survival was supported and who, where a poorer prognosis has been made, was left to die in isolation from loved ones due to COVID-19 restrictions. Each death was not just a hospital statistic, but a mother, father, son, or daughter to those grieving at home.

Respect for human life and the relief of suffering is integral to the nursing profession and, although we live in an increasingly secular society, the Royal College of Nursing (RCN) continues to reinforce the need for holistic care, stating in a report about its member survey about spirituality in nursing: 'Each person will have cultural, spiritual and religious beliefs that will shape the care you give' (RCN, 2010). Although care delivery must be client-centred, nurses too must deal with their own beliefs and feelings, while working to the Nursing and Midwifery Council (NMC) Code of Conduct (NMC, 2018).

Due to the overload and strain on services throughout the pandemic, doctors and nurses were not always able to respond to the individual needs of their patients as they would have wished. They often tried to offer that holistic support to patients grieving and dying alone in isolation from their families, while having to deal with their own emotional stress and burnout. This led many to question the political processes leading to ethical decisions being made that do not sit comfortably with their own consciences.

Pope Francis in *Amoris Lætitia* (2016) recognised how broken many of us are by everyday human life situations and that, although the Church is there to guide and inform us, as St John Henry Newman also argued, our individual conscience is paramount in informing our moral decisions.

This book by Teresa is excellent in highlighting that as doctors or nurses, we each have our role as the Good Samaritan, to give recognition to what our consciences tell us when faced with tough decisions, while recognising that we are also bound by our requirement to work within the NMC Code and guidance on conscientious objection. The NMC regulatory body for the nursing profession sets standards of care to protect the safety of patients. The role of nurses, working to NMC standards and to their consciences and duty of care, should not be to judge or discriminate or pass by on the other side of someone in need of care, but rather to question and to discern each individual situation to ensure the beneficence and non-maleficence of all levels of our care delivery in any situation, in any healthcare setting.

Mary Farnan, national secretary, Association of
Catholic Nurses of England and Wales.

A medical perspective

This book is about the 'Good Samaritan Nurse' who, like the gospel Samaritan, is moved by compassion not only to ethical, humane care but also to what springs from it: patient advocacy, vocation-driven respect for life and a belief that conscience gives insight into unethical practices.

Teresa Lynch is motivated by concern for Christian nurses in the hostile modern secular or anti-Christian environment. Nurses may feel helpless in an environment that created the Liverpool Care Pathway (LCP) (see Chapter 10) and continues to foster end of life 'care' through sedation and dehydration. Indifference to patients' needs and suffering may be injurious to nurses' health. Required participation in ethically tenuous practices, such as certain organ transplantation protocols, can be profoundly disturbing.

Although it may be a serious matter for nurses to challenge treatment decisions, the modern nurse is thrust centre stage into end of life decisions by her role in 'best interest' meetings and potentially as a palliative care nurse. In these settings, nurses can exert significant pressure on doctors' decisions and must be careful that their recommendations are always ethically based and motivated by genuine concern for the patient rather than to reduce the burden of difficult-to-nurse patients.

This may be increasingly difficult when a ward is poorly staffed, or nurses are pushed to perform duties above their grade. There is an ethical need both to support difficult patients as well as to ensure superiors are repeatedly appraised of inadequate staffing levels or failing morale.

The book importantly stresses that hydration and nutrition are basic humane care, not 'treatment' that can be withdrawn based on subjective quality of life or futility of treatment determinations.

The Good Samaritan comprehensively covers the areas that every ethically conscious nurse or doctor needs to navigate in the increasingly complex and treacherous modern medical environment. It could serve as a vade mecum to which a nurse or doctor can refer, not only for guidance in ethically contentious medical areas, but also the inclusion of relevant case law, medical association guidelines and Catholic Church teaching which gives a rich ethical and legal framework.

This book is unique as a guide to areas often skipped over in medical texts and deserves to be widely read and used as a sourcebook and guide for nurses and doctors.

Professor Patrick Pullicino,
retired consultant
neurologist.

Preface

Take care of him.
(Luke 10: 25–37)

The content of this book is aimed at nurses, midwives and other health professionals, but I hope that non-clinical health managers, policy makers and the public, may find exploration of the issues to be informative, thus empowering, for the future.

I wanted to author this book with the overall Christian theme of the parable of the Good Samaritan. The content is, therefore, written from a Christian perspective in line with this famous parable. The learning and expectations of this Christian parable apply to us all, whether lay people, health professionals, Christians, those belonging to other religions or those with no religious affiliation.

Although the term 'nurse' is used throughout the book, this can also be taken to include midwife and can relate to other health professionals, educators, managers and chief executive officers, in terms of their need to act as the Good Samaritan. Parliamentarians, too, need to remember their responsibility for listening to and protecting the public, including legal developments which may affect ethical treatment and care.

Consumerism and secularism

The concepts of the Good Samaritan and the 'good nurse' need exploration where consumerism and secularism appear to have an increasing dominance of contemporary life. Nurses, despite their intentions to heal and to act as the patient's advocate in line with their conscience and code of conduct, can find themselves working within a hostile culture. A common result of which is that the right of patients to ethical care and health professionals' rights to conscientious objection in practice are increasingly challenged. This is a radical change in orientation to care which is distressing to many practitioners.

They must work within the expectations of their code of conduct and conscience, resisting the pressure and expectation to act as a 'team player' where unethical practice is experienced.

NHS healthcare scandals

Long-standing National Health Service (NHS) care failures can be attributed to power corrupting some professionals who have power over life and death within, at times, understaffed settings. It is clear, that the greater the responsibility, the greater the expectation of accountability and transparency. Just 'obeying orders', however, is not a defence for any practitioner's action or lack of action which results in patient harm.

The press release for the New Charter for Health Care Workers (2017), states that: All these workers carry out their daily practice in an interpersonal relationship, marked by the trust of a person marked by suffering and illness, who resorts to science and the knowledge of a healthcare worker, who comes towards them to assist and heal them (Holy See Press Office, 2017).

The Preface of the Charter states that "The Charter certainly cannot amount to an exhaustive treatment of all the problems and questions that come up in the field of healthcare and sickness, but it was produced to offer the clearest possible guidelines for the ethical problems that must be addressed in the world of healthcare in general, in harmony with the teachings of Jesus Christ and the magisterium of the Church" (Pontifical Council for Pastoral Assistance to Health Care Workers, 2017). The work is divided into three major sections: "Procreating," "Living," and "Dying," each of which lays out authoritative teachings in medical ethics grounded in the traditional resources of the Church.

Patient advocacy and conscientious objection

The role of the patient advocate is enshrined as a professional expectation within the NMC code of conduct (standards of practice and behaviour) (NMC, 2018). The code is a means of educating nurses about this role expectation, which, it has been argued, is not for the faint-hearted. Moreover, the concept of conscientious objection must be understood, respected and cherished by all in healthcare.

The importance of educational, managerial and peer support cannot be underestimated in healthcare. Health professionals must understand that certain legal and professional developments can all impact on the right to conscientious objection in healthcare. These issues are explored throughout this book.

The code of conduct: patient protection and staff support

The nursing code of professional conduct affords protection to both patients and nurses by its required integration into practice. Members of the profession compile the code, together with members of the public and, when internalised and used in practice, it may allow the nurse to work against potentially unethical or defeatist care cultures.

It is vital to access required support and not suffer in silence when trying to act as the Good Samaritan for the benefit of patients and with the aim of preventing the occurrence of further NHS scandals, such as those discussed in Chapters 9–11. These reveal a microcosm of the wider picture of negative and disrespectful attitudes to vulnerable people, over the years. Together with a catalogue of inadequate managerial and ministerial oversight, equal culpability is clear.

Throughout the chapters, the Good Samaritan health professional can often be seen to be at risk of cultural indoctrination into unethical practice. The need for awareness of this danger is emphasised throughout the book.

Good people, of which there are very many in healthcare, may find it difficult to be immune to the contagion of peer pressure, which may be applied to get them to accept unethical practice. This type of pressure may become normalised and soon can be tacitly accepted as beyond question.

The conscience is a necessary and protective prompt in such care settings, despite attempts by some to devalue it and view conscientious objection as an inconvenience and unwarranted in healthcare.

The NMC code of conduct is a clear directive for practitioners who need to internalise it and understand its value in providing protection for patients and themselves.

Peer support can be an invaluable means of countering unwanted and inappropriate pressure for unethical practice in the work area.

I hope that anyone reading this book will benefit from the information and evidence presented about the important issues in healthcare, which include the often-difficult role of patient advocacy and that of a whistle blower.

Healthcare is a privilege to which we are called but acting as the patient advocate is not always an easy option in our increasingly secularized society which reaches into many areas. The recognized helplessness which can be induced in practitioners as a result of such a culture, need not be viewed as insurmountable by those placed in questionable, ethical situations.

The importance of a positive organizational culture, both in the hospital and training institutes should be reflected in practitioners' sound knowledge of professional and legal developments, their own human and legal rights and those of their patients.

The Duty of Care

Nurse education should include the concept of the duty of care. Those nurses who are against strike action need not be condemned but regarded as true Good Samaritans. Disregard of conscience and the professional code can only make the practitioner complicit in wrongdoing.

Nursing is a profession, like medicine, entered into by people who hopefully practise for the good of their patients. The argument that they practise out of the goodness of their hearts as their main drive, fails when we see the nursing union supporting strikes "in December of all times" (Murray, 2022). The understandable public goodwill for nurses since the COVID crisis is understandably sorely tested by the 19% pay rise demand, in such economically harsh times.

It is clear that many other people, like the nursing and medical professions, worked through the COVID crisis from the outset, when fear was at its height, devotedly as heroes and heroines to allow some semblance of normal life for us all. They too warrant pay rises but their salaries are not paid for by direct taxation.

Nurses must also be aware that simply carrying out higher orders that would harm a patient is no defence in law, further to the judgements at Nuremberg following the Second World War.

It is, therefore, incumbent upon educators and managers to provide the required educational support and signposting to assist those whose vocation and lifelong learning ambition is primarily to act as the Good Samaritan, to do no harm.

Conclusion

Individualised, holistic care approaches are the expected elements of a philosophy of patient care. Yet nurses must consider this important approach for their own self-care. Effective management of nurses' own physical, psychological, social and spiritual needs with the relevant support, can enhance their own wellbeing and the holistic care needs of their patients.

Introduction

The Parable of the Good Samaritan (Luke 10:25–37)

Just then a lawyer stood up to test Jesus.
'Teacher,' he said, 'what must I do to inherit eternal life?'
He said to him, 'What is written in the law? What do you
read there?' He answered, 'You shall love the Lord your God
with all your heart and with all your soul and with all your
strength and with all your mind; and your neighbour as yourself.'
And he said to him, 'You have given the right answer;
do this and you will live.'
But wanting to justify himself, he asked Jesus,
'And who is my neighbour?'
Jesus replied, 'A man was going down from Jerusalem to
Jericho and fell into the hands of robbers, who stripped him,
beat him and went away, leaving him half dead. Now by chance,
a priest was going down that road; and when he saw him, he
passed by on the other side. So likewise, a Levite, when he
came to the place and saw him, passed by on the other side.
But a Samaritan while travelling came near him; and when
he saw him, he was moved with pity. He went to him and
bandaged his wounds, having poured oil and wine on them.
Then he put him on his own animal, brought him
to an inn and took care of him.
The next day he took out two denarii, gave them to
the innkeeper and said, "Take care of him; and when
I come back, I will repay you whatever more you spend."
Which of these three, do you think, was a neighbour to
the man who fell into the hands of the robbers?'
He said, 'The one who showed him mercy.'
Jesus said to him, 'Go and do likewise'.

(Bible Gateway, 1993)

Ongoing required care

The parable of the Good Samaritan shows that Jesus wanted to emphasise to the lawyer the importance of how we must be towards our neighbour when asked to respond to the question 'who is my neighbour?'.

The question posed by Jesus had only one reply when He asked the lawyer, of all the people involved with the poor victim of robbery, who was a neighbour to him?

Caring has many elements and does not end with immediate care but is ongoing. The stages of the care process undertaken by the Good Samaritan in the parable, are a lesson for us all about the importance of assessing, planning, carrying out and evaluating care.

The Good Samaritan teaches us the important need for:

- immediate assessment of care needed and planning and implementing the care by treating and bandaging the wounds
- planning and supporting the victim's transportation to the inn
- staying with the injured man that night as part of the evaluation process of the care given
- arranging with the innkeeper for required, continuing care and providing money for this
- returning later to check on the man's progress and to see if any more money was owed to the innkeeper.

Who is my neighbour?

Jesus explains the renowned parable of the Good Samaritan. The Jewish victim is unaided by those reputedly 'good' people of his own culture, who pass by on the other side, leaving him alone and very vulnerable on the road to Jericho. This route was renowned for bandits. They do not want to act as his advocate and get involved. Perhaps they believe any intervention will be 'futile' or too 'costly' for them to implement. In the days of Jesus, stories were a commonly used method of allowing people to reflect on life and their own situations.

This parable can be seen in healthcare where the simple vocation to nurse can be questioned, compromised, or even devalued by those with opposing views on 'saving' patients often preferring to 'walk by on the other side'.

Patients have suffered discrimination, by being considered 'unworthy' of treatment often considered, unjustly, to be 'futile' and/or too 'costly'. Such attitudes need contesting by positive confrontation by the Good Samaritan health professional as the patient's advocate.

It has been suggested that our society is in the grip of narcissistic tendencies; where such selfishness dominates that it can result in a society that does not care enough for others. Such tendencies may reflect an aggressively secular culture which can infect bioethics, healthcare ethics and judgement. This attitude is not in line with a Christian orientation to life or the demands of the expected role of the Good Samaritan patient advocate.

An Anglican vicar with a Jewish heritage, suggests that the parable of the Good Samaritan is not just an encouragement to look after the vulnerable and stranded, it is a subversive dig at the failure of those who should have been first to help. The Samaritan is the New Testament's representative "other", disliked for being culturally and theologically different. To make a Samaritan the hero of the story is a withering critique of the established religious order (Fraser, 2022a).

The Good Samaritan in healthcare may need to be prepared to critique a health system which may favour some patients over others. Such people may be considered economically unproductive and can become victims of a dystopian, eugenic ideology of the survival of the fittest.

The following chapters cover the past, current and potential problems for health professionals who wish to act as the Good Samaritan or advocate for all patients, particularly the broken and vulnerable, in line with their code of conduct and conscience as a guide to compassionate practice.

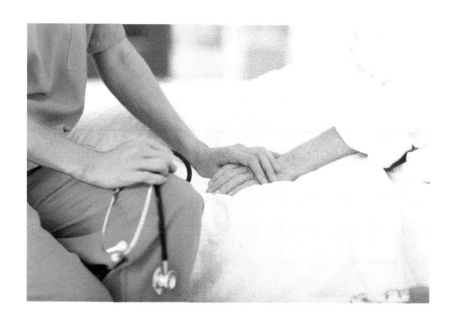

Chapter 1
Nursing history, philosophy and holistic care

The poor and the sick are the heart of God.
In serving them we serve Jesus Christ.

(St Camillus de Lellis, the patron saint of nursing)

Introduction

Themes within a care philosophy include holistic assessment and holistic care approaches provided by educated professionals with an understanding of the importance of effective communication and the principles of the nursing code of conduct (NMC, 2018). The nursing code expects nurse-patient advocacy, evidence-based practice, accountability and the right to conscientious objection in practice. These concepts are explored extensively throughout this and the following chapters.

The influence of St Camillus on healthcare

St Camillus was born in 1550. At the age of 25, he converted to Catholicism as the result of hearing a sermon. He twice tried to join the Capuchin friars but was rejected because of his poor health. Having had experience of hospitals due to his illnesses, he was determined to improve them. He offered himself to the hospital of San Giacomo in Rome and eventually became its bursar. Hospitals were often filthy and hospital staff inadequate. Like Florence Nightingale, he introduced many reforms. He founded a congregation of priests and lay brothers, the Servants of the Sick (later known as the Camillians), to serve the sick both spiritually and physically. He was ordained a priest in 1584 and he devoted the rest of his life to the care of the sick as a Good Samaritan until his death in 1614.

The United Kingdom Reformation and healthcare

The United Kingdom (UK) Reformation arose in the 1500s and could, more accurately, be termed 'the Great Revolt' against Catholicism. Apart from their persecution, Catholics at the time saw the dissolution of the monasteries have a negative impact on the care for the vulnerable which had been provided through their work. It is argued that the dissolution of the monasteries in the late 1530s was one of the most revolutionary events in English history (Barnard, 2011). This resulted in the destruction of holistic care, which had been provided for centuries by the religious orders. Thereafter, vulnerable and poor people needed a state-led source of support. The repercussions of the loss of the monastic care movement in the UK were immense and immeasurable in terms of social, physical, spiritual and psychological needs for the poor and vulnerable.

The charitable Church

The Catholic Church had established the world's first hospitals during the Middle Ages. The foundations of modern medicine are rooted in Her solicitude for the sick. She managed each patient as if Christ Himself. Thus, the Church sent orders of priests, monks and nuns to supply free healthcare for the poor and sick all over the world. Down through the ages, amid plague and pestilence, we find the Church in their midst, ministering to infected people despite great dangers. Above all, the Church cared for the souls of the suffering sick. She comforted, consoled and anointed the afflicted (Horvat, 2020a).

The nature of nursing

The generally accepted view of nursing is that its fundamental nature reveals a deep and profound concern for humanity that transcends contracts and the current ideology of the 'marketplace' within healthcare (Brown et al., 1992).

Nursing is difficult to define. It is a unique and complex discipline that can be considered as both a science and an art, both needing a depth of specialised knowledge and many skills.

Nurses have a privileged role; they care for some of the most vulnerable and share the lives of people for short to considerably lengthy periods. Nursing encompasses many different roles, including the important, fundamental role of nurturer.

Trust

As a phenomenon of human society, nursing is as old as humanity itself (Mellish and Wannenburg, 1992). Patients deserve high standards of quality care and rely on the nursing profession to meet this expectation. The nurse-patient relationship is formed by our commonality as human beings and based on the concept of trust. The general public trust the profession to deliver excellent care and nurses are privileged with this trust (Malone, 2005). We must not destroy such trust yet where it has been damaged, we need to be determined to repair it.

The history of nursing

The history of nursing goes back further than Florence Nightingale (who felt called by God to nurse). The Anglo-Saxon interpretation of the word 'care' was 'to make extra efforts for someone in need'. The word 'patient' comes from the Latin '*patiens*'. The term means endurance or suffering and refers to an acquired vulnerability and a dependence which is imposed on people by changing health circumstances.

Although the origins of nursing predate the mid-19th century, the history of professional nursing traditionally begins with Florence Nightingale. A well-educated daughter of wealthy British parents, Florence defied social conventions and decided to become a nurse. The nursing of strangers, either in hospitals or in their homes, was not then seen as a respectable career for well-bred ladies who, if they wished to nurse, were expected to do so only for sick family and intimate friends.

Florence believed, in a radical departure from these views, that well-educated women, using scientific principles and informed education about healthy lifestyles, could dramatically improve the care of sick patients. Moreover, she believed that nursing provided an ideal, independent calling, full of intellectual and social freedom for women, who at that time, had few other career options.

Florence Nightingale and Mary Seacole's legacies for healthcare

Nurses need to revisit the life and times of Florence Nightingale, whose mission for the vulnerable soldiers, wounded in the Crimean War, was thwarted and challenged by those some may have perceived as 'more powerful' and influential. They, however, were not considered as such by Florence herself. She was a strong woman with her female team in a man's world, dealing with the antagonistic attitude of the British camp authorities.

English officers seemed unable to accept the presence of working women in the camp. Even more telling was the antipathy of the military physicians, made worse because of Florence's personal contact and influence with the Minister of War and her huge influence with the British government. At first, they saw her opinions as an attack on their professionalism. But after fresh casualties arrived from the Battle of Inkerman in November 1854, the staff were soon fully stretched and accepted the nurses' aid.

The nurses would never have managed had it not been for the help of the orderlies, who were also under Florence's control. They idolised her and she cared for them in a special way. Thanks to Florence, the order was given to improve their working conditions. Fighting for the good of her patients, Florence grappled with the greatest enemy of all – bureaucracy. She was made to wait three weeks for a delivery of shirts and six weeks for lemons, needed to fight scurvy, this when the fruit was already stored in a nearby warehouse. In such situations, Florence was perfectly capable of ignoring rules. On one occasion, she even instructed orderlies to break open a door to get at the much-needed supplies. At last, some months after her arrival, relations with the military began to improve when officers realised that this 'intruder' never used her influence for personal gain: 'My aim is to ensure the best nursing care for the wounded' (Bostridge, 2011).

Florence saw religion as having two complementary strands of both rationalistic enquiry, the 'reason' of Unitarianism and practical service in the world. This was alongside a more contemplative practice of an inward seeking union with God. In Volume 4 of her Collected Works on Mysticism and Eastern Religions, Florence reflects deeply on the relationship between mysticism and pragmatism:

> *For what is mysticism? Is it not the attempt to draw near to God, not by rites or ceremonies, but by inward disposition? Is it not merely a hard word for 'The Kingdom of Heaven is within'? Heaven is neither a place nor a time. There might be a Heaven not only here but now…*
> *Where shall I find God? In myself.*
> *That is the true Mystical Doctrine.*

(Miller, 2021)

> *Like a fiery comet, Florence Nightingale streaked across the skies of 19th century England and transformed the world with her passage…*
> *We know Nightingale best as the founder of modern secular nursing,*
> *but that is only one-side of her many-faceted life.*
> *The source of her strength, vision and guidance was a deep sense of unity with God, which is the hallmark of the mystical tradition as it is expressed in all the world's great religions.*
> *This aspect of her life has been vastly underestimated, yet we cannot understand her legacy, without taking it into account*

(Dossey, 1999)

Scholars are finding that there is much more to the *Lady with the Lamp* than her famous exploits in the Crimea War. Nightingale in 1858, became the first woman to be made fellow of the Royal Statistical Society (Hammer, 2020). Her legacy is unforgettable for nursing but also as a first-class statistician which skill complemented her war work with nurses and patients in the Crimea.

Mary Seacole

Another 19th-century heroine of the Crimean War and true patient advocate, was Mary Seacole. She was a woman of Scottish, British and Jamaican heritage who, independently of Florence Nightingale, also paved the way for women to become highly qualified as nurses or physicians. Her wounded soldier patients loved her as they loved Florence Nightingale.

When Britain, France and Turkey declared war on Russia in 1854, many of the soldiers based in Jamaica were transferred to Europe. Seacole was excited to follow with a wish to join Nightingale's team to go to the Crimea and look after the troops she had known in Jamaica. Rejected, she resolved to travel to the Crimea independently.

Mary Seacole's bright personality lit up the war zone and brought comfort to the men under her care. By travelling to the Crimea, she had aimed to be of some use to the soldiers and discharge her keen sense of duty. Her interest was to give comfort and solace and use her skills to heal the sick and injured. Mary Seacole was more than a nurse; she was an adventurer. She was celebrated by *Punch* magazine as 'our own lifeline for suffering soldiers'; she was both ahead of her time and made history on her own terms and was literally, a self-made woman.

She was a 'doctress' who practised Creole or Afro-Caribbean medicine and learnt nursing and herbalism from her mother. She arrived in the Crimea and set up her own business, the British Hotel, which was a general store and a place where soldiers could come to be nursed. She also rode out to the battlefield to nurse soldiers and would perform operations. She was affectionately known by the troops as Mother Seacole, because of the care she gave them. After returning to London after the war Mary wrote her autobiography *The Wonderful Adventures of Mrs Seacole in Many Lands*, which was published in 1857 and is still in print today. She continued to practice as a 'doctress' in London and when visiting Jamaica.

She converted to Catholicism, having recognised the spiritual needs of the injured and dying soldiers during her time in the Crimean War (Vernon, 2021). She died in 1881 and was buried in the UK in the Catholic Cemetery at Kensal Rise.

Although Mary Seacole is celebrated today as a heroine of the Crimean War and a pioneering nurse and doctress who was greatly admired in her lifetime for her service, immediately after her death in 1881, her name and achievements slipped from public memory.

For a century, her fame and achievements died with those who knew her, but recently she has been remembered and restored to our history. In 2004 Mary Seacole was voted the top Black Briton in a poll of 100 people. She has once again become recognised by the public for her heroic achievements during the Crimean War.

Now, approaching a century and a half after her death, she has achieved iconic status and her experiences make her an impressive woman in any century. In 2016, after a long campaign, a statue of her likeness was unveiled in front of St Thomas' Hospital. The first statue of any named black woman in Britain, it serves to recognise Mary Seacole's many contributions not only as a nurse but also to the advancement of medicine (Florence Nightingale Museum, 2021–2022).

The wounded patient today

The Latin '*vulnare*' translates as 'to wound' and the Latin word for nurse is '*nutricula*'. This word logically reflects the expectation of the nurse to provide the care requirements for maintaining a helpless person's health and life. Statute law in the UK, however, through the Mental Capacity Act (MCA) 2005 (Department for

Constitutional Affairs UK, 2005), now defines assisted nutrition and hydration as 'medical treatment'. This change in outlook for the vulnerable, causes ethical and philosophical problems for nurses who regard such 'treatment', where needed, as basic and humane care. Such a belief has been a longstanding commitment for both doctors and nurses. Such a radical development in the concept of 'treatment', is considered as unjust and continues to be challenged by faithful adherents to the virtue of charity.

Professionalisation of nursing

Professions represent a highly skilled sector of the labour market with a defined body of specialised knowledge. This knowledge is transmitted to trainees who are prepared in institutions and faculties under the control of the profession; the knowledge base is extended through research.

There is a monopoly on the field of work, in that practitioners must be registered by the state as being suitable to practice the profession and there is agreement by employers that only those registered will be given a job.

There is autonomy in the organisation, development and definition of the nature of the work undertaken. This implies that only a member of the profession is competent to assess another professional's work. Lastly, a code of ethics prohibits the exploitation of clients and regulates interprofessional relations (Thomas, 2016).

Nursing's education structure changed over time. Dependence on hospital-based training schools declined and training schools were replaced by programmes in universities. In addition, more systematic and widespread programmes of graduate education began to appear. These prepared nurses not only for roles in management and education but also for roles as clinical specialists and advanced nurse practitioners. Nurses were setting up their own doctoral programmes, emphasising the knowledge, science and research needed to address the urgent nursing care and care-delivery issues.

A philosophy for nursing

'Philosophy' is commonly understood as the study of the fundamental nature of knowledge, reality and existence, especially when considered as an academic discipline. Any nursing philosophy, worthy of the profession, should promote a central and shared purpose, which should be an agreed, over-riding concern for preventing patient harm.

Rather than many works on nursing philosophy, there are many nursing theories and models adopted over the years in nursing's quest for 'professionalism'. The healthcare scandals that have characterised certain areas of healthcare reveal, among many other problems (and not all within nursing), the apparent disregard for a philosophy of care.

Public trust

The noted NHS scandals explored in later chapters damaged the trust of the public in several areas. Although the diminished public trust has been reinstated in many people due to the heroic efforts of the NHS staff in caring for patients suffering from COVID-19, nevertheless, the lessons from these care failings, which clearly do not involve nurses alone, must be learnt by all involved.

A new vision for nursing?

The scandals involving NHS care can be traced back for many years, occurring both pre- and post-2000. Nursing's regulatory body, at the time, introduced a new vision for nursing, which was approved by the government and known as 'Project 2000' (UKCC, 2000). Methods and procedures in nursing were becoming more knowledge-led. Instead of the former apprenticeship system whereby nurses were trained at hospitals, the aim of the Project 2000 scheme was to contract the training of nurses out to British universities and for them to achieve student status with periods of clinical, mentored experience.

This was intended, from the year 2000, to change the training and supervision of student nurses, ensuring that students would be educated to degree level and would be on an equal footing with other professions. Nursing would consequently be more questioning, autonomous and 'professionalised'. This was a worthy aim.

Philosophy of care and conscience

It is becoming clear that patient advocacy, nursing autonomy and accountability cannot be considered as mutually exclusive concepts. All these issues must be linked to ensure the highest ethical standards as part of a philosophy of holistic care.

The concept of conscience is an inescapable part of human nature, whether conscience is sensitive or blunted and whether the person is highly educated or not. It can guide practitioners in their expected role of the Good Samaritan or patient advocate.

Ethical dilemmas

Nursing has traditionally been considered as a vocational profession, with the public's perception of nurses as ministering angels at the bedside. A nursing philosophy cannot always bring easy answers to ethical dilemmas but can provide some of the intellectual and emotional rigour that nursing requires. The analytical attitude associated with philosophy may allow critical enquiry and the questioning of assumptions about complex medical and nursing issues.

Care requirements

Nurses with or without religious belief, generally enter the profession with a compelling drive to help others in need. The word 'vocation' comes from the Latin dictionary and means 'to be called – to be summoned'. Nurses are called to a privileged practice.

It has been explained that health professionals make decisions about those in their care by using cognitive capacity based on intuition and feelings. This capacity includes:

- perceiving the vulnerability of others that develops over time as a stable characteristic

- interpersonal orientation (focusing on the relationship between the patient and the professional)
- structuring moral meaning (evaluating decisions and actions)
- modifying autonomy (protecting the care recipient from self-harm)
- expressing benevolence (being motivated to act for the care recipient's benefit)
- experiencing moral conflict (identifying underlying feelings, intuition and perceptions of a situation compelling the professional to take some action)
- confidence in medical and moral knowledge.

(Lutzen et al., 1995)

Nursing care models

An important first step in the development of ideas about nursing was to try and identify the core concepts central to nursing, then to identify the beliefs and values around those. Historically, both the theory and practice of nursing had been heavily influenced and dictated by the goals of medicine a position perpetuated through the apprentice-style approach to nurse education. The 'medical model' focused on diagnosis, treatment and cure of physical disease. Growing concerns among nurses about the suitability of the medical model added impetus to the development of models for nursing (Pearson et al., 1996).

It was anticipated that models of nursing would capture, represent and articulate the particular concerns and purpose of nursing and develop that all-important knowledge base characteristic of professional status (Hodgson, 1992). There was also a return to the ideas of Florence Nightingale, a great nurse and one of the earliest and most influential writers on nursing.

Defining nursing by models

Initially, formal models of nursing were considered as ways of representing what nursing was, what it aimed to achieve and the different components of nursing that could then be taken apart, analysed and understood. The components of nursing – however defined – are complex and, as a result, several models were developed. Each offered a different way of thinking about nursing and each presented a different way of guiding nursing practice. So, a nursing model could be defined as 'a picture or representation of what nursing actually is' (Pearson et al., 1996).

Nursing models were supposed to be used extensively in practice and to guide the education of nurses. At a basic level, there are three key components to a nursing model:

1. A set of beliefs and values
2. A statement of the goal the nurse is trying to achieve
3. The knowledge and skills the nurse needs to practise.

(Pearson et al., 1996)

The process of nursing

In the 1970s, the idea that the nursing process comprised a four-stage, problem-solving method was introduced to enhance the delivery of individualised patient care. This was a method of applying nursing models to clinical practice.

The four accepted nursing care stages of the nursing process are: assessment, planning, implementing and evaluation of care. The values, beliefs and theories for care within a given model of nursing, could be used to guide these stages as exemplified by the Good Samaritan in the Christian parable.

It was important that the required stages of the nursing process were documented, but this did not always happen as producing documentation can be time-consuming and time is a precious commodity in healthcare. Despite having fallen out of favour, nursing models may incorporate fundamental concepts, values and beliefs about contemporary nursing.

When nursing models entered widespread use in British nursing from the 1970s, they represented specific values and beliefs about nursing held by individual nursing authors. Subsequent critical analyses have suggested that models of nursing are narrow perspectives that fail to capture what nursing is

(Hardy, 1982). Many textbooks and journal articles were written which attempted to explain what these models were and how they could be used. However, the models were heavily criticised, particularly for the documentation involved.

Nursing – a unique body of knowledge

Patients need an individualised approach to their care needs, regardless of models, pathways, or other structured approaches to nursing care, or whether in pursuit of a body of nursing knowledge as occurred with developed models of nursing.

Care pathways

The introduction of care pathways to the UK healthcare setting, heralded a significant move away from the nursing process and were believed to be a potential threat to the ideals of individualised care. This was seen in the implementation of the Liverpool Care Pathway (LCP). An understanding of the importance of individualised patient care can be reflected in holistic care approaches.

Holistic care needs

Holistic care is a successful method of thinking critically about the individual care needs of patients in the education of both student and qualified nurses. The process, including patient data collection, assessment, care planning, implementation and evaluation phases, makes it possible to consider all patient needs and nursing practice, through reasoned judgement and helps nurses to gain critical thinking and effective problem-solving skills. However, students may encounter difficulties initially with this process of nursing and need effective mentoring to understand the process.

It is worth noting that sometimes it is not so much a matter of whether the care patients receive maximises their subjective well-being but whether it minimises the damage they have suffered (Booth, 1985).

The term 'holism' suggests that one is essentially whole and not simply made up of component parts. It is recommended that a holistic model of medicine and nursing must address all three aspects of the person: psyche, soma and spirit.

The Good Samaritan – a model for holistic care

In his first encyclical, Deus Caritas Est, Pope Benedict XVI points four times to the significance of the parable of the Good Samaritan as the model for holistic care. He writes that the parable, '... remains as a standard which imposes universal love towards the needy... whoever they may be' (Pope Benedict XVI, 2005a).

This masterpiece of literature, Pope Benedict says, sets out 'the programme of Jesus' for social and personal healing that He himself adopted and implemented and that Jesus calls all his followers to do the same. (Pope Benedict XVI, 2005b).

The phenomenon of caring

The term 'cure' comes from the Latin, via the French curé (which in France is still the Priest). The Norman conquest of England resulted in Anglo-Saxon becoming the language of the conquered, French the language of the conqueror. The different terms are suggestive of an original class difference in the origin of care and cure. The higher orders 'cured' while the lower orders 'cared'. Differentiation of 'care' and 'cure' is problematic, in no small part due to the difficulty in defining the concept of 'care'. Many physicians quite properly reject the clear implication that their focus is on 'cure' not 'care' and they can rightly claim that they are as caring as any caring nurse within their team.

Though the meanings of the terms have developed in their separate ways, the relationship to power seems to have remained with 'cure' continuing to exert a more direct relationship of power and control. While doctors are renowned for often feeling a sense of failure when unable to 'cure'.

The American nurse anthropologist, Leininger (1978), examined the concept of caring as part of the central essence of nursing. Dunlop (1986), explored whether a 'science of caring' was possible. The feminist grounded theory study by Wuest (1997), acknowledged that little was known about the process of women's caring or the effects of caring on women but concluded that the existing social structure creates and intensifies problems for women caring.

The caring professions have generally been haunted by a feeling, influential on attitudes, that those who admit to fears of being 'unable to cope' may be seen to be weak and unsuited for their role.

Care dimensions

The four phases or dimensions of care have been described as: 'attentiveness, responsibility, competence and responsiveness' (Sevenhuijson, 2000a). Caring can be considered as the one true, moral concern.

Many of those who enter the professions are ethical people of great sensitivity – a characteristic desirable for delivery of empathic care but one which may render professionals vulnerable to the painful effects of suffering. Care is perhaps the most basic element of a patient's treatment that a nurse can provide, yet it is the most essential. The impulse to care, together with the desire for nurses to put the interests of others' well-being before their own, can be a clear statement of their own ethical position.

The UK Nursing and Midwifery code of conduct: standards for conduct and behaviour

The NMC's code of conduct expects nurses to make sure that people's physical, social, spiritual and psychological needs are assessed and responded to in the following ways:

- Pay special attention to promoting well-being, preventing ill health and meeting the changing health and care needs of people during all life stages.
- Recognise and respond compassionately to the needs of those who are in the last few days and hours of life.
- Act in partnership with those receiving care, helping them to access relevant health and social care, information and support when they need it.

(NMC, 2018)

15

The developed role of the nurse

One development in nursing which was unquestioned was the introduction of the developed (or extended) role of the nurse. This is generally understood as technical tasks being historically delegated by the doctor to the nurse or the phlebotomist, someone who can be greatly skilled in taking blood (venepuncture).

Developed nurse roles now include, for example, cannulation and venepuncture, both of which involve technical skills and often require lengthy efforts and perseverance for an effective, safe outcome. From September 2019, UK nurse training prepares nurses, on qualifying as a registered nurse (RN), to be competent in both these tasks, as well as in male catheterisation.

Important concepts in nursing

Nursing incorporates concepts of autonomy, accountability and patient advocacy (Esterhuizen, 1996). These concepts are documented as mandatory in practice in the current code of conduct for nurses (NMC, 2018). Despite the emerging changes in the amount of nurse involvement in decision-making, the changes have often been slow and variable between clinical settings. In most Western medical practices, it is clinicians who maintain the legally approved monopoly over central tasks such as diagnosis and therapeutic measures (Bucknell and Thomas, 1997). There has, however, been increasing interest in the concept of nursing 'autonomy' in clinical practice.

Autonomy

Nurses have long wished to increase their autonomy with the other professions, particularly medicine. Traditionally, nurses had limited scope to develop a sense of autonomy, but this is changing in certain areas of their work. Studies highlight the position of nurses in hospital care and their need to develop more autonomy and equal decision-making with medical colleagues. The code of conduct states that:

> All nurses must act first and foremost to care for and safeguard the public. They must practice autonomously and

be responsible and accountable for safe, compassionate, person-centred, evidence-based nursing that respects and maintains dignity and human rights.

(NMC, 2018)

Developed nurse roles

Despite the search for and success in achieving autonomous nursing practice in some specialist areas, nurses will receive treatment orders to carry out, all of which may impact the quality of a patient's life. These may range from management of wounds to those orders relating to patient resuscitation or treatment omission. Orders may be associated with requests for nurses to assist clinicians lacking appropriate expertise. Other progressive developments in nursing include the introduction of roles such as clinical/advanced nurse practitioner and nurse specialist, consultant nurses and the nurse physician associate. The work undertaken in nurse specialist roles includes managing patient consultations in clinics, reviewing test results, chronic disease management and sharing such nursing expertise with medical colleagues, both formally and informally, in medical training and clinical settings. Other roles, such as drug prescribing, are now within the province of advanced nurse practitioners and certifying sickness has been discussed as another remit for some nurses for the benefit and convenience of patients.

Nurse-led clinics

The results of a study exploring the effectiveness of nurse-led advanced practice for patients with cancer, support the effectiveness of nurse-led clinics in improving self-reported responses such as distress levels, satisfaction, quality of life including concerns about vomiting, and depressive symptoms. The effectiveness of nurse-led clinics needs further evaluation with stronger trials and wider focus on nursing-sensitive clinical outcomes and costs (Molassiotis et al., 2020). This study recommended future studies be conducted which should focus more on the costs and effectiveness of different models of care administered by advanced practice nurses.

All practitioners must respect their autonomy. We are entrusted to it by our patients and the profession. We must never let down these groups by an overreach of our power for which we are accountable.

Accountability

The nursing code of conduct has the following expectation of nurses:

> Being accountable means being open to challenge. It means being held to account for your actions and being able to confidently explain how you used your professional judgement to make decisions – even in complex situations.
>
> (NMC, 2018)

The emphasis on nursing can focus too much on responsibility being the sole remit of nurses with their constant involvement with patients. Voicing concerns to management about systemic problems can be difficult for nurses. The code of conduct also says: 'Be accountable for your decisions to delegate tasks and duties to other people' (NMC, 2018).

Meanwhile, the less technical, expressive skills which historically have been expected of nurses, are consequently often denied to their patients where there are shortages of both trained nurses and care support workers. It is well known that nurses find this upsetting as they have, for many years, complained of not being able to devote more time to their patients to provide holistic care and feeling powerless as a result.

Patient advocacy

The ideal of service and the picture of the autonomous and accountable nurse that is portrayed in the nurses' code of conduct (NMC, 2018) is not always reflected by reality. The promotion of nursing is long overdue, not only as unique and irreplaceable, but equal to medicine in perhaps less obvious but nevertheless significant ways such as the role of the patient advocate (see Chapter 2).

This role of the patient advocate is considered so essential as to be included in the expectation of the code of conduct:

'the nurse must promote the interests of patients and clients' (NMC, 2018).

Communication

The importance of nurses needing to develop their communication skills for patient care and also to have their voices heard as an apparently 'subordinate' group in healthcare is supported by the nursing literature. Having good communication skills is essential to collaborating on teams with fellow nurses and colleagues from other disciplines. It is also important to patient-centred care. Nurses who take the time to listen and understand the concerns of each of their patients are better prepared to address issues as they arise, resulting in better patient outcomes.

Effective nurse-patient communication is an essential aspect of health care. Time to communicate, however, is limited and subject to workload demands. Little is known about how nurses manage this 'lack of time' when caring for patients with developmental disability and complex communication needs, who typically communicate at a slow rate (Hemsley et al., 2012).

Nurses may also need to overcome their own psychological barriers when speaking to patients and family members about death, disease, and other sensitive topics.

One important source of moral difficulty for nurses often cited is the perceived inappropriateness of medical treatment. Some factors are inevitable in nurses' disagreements about doctors' decisions on treatment issues: different ethical issues may be perceived and a lack of understanding of each other's point of view leads to conflict. Nurses may raise more questions about the benefits and burdens of therapy they are asked to administer (or omit) due to their closer relationships with patients.

Critical thinking

Critical thinking in nursing can best be described as that higher order reasoning used in reaching professionally informed judgements. Professional judgement develops and matures with the acquisition of greater knowledge and the reflective analysis and evaluation of actual practice experience.

Collective responsibility ought to be taken for patient management and all practitioners need to understand the importance of critical thinking for reflection in and on their practice. This discipline is invaluable for all qualified nurses taking on the developed nurse roles, which all trained nurses must now do.

Reflection in nursing

Reflection can be defined as the process of thinking about our actions, either while in operation or after the fact (Taylor and White, 2000). A general description of 'reflection' is the examination of personal thoughts and actions. Nurses are constantly being reminded of the need for reflective practice.

Critical reflection

This is a concept commonly mentioned in the literature, which refers to the ability to uncover assumptions about self and others and the workplace to encourage 'reflective' practitioners.

Reflective practice

Nursing has developed a formalised concept of reflective practice in keeping with its role with patients and the expectation of nurses as professionals with a mentorship responsibility for less experienced nurses. Reflective practice is important for several reasons.

Much development in the encouragement for 'reflective nursing practice' has derived from the recent initiatives for the continuing efforts towards improvements in care quality.

This drive, known as 'clinical governance', is accepted by organisations engaged in healthcare and all health team members, under the gaze of the UK National Institute for Health and Care Excellence (NICE).

Nurses are responsible for providing care to the best of their ability to patients and their families in line with the imperatives of their code of professional conduct (NMC, 2018).

Therefore, nurses must focus on necessary skill components (their knowledge, attitude and behaviour) to ensure that they are appropriately skilled to meet the demands made upon them.

RCN study on the lived experience of nursing in Northern Ireland during the coronavirus pandemic

A qualitative survey was commissioned by the RCN Northern Ireland, which aimed to identify nurses' experience of delivering care and treatment during the coronavirus pandemic across a range of settings during the period of April 2020 to March 2021. One of the survey findings highlighted the importance of reflective practice:

Reflective practice and adaptable support (4.2)

The COVID-19 pandemic revealed that time to reflect, support from peers and line managers and flexibility in the face of changing circumstances were highlighted as effective ways to support nurses to get on with their jobs and adapt to new ways of working during the height of the pandemic. Post the immediate 'crisis' in March to April 2020, stories reflected the need for proactive rather than reactive support. Opportunities for reflective practice opportunities during the May to September 2020 period were said to be vital in supporting the workforce to make sense of the crisis phase and build resilience and learning from the experience.

(RCN, 2020/2021)

Reflection, self-reflection and reflection-on-action

Reflection and self-reflection are crucial aspects of refining personal, professional ethics (Grace and McLaughlin, 2005). Some of the literature on reflection focusses on identifying the negative aspects of personal behaviour, which is aimed at improving professional competence.

Reflection-on-action

This is perhaps the most common form of reflection. The aim is to value strengths to develop different, more effective ways of acting in the future, without neglecting work on those areas of behaviour that require attention.

Reflection-in-action – clinical supervision

This is the hallmark of the experienced professional who examines his or her own behaviour and that of others within a given situation. This is now formalised by the introduction of clinical supervision (clinical support for nurses). This supervision enables supportive reflection and development of enhanced communication skills (see Chapter 7).

This is another excellent means of critical reflection which supports the process of professional and personal development and is an invaluable part of the revalidation process for nursing re-registration. Nurses generally agree that this form of reflection is an invaluable tool for improving practice and professional development in a supportive and constructively critical way.

Nursing invisibility

In 2001, the findings of one nursing study (Rodney and Varcoe, 2001) included the point that,

> Nursing services remain largely invisible to other providers, to administrators and policymakers and to theorists in fields such as bioethics and health economics. What remains invisible is all too easy to dismiss and what does get measured does not necessarily reflect the full worth of nursing services.

The authors of the study also argued,

> *... the invisible, paradoxical processes involved in the day to day rationing of nursing and other resources must be explicated, that economic enquiry needs to be supported by expertise in*

ethical enquiry, that the nursing profession must examine values concurrently with costs, and that a failure to shed light on the values inherent in nursing practice, distorts the economic evaluation of the true costs of healthcare.

(Rodney and Varcoe, 2001)

Taking nursing forward

Ashworth (2000) argued that nurses who can take nursing forward and collaborate with others to the ultimate benefit of all concerned are those who adopt the following stance:

- Recognise that nursing is equal in importance to medicine for people's health even though these overlap in places.
- Are confident of nursing's value and therefore of the legitimacy of their roles as full members (and sometimes leaders) of healthcare teams.
- Can identify and pursue in their own context what is essentially nursing, whether they achieve it by direct care or through others, and whether or not, their activities include some which are performed by doctors or other health workers in other contexts.

Ashworth argues that unless nurses have vision and a clear sense of direction and are confident and articulate about the value of all nursing aspects of their role not just the technical ones, then the nursing aspects will be steadily eroded as nurses are given further tasks by others. Nurses can do almost anything with appropriate preparation; the question is whether they should and their decision in this is crucial to patients' welfare (Ashworth, 2000). This view can apply to doctors, managers and anyone with a position of power in healthcare.

Holistic healing

Retelling the Good Samaritan, St Pope John Paul II tells us that the parable of the Good Samaritan,

*... not only spurs one to help the sick, but also to do all
one can to reintegrate them into society. For Christ, in fact,
healing is also this reintegration: Just as sickness excludes
the human person from the community, so healing must
bring him to rediscover his place in the family,
in the Church and in society.*

(Arbuckle, 2007)

In addressing the two aspects of sickness – disease and illness – the parable of the Good Samaritan removes the social stigma and poverty that entrap the victim. Healing requires us to stand in a certain relation to the wounds – we must come close. The Lord does not heal from a position of detachment and safety. What is effective is the 'sharp compassion' meaning that the best instrument of healing is the ability to suffer with others.

Christ as doctor, finds poignant, modern expression in T.S. Eliot's *Four Quartets*:

*The wounded surgeon plies the steel
That questions the distempered part
Beneath the bleeding hands we feel
The sharp compassion of the healer's art.*

(Eliot, 1941)

Caring for the sick was a central activity of Jesus' public life. Healing involved repairing physical ailments – and removing demons from those who had been possessed, giving them hope, an intrinsic part of care and cure.

A Cardinal's advice for student health professionals

Vincent Nichols, Roman Catholic Cardinal of Westminster, said in his address to students of the Catholic Medical Association (CMA):

*Be the healing touch of Jesus. Release from captivity
the sick who can suffer an acute sense of loneliness even
when surrounded by hospital staff and fellow patients.
The way you relate to your patients is extremely important –
it has immense therapeutic value. So, love your patients.
It is never just a body before you with whom you tinker,
as if a crashed computer. Rather, always before you,
is someone, a person, a body and soul, made in
God's image. Let this person meet in you – Jesus –
whether or not you mention His name.*

(Nichols, 2014)

Conclusion

Florence Nightingale would recognise the wounded today in healthcare, as the Good Samaritan that she was. She was clear that enabling staff to feel and always be compassionate towards patients in their care requires action on multiple levels.

Individual experience

At the level of the individual, one of the most powerful resources that nurses consistently cite is patients' stories. In cases where professionals themselves, or their loved ones, become patients, the nature of their personal experience of care very often has a profound effect on how they carry out their clinical practice.

Nursing philosophy

Nursing has come a long way in its attempts to be recognised as a profession and needs a philosophy to be recognised as such. Nurses can heal patients by their philosophical approach of holistic care as advocated by Florence Nightingale and their code of conduct to care for their patients' physical, mental, spiritual and social needs. They care through the development of a therapeutic relationship which promotes the possibility of healing even where physical cure may not always be possible.

Nurse education

Educating nurses on an ongoing basis about professional values and standards is essential for the Good Samaritan care culture. Nursing requires skills at various levels before nursing competence is assured. Any skills, but particularly those required for nursing competence, have accepted components: knowledge, attitude and behaviour, some of which are difficult to assess for ongoing competence in the care of all patients.

Education plays a vital part in nurse development, whether in pre-registration or post-registration learning. The curriculum needs to ensure that nurses:

- Are aware of the importance of the practical implications of a formulated moral principle in their daily professional practice.
- Require ongoing educational activity, which should place the patient at the centre of all learning theory and practice as part of the philosophy of nursing,
- Are competent in both the expressive and technical care skills.

A timely exploration is required into the strategies that nurses adopt for dealing with certain orders that they may oppose in their role as patient advocate. Some orders may be irreconcilable with the nurse's ethical and moral stand for patient advocacy (see Chapter 2).

The compassionate care of patients must be central to nursing, irrespective of its definition. Exercises in which staff are asked to roleplay or write a narrative imagining themselves as patients can be useful. Optimum educational preparation for interaction with patients will include the important concepts of philosophy, cultural competence, autonomy, accountability, nursing reflection, holistic care and patient advocacy.

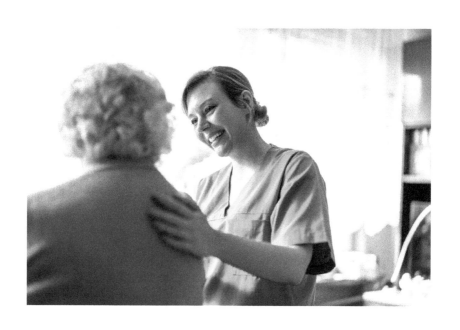

Chapter 2
Nurse-patient advocacy, ethical principles and moral distress

The Lord says, I love justice and I hate oppression and crime

(Isaiah, 61:8)

Introduction

All nurses, whatever their faith background, are closer to their patients than any other members of the multidisciplinary team. They are thus in a good position to act as the patient's advocate, in line with the expectation of the nursing code of conduct and cannot 'pass by on the other side' as the Good Samaritan could have done. He chose instead not to leave the victim abandoned to certain death.

Advocacy

Advocacy has been described as 'pleading the cause of another' and is particularly applicable to the world of nurses and their patients.

Results of a study analysis in 2003 revealed that advocacy has three essential attributes – valuing, informing and interceding – and each attribute is a helping strategy used in nursing. It is argued that only when all three attributes are present can advocacy be realised (Baldwin, 2003).

Required for advocacy are vulnerable populations and nurses willing to take on the responsibility for advocacy. This is a concept of such importance that the expectation for nurse advocacy has entered the nurses' ethical code of conduct: 'You must act as an advocate for those in your care' (NMC, 2018).

Evidence suggests that nurses' understanding of patient advocacy determines whether and how they will advocate for their patients (Kohnke, 1982). A recent study of RNs in Ghana explored nurses' understanding of patient advocacy. It revealed that the nurses described patient advocacy as promoting patient safety and quality care which includes the following: protecting patients, being the patients' voice, provision of quality care and interpersonal relationship as well as educating patients. The nurses had adequate understanding of patient advocacy and were willing to advocate for patients. The study concluded that there is, however, a need to research into barriers to patient advocacy in the clinical setting. This study made significant contribution to the understanding of patient advocacy and its positive effect on the provision of quality patient care (Nsiah et al., 2019).

Two of the study respondents, each with over six years of experience post-registration, summed up their view of patient advocacy:

"What I understand is that you take good care of them".
"Patient advocacy is about how as a nurse you speak up for your patients to ensure that they get the best... there are times you have to speak up for the patients when it comes to taking critical decisions".

(Nsiah, 2019)

Advocacy is everyone's responsibility

There is a pressing need for patient advocacy today, particularly as the NHS healthcare scandals are now becoming known, some of which have occurred over many years in many care settings. Many are yet to be addressed and managed to the satisfaction of those who suffered as a result.

Advocacy is not restricted to nurses, doctors, or lawyers. Patients' relatives also sometimes find themselves in a position where they need to act as the advocate for their loved one. This, sadly, is not what they will have expected, nor have realised the role to be so challenging. Nor would their loved ones have ever thought they would fear going into hospital due to the NHS scandals where many patients with non-terminal conditions never returned home and worse, no adequate (true) explanation has ever been provided for their deaths. This has required broken-hearted relatives themselves, over many years, to instigate inquiry and at the same time to cope with unresolved grief. Such tragic stories are narrated by relatives of people at all stages of life from babies to children, pregnant women and elderly people as the following chapters record.

Patients warrant educated practitioners, all of whom must be aware of legal developments which may impact on professional ethics in their day-to-day practice. They must be aware of their rights to conscience and how to exercise those rights. They also need to be aware that where systemic problems exist they need to support each other in movement for required change.

Advocacy is not for the faint-hearted

Nurse-patient advocacy has been described as: 'not a slogan, nor a hobby, nor to be entered into by the faint-hearted' (Copp, 1986). This description of patient advocacy can be related to the problems that nurses can face in ethically challenging workplaces. It can be argued that nurses' advocacy for patients is difficult to maintain in a climate where certain legal developments and some professional guidance relating to patient care need to be contested. Often a nurse's attempted role as patient advocate has not been given the required support by colleagues and the organisation. Such examples are seen in the healthcare scandals detailed in Chapters 9–11.

A lack of support can have damaging consequences for patients and nurses, one of which may be nurses leaving the profession. Family members often need to act as the patient advocate and must be respected and supported in this role.

Nursing – a moral endeavour

Literature in the field has reflected for a considerable time on the moral development of nurses and how ethical decisions are made. Nursing is by nature a moral endeavour. Writers argue that a difficult balance is being struck by nurses in technological environments (Gadow, 1984). The issue is whether the medical, technical arena disables humanistic caring. This is by no means a clear-cut position; nurses are involved in a paradoxical relationship, balancing technical expertise and humanistic caring within an environment that may not be supportive of caring activities.

Safeguarding as part of patient advocacy

There is an expectation of annual, mandatory staff attendance at certain training programmes in the NHS, as well as the voluntary and private sectors. These programmes include issues of patient safety in areas such as cardiopulmonary resuscitation (CPR), infection prevention and control, fire safety, moving and handling patients and loads, equality, diversity and human rights and adult and child safeguarding. All these topics are concerned with patient safeguarding, which is an inescapable part of nurse patient advocacy.

Advocacy is not a new expectation of nurses

Patient advocacy is argued to be a modern idea (Hanks, 2008), but its first movements had been exemplified by the monastic, caring tradition. Florence Nightingale's work in defence of her soldier patients during the Crimean War, to improve the terribly unhygienic and deprived conditions, reflected her mission for patient advocacy.

Patient advocacy is an ideal in nursing practice but providing a single definition for the term 'advocacy' is difficult. Nurses who have effectively performed their role as advocates can still be vulnerable to complications such as fear, anger, frustration, hopelessness and a sense of separation from their peers (Hanks, 2008; Tomaschewski-Barlem et al., 2015). Doctors too, who have attempted to act as the patient advocate, for example by whistleblowing, have suffered the consequences, as have some nurses who have been forced to leave a well-loved care area.

Patients' needs for advocacy

It has been argued that patient advocacy helps to provide effective nursing care (Davoodvand et al., 2016) and improves the quality of patient care (Negarandeh et al., 2008). Patient advocacy is an extremely important role for nurses, as often the patient or client is vulnerable and may have experienced or is currently suffering from varying degrees of distress.

Examples of patient advocacy

Apart from the obvious duty and goal of nurse-patient advocacy, to safeguard and protect patients from unethical and illegal acts, many other opportunities arise in nursing for patient advocacy, such as:

- Educating patients as a means of patient empowerment.
- Ensuring compassionate care for helpless patients, representing their needs in team meetings.
- Protecting research participants in clinical trials.
- Ensuring the support and protection of organ donation volunteers.
- Ensuring access to effective healthcare.
- Defending the patient's universal rights.
- Explaining to patients the holistic model of care
- Protecting the patient's potential benefit with their informed decision-making.
- Supporting patients in their need for making a complaint about treatment or care.
- Explaining the definition of treatment today and its implications for potential denial of treatment or investigation.
- Educating learners in the need for patient advocacy as part of code of conduct compliance and ethical care.
- Helping patients understand side effects of treatment and how these can be managed with nursing support.

Management issues, nurse-patient advocacy vs patient autonomy

The nurse is in a close position to patients to act as their advocate and to promote their needs, including the most fundamental need for food and fluid. Nurses who do not, or cannot, enact the role of advocate can lose the trust and respect of the patient and their family. Both the nurse and the patient can subsequently experience moral distress. This can sometimes result in nurses leaving the profession.

The nurse advocate may sometimes need to address the systemic problems of managerial and professional issues which impact on the quality of care, but such effort can be stressful and non-productive and will need support. Advocacy is everyone's business.

Patient autonomy vs the nurse as patient advocate

Problems for the nurse wishing to fulfil the role of the patient's advocate may conflict with the respect due for patient autonomy and the following interlinked issues:

1. Healthcare settings are considered as a *marketplace* with expected nursing compliance as a prevailing culture.

    Other team members may need to understand that in addition to illustrating the professional power of nursing, practitioners who strongly advocate for patient autonomy need to be mindful of developments such as the Mental Capacity Act (2005). This exhorts professionals to respect patients' decisions, no matter how 'eccentric'. The Act also considers assisted food and fluids as 'medical treatment', which patients may not have understood when drawing up an earlier advanced directive. Nurses must be aware of the encroaching, 'modern' bioethicist ethos of 'futile care'. The nurse, therefore, as the Good Samaritan patient advocate, has a duty of care to ensure patient understanding on these critical issues.

2. An age of *secularism*, where patient autonomy (though an important concept) can appear as the ultimate arbiter of care.

    Patient insistence on self-autonomy may conflict with a nurse's perception of true advocacy and thus optimum care for patients. Such conflict can derive from the perception by many patients about their right to autonomy, so this requires nurse-patient communication and education about possible harms. Many patients may not fully understand potential clinical developments, either presently, or into the future, despite having planned for a future scenario where they may not be self-sufficient in relation to past decisions.

3. Patients do not always understand the complexity of their *perceived autonomy* vs appropriate treatment and care.

   Patients may believe their wish for autonomy guarantees their true benefit. Nurses must, in conscience, help patients to understand that their rights to autonomy must confer real benefit, not harm. Challenging medical orders and the team consensus is always a formidable task for the lone nurse, whether or not they were ultimately successful in the role. Nurses who have attempted to perform the role of patient advocate at a time when practising within a hostile or defeatist culture, or with a practitioner or manager in a more 'powerful' position, never forget it but can benefit by knowing that they made the effort on behalf of their patients often with success.

Patient need for understanding of the implications of 'eccentric' decisions

The medical and nursing goal of treatment and care should be to help in the alleviation of suffering. Hence the need for vigilance among health professionals in their discussions with their patients to ensure understanding of the implications of possibly 'eccentric' decisions being made. Such patient decisions, according to the Mental Capacity Act (MCA, 2005), must be respected (see Chapter 5).

Patient advocacy – the role of family and friends

Bless the families
who daily support those they love
Amen

(Stack, 2022)

The role of patient advocate is not the sole province of the nurse. All involved in healthcare must be mindful of this key role and should acknowledge the input of relatives and friends who wish to act on behalf of their loved ones. This role for them can be daunting, therefore, any support from professional caregivers in their role is vital.

When elderly or disabled people enter hospital as patients, they may be in a very vulnerable state. The healthcare staff – nurses, doctors and paramedical staff – have distinct roles and responsibilities but together they should ensure that the patient's needs are met.

The patient's next of kin and close friends also have an important part to play. They should be consulted when the healthcare team is formulating a care plan for the patient at the time of admission and in relation to discharge planning. Friends and relatives may be needed to act as the patient advocates in an official or unofficial capacity.

The following prompts can be helpful for family or friends

- The care plan requires your contribution so that the patient's needs may be met.
- Never be hesitant to ask questions or make suggestions on behalf of your relative or friend.
- You should feel free to ask questions of any team member as you see fit but the nurse in charge should be the most appropriate.
- It will help the team to know that someone is there to keep an eye on the situation.
- Tell the team that you want to be kept informed about any changes in the care plan, from admission to discharge. (It is important, when possible, to first get the patient's consent for this and then confirm a clear agreement with family/friends as to who is the trusted person/next of kin.)
- The staff will then identify role and responsibility as friend or next of kin.

Situations that may arise and questions that may be useful

A. Feeding and hydration

Is the patient able to take anything by mouth?

- Is it safe for the patient to eat? If so, could I help with feeding?

- Is there a 'nil by mouth' notice by the bed? If so, ask:
  - o   How long has the notice been there and why is it there?
  - o   How long will the order notice last?
- Where is the fluid intake chart? If there is no chart, and the patient cannot take food or fluid without assistance, you should raise the question of hydration by a drip into a vein or under the skin.
- If the drip has been removed, ask why.

What are you doing about hydration?

- A lack of fluid intake is a cause for concern, as no one can survive more than about a week without fluids of any sort. Dehydration can add to the patient's discomfort, causing thirst, confusion, severe agitation, delirium, kidney failure and ultimately death.
- You may be told that the patient will not suffer from thirst, but this opinion is not universally accepted. It depends on the clinical situation.
- Hydration by means of a drip under the skin is simple to insert in hospital or at home as a prevention of thirst and delirium due to dehydration.

What are you doing about feeding?

- Hydration should always be provided while checks and required investigations are performed on the patient's safe swallow reflex, e.g., in the case of a stroke. Most doctors advise that decisions about feeding should be taken sooner rather than later as malnourishment adds to the patient's problems.
- If swallowing is a problem, the patient should be expertly assessed by a speech therapist and investigated with the appropriate technology (i.e., video fluoroscopy) and reassessed at least weekly.
- Oral feeding can often be maintained using specially thickened feeds. The advice of a dietician is helpful.
- If no food can safely be given orally, feeding can be achieved via a tube, either passed into a central vein (Peripherally inserted central catheter – a PICC line) or passed into the stomach either via the nose (naso gastric-NG tube), or directly into the stomach.

The latter is called a percutaneous endoscopic gastrostomy (PEG) tube. This requires a small procedure under local anaesthetic and sedation. The advantages and disadvantages of this procedure should be discussed with all concerned. It carries an exceedingly small risk.

- If the doctors advise tube feeding, accept their advice, because without food or fluids, a patient will inevitably die. If this matter is not raised, do so yourself.

B. Undue drowsiness

- This can be due to several factors but the first thing to check is whether the patient has been given a sedative, or medication such as morphine for any reason.
- You are entitled to make enquiries about these matters. If sedation or other medication has been given, ask 'Why?' Keep on asking until you get an answer.
- You may need to speak to one of the doctors and, if necessary, speak to the consultant if you are still not happy about the situation.
- Seeking a second medical opinion is a right of patients and relatives.

C. Pain control

- If the patient seems to be in discomfort or pain, report this to the nurses and ask them to assess the situation. There may be a simple explanation, such as a need for the toilet, or the need to be turned in the bed, or the need for a drink or some food. Abdominal pain is sometimes due to severe constipation, which can be overlooked and can make the elderly unwell and confused (see chapter 15). A urinary infection can also cause discomfort and confusion and is a particular risk for those with indwelling bladder catheters.
- Sometimes patients are given morphine for reasons other than pain as it is also an effective medication to relieve coughing and shortness of breath. However, this drug can cause constipation.

- If the patient has been prescribed pain medication, check what drugs are listed and find out why they have been used. Some patients may have what is known as neuropathic pain. This requires nerve painkillers rather than opioid drugs. Hospitals have been criticised for overusing strong painkillers. These are usually given via a syringe driver which can be dangerous but may be valuable for patients who are terminally ill and whose pain cannot be controlled with simpler medication.

Further questions that may arise on care and symptom management

- How could the patient be made more comfortable?
- What can be done about…?
- Would it be a good idea to try… e.g., pressure-relieving mattress?
- Is mouth care being provided?
- Would it be a good idea to contact: a speech therapist (in the event of swallowing/speech problems), dietician, a consultant for elderly care, physiotherapist, occupational therapist, minister of religion, discharge planner?
- In the event of a negative response, ask: 'What grounds do you have for not contacting these people?'
- How do you know that the patient is not experiencing hunger and thirst?

The ideal situation is that from the outset, there is effective communication between staff and the patient's family and friends.

Ethical principles

Physicians are primarily guided by the Hippocratic Oath, which although not a mandatory oath taken at qualification today, nevertheless, can act as a guide for doctors together with their code of conduct and Guidance for Good Practice (GMC, 2022).

Nurses are guided by their own code of conduct, which states: 'You will act as an advocate for the vulnerable, challenging poor practice and discriminatory attitudes and behaviour relating to their care' (NMC, 2018).

There are many factors related to ethical principles. These include types of ethical perspectives, ethics in clinical practice and the patients' own interpretations and understanding of ethical principles.

Ethical perspectives

Utilitarianism

The utilitarian ethical perspective emphasises the global community and the need for a redistribution of 'scarce' healthcare resources (J.S. Mill's utilitarianism – *Greatest Happiness Principle*). Such a view of ethics could be said to work to the detriment of a chronically ill or severely disabled patient. Such an ethical view can also impact strongly on the nurse trying to care for these patients, as patient advocate, where treatment may be perceived as 'futile' by the team. The Good Samaritan nurse who cannot agree may consequently be considered, unfairly, as not a 'good team player'.

Kantian principle of autonomy

Whereas the Kantian principle (categorical imperative) of autonomy and free, rational choice can apply to a person with capacity, how do we care for those who cannot so choose? How do we best preserve a person's dignity when they are unconscious? How can we respect a person's choices when they cannot articulate their choices to us, where their capacity is for any reason, impaired, either temporarily or permanently? (Fullbrook, 2007).

'Health' can be a subjective concept and does not always lend itself to the expected norms of a society which may be concerned about economics rather than care.

Ethical principles in clinical practice

The four well-established ethical principles which relate to the needs of patients and that healthcare providers can use to apply principles of legal and ethical behaviour are *beneficence, non-maleficence, justice and respect for autonomy* (Beauchamp and Childress, 1994). These four, along with other ethical principles, in particular relation to research subjects, are fully discussed in Chapter 5.

Ethical principles offer a common, basic, moral analytical framework and a common, basic moral language. It is suggested that although they do not provide ordered rules, these principles can help doctors and other healthcare workers to make decisions when reflecting on moral issues that arise at work (Gillon, 1994).

Distinct cultures may value certain virtues more than others but generally 'virtues' refer to common examples such as '... honesty, kindness, patience, civility, compassion, diligence, self-reliance, loyalty, fairness, courage, tolerance, temperance, self-control and prudence' (Capsim Management Solutions Inc., 2020). Such virtues are particularly important in any care setting.

Costs vs compassion

How can we act as the Good Samaritan? Some 'costs' (which may often be minimal) can be seen as an obstacle to ethical care in ensuring effective, compassionate care. This may be reflected in denial of patient hydration at the stage of 'end of life' which is obviously unethical practice. Generally, issuing a prognosis of 'dying' is notoriously difficult particularly when patients have a long-standing illness such as chronic heart and lung conditions (see chapter 4).

The 'good nurse'

Despite an abundance of theoretical literature on virtue ethics in nursing and healthcare, little research has been carried out to support or refute the claims made. One claim is that ethical nursing is what happens when a good nurse does the right thing (Kelly, 1993). What little empirical data that has emerged suggests that the meaning of a virtuous, good nurse is anything but simple or obvious and such an extremely complex notion requires more investigation (Smith and Godfrey, 2002).

The purpose of a descriptive, qualitative study by Smith and Godfrey (2002) was to examine nurses' perceptions of what it means to be a 'good nurse' and to do the right thing. Their study involved 53 nurses who responded to two open-ended questions:

Question (1) A good nurse is one who...?

Seven categories emerged from responses received: personal characteristics, professional characteristics, patient-centredness, advocacy, competence, critical thinking and patient care.

Question (2) How does a nurse go about doing the right thing?

The study participants' responses to this question were interesting. They viewed ethical nursing as:
... a complex endeavour in which a variety of decision-making frameworks are used. Consistent with virtue ethics, high value was placed on both intuitive and analytical personal attributes that nurses bring into nursing by virtue of the persons they are.

The study recommended further investigation to determine just who the 'good nurse' is and the nursing practice and education implications associated with this concept (Smith and Godfrey, 2002).

Does the code of conduct guide nursing practice?

An international study by Norberg et al. in 1994, reported that expert nurse respondents were able to make morally responsible decisions based on autonomy and beneficence, but were willing, however, to alter their decision on receiving medical orders, or at the request of a family member, even though they perceived them to be contrary to the principles of their nursing code. Although the original decision made by the nurses was in accordance with their nursing code, they seemed unwilling or unable to maintain their original ethical stand.

The study concluded that this outcome may relate to a lack of assertiveness on the part of nurses for historical, gender and/or educational reasons (Norberg et al., 1994). This result leads to the question of whether codes of conduct can guide nursing practice?

Moral distress

'Moral distress' is an umbrella concept that describes the psychological, emotional and physiological suffering that may be experienced when we act in ways that are inconsistent with deeply held ethical values, principles or moral commitments.

Moral distress in healthcare has been identified as a growing concern and a focus of research in nursing and healthcare for almost three decades

The inherent problems for the nurse wishing to act as the patient advocate have been well documented. Moral distress has been examined in *Moral distress, advocacy and burnout: theorising the relationships* (Sundin-Huard and Fahy, 1999), *Dilemmas of Moral Distress* (Jameton, 1993) and *Moral distress in Nursing Practice* (Wilkinson, 1987). The importance of such works needs to be discussed within training programmes to help nurses understand the need for support when embarking on the role of patient advocate.

Researchers and theorists have argued that moral distress has both short- and long-term consequences. Moral distress has implications for the delivery of safe and competent, quality patient care and implications for satisfaction, recruitment and retention of healthcare providers.

Moral constraints on nurses

The philosopher, Andrew Jameton, noted moral distress to be present among the nursing students that he was teaching. He recognised that the nursing role is morally constrained in a significant way.

Jameton's original account of moral distress focused on the way in which institutional policies and practices can lead nurses to do things that they believe to be morally wrong. Nurses need to become more aware of the importance of the practical implications of a formulated moral principle in their daily professional practice, although they are often constrained in following their own moral decisions.

Psychological disequilibrium

Nurses taking stock of how they had performed in relation to their inability to act, experience what has been referred to as 'psychological disequilibrium'. Associated with this state is goal disruption which can influence the thoughts and actions of the person for whom the ultimate goals are survival and the regaining of a sense of equilibrium (Wilkinson, 1987). It is argued, however, that a possible outcome of the experience of repeated psychological disequilibrium, inherent to adult life, is the development of psychological resilience (Buckle-Henning, 2011).

Some situations can make it nearly impossible for a nurse to pursue the right course of action despite professional codes, conscience and the supposed 'strength' and will for patient advocacy. The result is that many nurses begin to feel that they lack the courage to do the right thing or to raise concerns about poor standards of care. Nurses must choose to defend patients' well-being, accessing required managerial, educational and peer support to help them in their role as moral agents.

Cultural diversity, sensitivity and competence

During the last two decades, there has been a growing emphasis on the delivery of healthcare to meet the needs of patients in ethnic minority groups. It is commonly understood that patient advocacy is a moral imperative in healthcare but understanding cultural diversity needs to be considered as equally important and as part of patient advocacy. Therefore, in this regard, nurses must be provided with the time and the autonomy and knowledge to act as patient advocates

(Purba, 2020). Learning about how cultural differences may impact healthcare decisions and being able to reflect care in line with a patient's culture can allow for cultural competence in health professionals.

Nurses' experience of cultural diversity

Cultural sensitivity, though an expected component of holistic care, is not always easy to achieve in healthcare settings. An exploratory, research study investigated nurses' experiences in caring for culturally different patients (Boi, 2000). The results found that the nurses shared similar experiences and the same problems that impeded safe, holistic and effective care. Recurrent issues raised were the problems of language barriers, which were worsened by a lack of knowledge of the patient's culture. Holistic care was not, therefore, perceived as possible and there was inability to deliver a high standard of care.

The 2000 study by Boi, suggests that there is a need for courses to address the issues of diverse cultures, health beliefs and practices. It is hoped that these findings will increase healthcare professionals' awareness of how best to care for culturally diverse patients. It is not suggested that nurses ought to have expert knowledge about all ethno-cultural groups but that they have an awareness of cultural flexibility and accept and understand each patient as an individual. Undergraduate and post graduate nurses need a basis of understanding to meet the needs of culturally diverse patients.

Experience of culturally diverse patients

There is less research emphasis on the views of the patients from ethnic minorities themselves. One study by Hamilton and Essat (2008), included six community groups, some of mixed ethnicity and some of specific ethnic identity. The aim of the study was to try and understand the patient's perspective. Data were analysed using a thematic approach and three themes were identified as representing the views of the participants:

- knowledge of cultural and religious practices was essential for nurses for them to understand the basis of their beliefs and practices
- actions and behaviour of nurses either confirmed or ignored their specific requirements
- inherent communication problems for those who had difficulty in communicating in English.

Overall, patients reiterated their need to be treated with dignity and respect. For nurse educators, the challenge is to develop not only the knowledge base of student nurses but also to help them translate that into practice that demonstrates cultural understanding and sensitivity (Hamilton and Essat, 2008).

The culturally sensitive nurse as patient advocate

The diversity that exists within the NHS should be harnessed, particularly during time of a pandemic. With approximately one in eight NHS staff reporting a non-British nationality, some may be able to translate/interpret health communications during periods of crisis – a role historically undertaken by interpreter/translation services (Public Health England, 2018). The private sector has had interpreters on the pay roll to meet the needs of patients from diverse ethnic groups for many years.

The studies reveal that cultural sensitivity can be considered as an integral part of patient advocacy and to achieve nurse competence in this issue in theory and practice, educational programmes are vital for pre- and post-registration nurses. The importance of acknowledging diversity is today included in NHS mandatory training for all staff. This can only provide a superficial approach. Therefore, cultural diversity training courses are essential for all health professionals in clinical practice.

Conclusion

Attempting advocacy by required action (individually or in a group) can be draining, time consuming and upsetting within any environment where maleficence exists, albeit in subtle form.

Patient advocacy must be part of the daily responsibility of those at the 'top' and the 'bottom' of the workforce. Christians and non-Christians and everyone who cares for the dignity of human beings – must be vigilant.

Those who can, must speak out. Those who have a duty to teach and be active in the public square, must acquire the knowledge that will put them in a position to discharge their duties

(Cole and Duddington, 2021a).

Acting against evil

Action is the factor that is most effective and brave at minimising the danger and evil in the world, or any area where there are dependent, vulnerable people.

Why is action important?

Action, in this situation is about doing things to act against the evil acts of others as the patient advocate. The action necessary to thwart evil acts is probably the most dangerous and the most rare and brave as seen in warfare. It is an action the evil doer is not expecting, as it is so rarely done. This applies in managing bullies who generally crumble when confronted. In each case, any counteraction in some way makes it harder for evil to succeed. The result of the action is why action is important.

Recognising the need for action

There are lots of things we can do to make the world less dangerous. When people lie and they are not called to account, the world is rarely safer. Lies are more dangerous when they are spoken by more powerful people. When such a 'code of silence' becomes part of an institution, it has become, by definition, corrupted.

In politics, there are many dictators. In non-healthcare professions, there are always allegations of corrupt behaviour: for example, in police forces or in businesses. One example is reflected in the unnecessary economic crash of 2008, due to those who were aware of their wrongdoing but felt inviolate and which eventually affected so many innocent and helpless people. How will history judge recent healthcare scandals and the ruinous effects of lockdowns during the COVID 19 pandemic?

Maintaining the status quo or patient advocacy?

Nurses may feel that they require extra support and understanding from supervisors, friends and colleagues when experiencing difficult ethical dilemmas and challenges. They must understand their right to this. They must not be afraid to seek independent counselling to support them through difficult ethical issues. Discussing fears with someone else often puts events into perspective, confirms resolve and provides courage for the nurse to proceed with the aim of fulfilling the duty of patient advocacy.

This, in summary, means representing and educating patients of their rights, including to consent, working for their true benefit, and never allowing their care to be compromised. This may occur due to elements of fear, ignoring conscience, conviction, intuition, and the protective nature of the code of conduct for both patient and nurse.

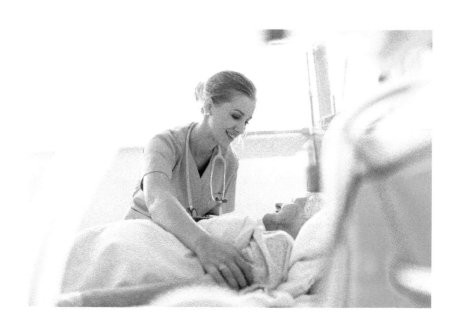

Chapter 3

The nurses' code of professional conduct, empathy and compassion

When Jesus saw the crowds, he had compassion for
them, because they were confused and helpless,
like sheep without a shepherd.

(Matthew 9:35–10:8)

Introduction

The particularly vulnerable nature of the sick allows for the possibility of exploitation, which is why the medical and nursing professions are bound by ethical codes.

The Hippocratic Oath

The Hippocratic Oath was modelled on priestly vows, effectively elevating medicine above such mundane activities as trade and thereby establishing the idea of transcendent commitment as central to the Western ideal of professionalism (Baker, 1997). The wording of the original Hippocratic Oath lost some of its relevance in calling upon Greek gods and opposing performance of surgery, but not in terms of its ethic, as in the famous Latin phrase: *'Primum non Nocere'* meaning - 'First do no harm'.

John Gregory viewed the practice of medicine, as an art rather than a trade. Teaching his students in the eighteenth century, he asserted that the virtues of the physician include: 'humanity, patience, attention, discretion, secrecy and honour' as well as 'temperance and sobriety', 'candour', and, above all else, 'sympathy'. Gregory also forged the ethical concept of a professional, i.e., someone who lives primarily according to fiduciary obligations of service to patients rather than primarily according to the dictates of self-interest. Gregory thus helped to invent medicine as a fiduciary profession, a legacy that persists into our time. Gregory did so in response to the state of disarray in the medicine of his day, a disarray that he meant to set to rights by using the tools of moral philosophy and philosophy of medicine (McCullough, 1998).

Tenets of Gregory's code were later to be employed in the successful prosecutions of doctors at the Nuremberg medical war crime trials after World War II. A belief that murders and torture are crimes that must be prosecuted and punished was indisputable but, as chief prosecutor General Telford Taylor declared in his opening statement of the trials; 'This is no mere murder trial'. He insisted that the court, 'act as an agent of the United States (US) and as the voice of humanity, stamp these acts and the ideas which engendered them, as barbarous and criminal' (Military Tribunal no 1, 1950).

Modern medicine

Towards the end of the 18th century, the role of physicians in dealing with disease in individuals as well as population groups (as in the great epidemics) led to the drafting of codes of professional conduct exemplified by that produced by Thomas Percival in Manchester. His proposals, published in 1803, laid the foundations for modern medical ethical standards in the UK

Over the centuries, the Hippocratic Oath has expressed the ideals of the medical profession, although nowadays other versions have supplanted it for graduating medical students – if they take any oath at all. Of note, in the modern version of the oath, there is no prohibition against abortion; there is no promise by the physician to 'do no harm' or never give a 'lethal medicine' as in the original Hippocratic Oath. This reflects the legal and professional changes affecting medicine over the years.

Is the oath still relevant?

A philosopher at the University of San Francisco argues in his recent book, *Hippocrates' Oath and Asclepius' Snake: The Birth of the Medical Profession* (Cavanaugh, 2017), that the oath is still relevant in establishing the fundamental ethics of the medical profession – to help and not to harm the sick (or the well). Steeped in Hellenic culture and philosophy, Cavanaugh argues that deliberate iatrogenic harm, especially the harm of a doctor choosing to kill (physician-assisted suicide, euthanasia, abortion and involvement in capital punishment) amounts to an abandonment of medicine as an exclusively therapeutic profession (Cook, 2019).

Accountability and a code of ethics

Accountability and a code of ethics are viewed as pre-requisites of a profession. However, nurses' use of codes of conduct (in relation to the issue of patient advocacy) appears to have been minimally studied. The ethical values of the nursing code can be seen to comply with religious principles which transcend nations, as they are universal principles.

Any code of ethical conduct, to achieve its purpose, must be understood, internalised and used by professionals in all aspects of their work. It must be explained throughout nurses' study and work lives. The code of conduct for nurses (NMC, 2018) is compiled and reviewed by the NMC and invites contributions from the public. Therefore, the code and taught ethical principles should help nurses in their attempts to maintain their own moral integrity, central to their moral experience of everyday practice with their patients.

The code in practice

The Nursing Code of Professional Conduct: standards of practice and behaviour (NMC, 2018) is compiled by the NMC in collaboration with the public. It presents the professional standards that nurses and midwives must uphold to be registered for practice in the UK and its principles are integrated into nursing's professional revalidation process. The code contains a series of statements that taken together signify what good practice by nurses, midwives and nursing associates looks like. It puts the interests of patients and service users first, is safe and effective and promotes trust through professionalism.

The UK nursing code is created with the assistance of members of the public and states that the nurse will:

- act as the patient's advocate
- be evidence-based in practice
- protect patients.

The code has four main principles:

- prioritise people
- practise effectively
- preserve safety
- promote professionalism and trust.

(NMC 2018).

Practise effectively

Always practise in line with the best available evidence, to achieve this, you must:

6.1 Make sure that any information or advice given is evidence based including information relating to using any health and care products or services.

6.2 Maintain the knowledge and skills you need for safe and effective practice.

(NMC, 2018)

Act as an advocate for the vulnerable

The code is essential reading to ensure the patient's expressed needs among others, for patient safety, trust, advocacy, effective communication and comfort. Knowing what the public believe is important in helping in formulating and reviewing the code, is educational and essential to interpret in practice by all nurses, 'challenging poor practice and discriminatory attitudes and behaviour relating to their care' (NMC, 2018).

There are conflicting opinions on the possible assistance afforded to practitioners by ethical codes in the management of ethical conflict. Codes of conduct for health professionals have existed and have been institutionalised within the nursing discipline since the end of the 19th century. Up until the early 1970s, ethical nursing codes advocated subservience to the medical profession.

It can be difficult for some nurses to implement their code's principles, particularly in terms of patient advocacy. Studies reveal that attempts to adhere to the ethical principles of the code can be undermined by fear of undue stress in the workplace and wanting to be considered by the majority as a 'team player'. This can occur when processes are in operation such as: reacting, distancing, hesitating for a long time about what to do and fearing the physician's anger or disciplinary measures (Kelly, 1998).

Florence Nightingale said: 'Apprehension, uncertainty, waiting, expectation, fear of surprise, does a patient more harm than any exertion' (Nair, 2017). Nurses who have incorporated the code into the psyche may find less fear and are more prepared in expressing its principles when in a situation of ethical conflict, so that advocating and protecting patients can become the norm. It is debatable whether the code of conduct for nurses is accepted as the cornerstone of nursing when examining the failures in NHS care over the years. These failures, however, cannot be attributed to nurses alone.

The nursing code: protection for patients and nurses

It should be apparent to nurses who carefully study their code of conduct that it can act as a protection for their patients and themselves. The code is approved by Parliament as part of the NMC's political endorsement as a professional body.

Nursing revalidation and the code of conduct

It is argued that little is done to provide nurses with the skills they need to reflect on codes of conduct effectively, in our complex, hierarchical healthcare systems. How can we prepare nurses to take on the complex and the sometimes-dangerous role of being truth tellers in the clinical setting and of understanding truth as nurses? (Drought, 2007). Even less attention is directed towards helping nurses to develop strategies for managing the emotions that clinical situations may engender.

Good nursing

The Nursing Code of Conduct contains a series of statements that when taken together, signify what good nursing and midwifery practice looks like. The code requires nurses to ensure holistic care, to make sure that the physical, social, spiritual, psychological and sometimes practical/financial needs of their patients are assessed and responded to in the following ways.

- Pay special attention to promoting well-being, preventing ill health and meeting the changing health and care needs of people during all life stages.
- Recognise and respond compassionately to the needs of those who are in the last few days and hours of life.
- Act in partnership with those receiving care, helping them to access relevant health and social care, information and support when they need it.

(NMC, 2018)

Nurse re-registration and the integration of the code of conduct

Today, the importance for nurses to be revalidated in their practice on a three-yearly basis has seen the important incorporation of the principles of the nursing code of conduct (NMC, 2018). The code's principles must be addressed in regular care reflection and recording of clinical experience as a personal and professional record.

Ethical dilemmas

The principles of the code of conduct advise the promotion and safeguarding of patients' interests, yet nurses are often faced with ethical dilemmas. The normally expected outcome is for a clear benefit to patients in need. The nursing revalidation process reinforces the duty to maintain fitness to practise within an individual's scope of practice. This is an improvement on past accreditation systems for qualified nurses. The process of revalidation for practice now:

1. Incorporates the need for reflection on the code of conduct in day-to-day practice and personal development
2. Encourages engagement in professional networks and discussions which can help to reduce professional isolation
3. Enhances employer engagement in NMC regulatory standards
4. Increases access and participation in continuing professional development.

Theoretical and clinical knowledge

The reflective account of theory and practice attained is completed in line with the NMC's documented format. This record can be verified and confirmed by another registered, experienced nurse or manager to allow for revalidation. This is an attempt to allow more scrutiny of the theoretical and practical continuing professional development attained and the associated documented reflections by the nurse.

Effective practice

One of the four principles of the nursing code of conduct is to practise effectively (NMC, 2018). This requires all registrants to ensure their practice is in line with the best available evidence and inherent in this is the need for nursing, midwifery and care staff to continually refresh their knowledge of the best available evidence to enhance outcomes and experiences for patients. An important, wider benefit of organisations which promote and value evidence-based practice is that such environments correlate with increased levels of staff job satisfaction. Nurses and midwives who are engaged and empowered to deliver research-informed care may also experience increased cohesion in team structures (WHO, 2017).

The nursing code of conduct states that nurses must provide holistic and non-discriminatory care and be evidence-based. The code describes registrants' personal responsibility for keeping up to date with the best available evidence and for this evidence to inform their practice. However, to enable this, the system, organisations and teams need to ensure that relevant, actionable evidence can be identified and presented in a way that practitioners can engage with and use to influence their practice – establishing an environment that facilitates this way of working. To achieve this aim, NHS England and NHS Improvement have published a guide to and examples of good practice in the NHS and is titled: *Leading the acceleration of evidence into practice: a guide for executive nurses* (NHS England and NHS Improvement, 2020).

The NHS guide is aimed at helping executive nurses to think about how to use the practical advice in organisations for implementation of the outcomes of research within practice. This initiative, it is hoped, will improve care, experience and outcomes for patients. The overall aim is to ensure the recognition and understanding of the importance of nursing research. This is a worthy aim which needs to be linked to patient focused care, as an equally commendable goal.

Adherence to the code of conduct in practice

Studies have confirmed that although ethical codes are recognised, nurses have not used them proactively to inform decision-making (Whyte and Gajos, 1996) but cite personal experience and the culture of the healthcare setting as roots of moral commitment in their work (Wilmot et al., 2002).

Moral problems

Twenty-five years ago, a literature review examined moral problems experienced by nurses when caring for terminally ill people. The results showed that nurses did not view important, societal issues such as euthanasia as being morally the most problematic. Rather, situations such as verbally aggressive behaviour of colleagues towards patients, keeping silent about errors and medical treatment given against the wishes of patients were the most troubling areas. Moral problems occurred especially when nurses experienced feelings of powerlessness in relation to the well-being of patients. Moreover, these moral problems proved to be related to institutional organisation, leadership and collaboration with colleagues and other disciplines. Nurses had a limited awareness of the moral dimensions of their practice (Van der Arend and Van den Hurk, 1995).

Another study, over a decade later, had concluded that nurses were troubled for years after experiencing individual incidents in practice when they had felt that they were thwarted in acting as the patient's advocate (Wolf and Zuzelo, 2006). More qualitative studies (which deal with words and meanings) are needed that give a clear picture of nurses' views on the content and functions of an ethical code which is now central to the nursing revalidation and re-registration process.

Helping those in need

Jesus spent his short life ministering to those without power, advantage, or rights. He also knew those who were rich and powerful, to whom He ministered in other ways. Both groups required His message of truth, justice, mercy, healing and peace. What was anathema to Jesus, according to St Matthew, was the strict adherence to the law by the 'great and good' and yet Jesus observed that they were indifferent to those in desperate need: 'They tie up heavy, burdensome loads and lay them on men's shoulders, but they themselves are not willing to lift a finger to move them' (Matthew 23:4). Jesus went on to caution His followers to 'practise and observe everything they tell you. But do not do what they do, for they do not practice what they preach' (Matthew 23:4).

Are we, as practitioners, perhaps feted for our good works, but sometimes oblivious or indifferent to the obvious needs of the most vulnerable? The recent healthcare scandals would confirm this in some areas. Jesus' admonition to the religious leaders of His time needs to be issued today by practitioners to those who treat patients with injustice. They must not walk by on the other side.

The nurse who wishes to act as a Good Samaritan must heed the words of Jesus, to achieve required justice for patients, despite the personal and professional cost sometimes involved when acting as the patient's advocate.

The nurse as link between the patient and the healthcare system

Many studies have referred to the failure to define and explain the concept of nursing advocacy and even the studies' results were not in agreement. Need for justice is one of the basic human needs (Johnstone, 2011). Therefore, it is suggested that nurses can provide justice for their patients better than anyone else (Roush, 2011). Nurses, more than anyone else, are in contact with patients and their problems and are the link between the patient and the healthcare system (Hanks, 2008; Maryland and Gonzalez, 2012).

The catalogue of NHS care scandals becoming known, reveal that despite nurses' close contact with patients, problems can be systemic and hard for one profession alone to challenge, let alone cure. Such situations have been described as insurmountable by some nurses involved.

The power of nurses

Beliefs about nurses' powerlessness, can be replaced by a conviction for change and with support, the status quo can be challenged by nurses with empathy and compassion for the welfare of their patients. Nurses together, as Good Samaritan patient advocates, can effect much change for the improvement of ethically questionable care areas.

Empathy and compassion

I have drunk at the clear and pure waters at
the source of the fountain of life and my thirst was
appeased. Never could I be thirsty, never more could

I be in utter darkness. I have seen the light. I have touched compassion which heals all sorrow and suffering; it is not for myself, but for the world.

(Blau, 1995)

Virtues and values

Educating nurses on an ongoing basis about professional values and standards is essential. Nursing practice requires skill at various levels before nursing competence is assured. Competence in caring for patients means consistency of skilled effort and effective outcome. Skills required are a balance of both technical and expressive components, of which empathy and compassion are essential virtues. Attributes and values associated with compassion have been listed as: *trust, empathy, sensitivity, advocacy, dignity and respect* (DH, 2012).

It is generally agreed that care, compassion and effective communication are essential elements of nursing, which must be demonstrated by all nurses and nursing students. These requirements form the basis of the first essential skills cluster, which stipulates key skills and behaviours that must be demonstrated to meet the standards for registration with the NMC (Bloomfield and Pegram, 2013).

Such elements appear to be lacking when examining the toll of the NHS healthcare scandals in past and recent times, despite the code of conduct and developments in nursing for critical thinking and the accepted forms of critical reflection. Why there has appeared, at times, to be a lack of care, compassion and effective communication is complex and needs analysis.

Compassion

Imagine a world without the countless individuals who risked their own lives to save others during wartime (i.e., the thousands of Holocaust martyrs listed as the Righteous Among Nations). Imagine a world without those who have run into burning buildings or executed other heroic feats of rescue during times of trauma. It is unthinkable.

And what about the concept of compassion in modern everyday life? If this quality has the power to inspire courageous deeds, it must also encourage all sorts of positive behaviours that have both individual and societal benefits (Longczak, 2019).

Compassion can unite the world. Compassion has been described as nursing's most precious asset (Schantz, 2007). The virtue of compassion takes its name from two Latin words, *'com'* and *'passio'*: to suffer with. In its traditional form, it has been a cornerstone of Judeo-Christian ethical traditions which have held it up as the highest virtue: to enter suffering with others and respond to them. It is an ultimate expression of what it means to be human. All the following qualities are expected of healthcare professionals and can define compassion: sympathy, condolence, fellow feeling, humanity, kindness, mercy, pity, sorrow, tender-heartedness, tenderness and understanding (Spooner, 2001).

There are many definitions of compassion – it can be defined as 'to actively promote the other's welfare'. Compassion can be considered an integral element of professionalism, which can be demonstrated by attitudes and behaviours and are the two components recognised as being inherent to a skill, with knowledge accepted as the third component.

Compassion, in simple terms, is 'a deep awareness of the suffering of another coupled with the wish to relieve it' (Chochinov, 2007). Compassion is like dignity; 'People can't necessarily define it, but they know when it isn't there' (Lewis, 2006). The concept of compassion in the Christian tradition is seen in the parable of the Good Samaritan (Luke 10: 25–37) who, at personal cost and with an enduring commitment, responded with compassion to the victim of violence and robbery (Fleming, 2019).

St Thomas Aquinas, following the work of Aristotle and Cicero, noted that the virtues are inherently connected. Compassion is a virtue, a stable, consistent and a morally praiseworthy character disposition (Fleming, 2019).

A study of virtues in palliative care nursing

A recent study by Sinclair et al. (2017) examined how patients with advanced cancer, in palliative care, feel about the virtues of sympathy, empathy and compassion expressed by their health professionals.

The aim of the study was to investigate understandings, experiences and preferences of sympathy, empathy and compassion to develop conceptual clarity for future research and to inform clinical practice.

The research results

- Sympathy was described by participants as an unwanted, pity-based response to a distressing situation, characterised by a lack of understanding and self-preservation of the observer.
- Empathy was experienced by participants as a response that acknowledges and attempts to understand an individual's suffering through emotional resonance.

Empathy has long been seen to be an essential feature of the nurse-patient relationship and can be seen to prefigure compassion.

- Compassion – patients in the study reported that unlike sympathy, empathy and compassion were beneficial, with compassion being the most preferred and impactful. Compassion enhances the key facets of empathy while adding distinct features of being motivated by love, the altruistic role of the responder, action and small acts of kindness (Sinclair et al., 2017).

In caring for anyone, young or old, there needs to be a basic moral awareness, in line with the Hippocratic tradition, 'to do no harm' and in the example of Jesus: to do unto others what we would have done to us. An absence of any empathy is equated with psychopathic states perhaps traceable back to a lack of early empathy experienced by some individuals.

Compassion fatigue

A subjective view of some nurses sees them as sometimes to be lacking in compassion for their patients. This view of poor practice is explored in the related incidents in the book's chapters.

Most nurses enter the profession intending to help others and provide empathetic care for patients with critical physical, mental, emotional and spiritual needs. Empathic and caring nurses, however, can become victims of the continuing stress of meeting the often-overwhelming needs of patients and their families, resulting in compassion fatigue.

It is argued that a lack of compassion towards oneself is likely to preface a lack of compassion towards patients (Gilbert and Procter, 2006). In the practical circumstances in which staff caring for patients feel under pressure, it is often difficult to give them time, often the one thing that makes patients feel cared for. The problem of affording time to care for their patients may be because nurses, due to the current system of nursing, take on those roles which have been devolved from medical staff. These tasks can be technically time consuming. An example would be attempting to take blood from patients or place a cannula. Time management is a skill, developed over time by nurses who must learn to assess and prioritise patient need and any subsequent required action. This may include the wise delegation of important and often basic care.

Wise delegation of care

Where delegation is concerned, the responsibilities of nurses, midwives and nursing associates don't change in circumstances where the person delegating and the person accepting a delegated task are both registered professionals. As a registered professional, whether delegating a task, or receiving a delegated task, you are accountable for your conduct and practice.

The expectation of the code of conduct is that people on the NMC register will:

- only delegate tasks and duties that are within the other person's scope of competence, making sure that they fully understand the instructions.
- make sure that everyone they delegate tasks to are adequately supervised and supported so they can provide safe and compassionate care.

- confirm that the outcome of any task delegated to someone else meets the required standard (NMC, 2018).

Detachment and compassion

It is argued that one achieves something like caring in its emergent form as it is applied in the public world: a combination of closeness and distance, which always runs the risk of tipping either way (Dunlop, 1986).

Compassion can become problematic for staff in settings when displays of emotion are treated as a failure to maintain an appropriate professional distance or authority, though this is not necessarily unique to any one profession or role within healthcare settings. This is particularly relevant to those in roles that place a high value on 'the detached professional'. Such attitudes are more commonly and historically, associated with doctors but perhaps are increasingly prevalent in nursing.

Conclusion

The code of conduct contains a series of statements that taken together can show good practice by nurses and midwives. It puts the interests of patients and service users first. It promotes patient safety, advocacy, evidence-based practice and trust through professionalism.

Nurses gain experience in focusing on their patients' holistic needs, whether they are immediate, medium, or long term. This allows for a professional, effective, yet balanced and caring relationship.

My nursing experience reveals that the more we are consistently committed to the code of conduct and the virtues of empathy and compassion, the more we can sustain the effective performance of such virtues. The less we are consistently committed to the code and these virtues, the less able we are to sustain consistently their application in the long term. As a result, compassion fatigue can hijack our energy and commitment.

We have a duty to manage our own holistic needs (see Chapter 17). This helps us to maintain a consistent commitment to the expectations of the code of conduct and essential virtues of empathy and compassion for each patient as an individual.

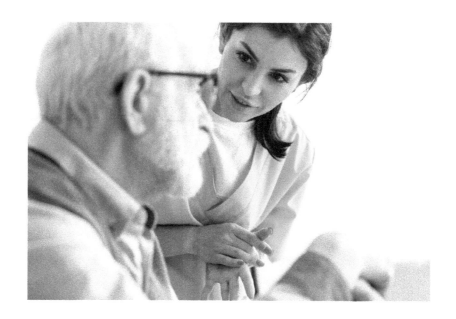

Chapter 4
The government end of life care strategy

If men define situations as real, they are real
in their consequences.

(Thomas and Thomas, 1928)

Introduction

The term 'end of life' is rather unrealistic, as we well know that prognosis-giving is notoriously difficult particularly for patients with non-cancer conditions. There is a risk that such 'labelling' is fraught with danger to vulnerable, elderly people. This is supported by the 'Thomas Theorem' in sociology which was formulated in 1928 and concluded that the interpretation of a situation causes the inevitable action.

'End of life': a self-fulfilling prophecy?

There is a clear need for a network of support and information for nurses working in ethically challenging clinical work environments. Such support must strengthen nursing resolve for defending vulnerable patients' lives. Some environments can be hostile to a pro-life ethos of care. Those nurses and patients' relatives who wish to act as the patient's advocate in an aggressively secular culture can experience opposition from some staff. This can happen in response to basic, warranted questions about patient treatment and care being planned, given, or omitted.

Holistic needs assessment is an opportunity to explore the considered needs for, and with, patients. An agreed plan can be owned by the patient and re-evaluated with their healthcare practitioner. The Macmillan charity have forms which can allow a personalised care and support plan. These can be adapted for patients with or without cancer. A care plan known as a 'continuing care plan' will include needs for care throughout the continuum of the disease.

'End -of -life' care

The term 'end of life care' can appear daunting to some patients. The term appeared at the time of the government's End-of-Life Care Strategy (Department for Health and Social Care, 2008). This strategy was introduced on the understanding that elderly people may not be in the dying phase but certainly would be, within about a year (notwithstanding that people are generally living longer today). Therefore, planning would be necessary for this time by the person's GP and 'end of life' choices would require documenting for all to be aware.

The government defined 'end-of-life' within their care strategy in 2008

The definition of the beginning of end-of-life care, is variable, according to individual person and professional perspectives... For some, the start may be at the time of diagnosis of a condition which usually carries a poor prognosis... For others, it will be at a point when there is deterioration in a chronic illness and it becomes apparent that the likely prognosis is measured in months or possibly a year or two. Alternatively, it could be an elderly person who is becoming increasingly frail.

(DH, 2008)

Questioning nurses

Apart from the need for patient consent to a procedure and for this to be documented wherever possible, as stated within the nursing code of conduct, nurses with concerns over proposed treatment or its omission must question, clarify and establish the ethics of care on behalf of their dependent patients.

No patient should be told 'there is nothing more that we can do' as there is always something to be done, for example, treating symptoms. There are limits to active treatments when prognosis is not hopeful. But where symptoms are to be alleviated, there is still treatment in terms of effective symptom control to promise patients. Moreover, issuing a prognosis is even more difficult where there is no cancer diagnosis. People may just be elderly, frail, or living with dementia or chronic conditions, such as heart and lung disease when prognosis is notoriously difficult.

The Gold Standard Framework is an anticipatory approach to 'end of life' care

The Gold Standard Framework (GSF), as part of the government strategy, is described as a model that enables good practice to be available to all people nearing the end of their lives, irrespective of diagnosis. It is a way of raising the level of care to the standard of the best. Through the GSF, palliative care skills for patients with cancer can now be used to meet the needs of people with other life-limiting conditions (Department of Health and Social Care, 2008).

The GSF both influences national policy developments and helps put policy into practice on the ground, supporting grassroots change in line with the following: NHS long-term Plan, NICE guidance, Enhanced Health in Care Homes, DH End of Life Care (EOLC) Strategy, Care Quality Commission (CQC) and Skills for Care (see https://www.skillsforcare.org.uk/Funding/Funding. aspx).

The EOLC strategy was endorsed by NICE:

This quality standard covers care for adults
(aged 18 and over) who are approaching the end of their life.
This includes people who are likely to die within 12 months,
people with advanced, progressive, incurable conditions
and people with life-threatening acute conditions. It also
covers support for their families and carers. It includes
care provided by health and social care staff in all settings.
It describes high-quality care in priority areas for improvement.

(NICE, 2004)

Such conditions, in terms of prognosis, can commonly surprise and confound doctors and nurses. Hence the need for caution with a label of 'life-limiting' conditions.

People with 'life-limiting' conditions

Many patients live good lives with chronic medical conditions. These are people who do not have cancer but simply are old and frail and/or living with dementia, of which, it must be understood, there are very varying degrees. However, the GSF has been introduced to many GP practices in the UK and is being used as a framework for patients with 'end of life' care needs, regardless of diagnosis (Hansford and Meehan, 2007).

This situation encouraged use of the LCP which was instituted for patients needing palliative care and then extended for patients with non-terminal illness. The LCP was not a perfect concept in palliative care, but the LCP (or its similar practices of sedation and dehydration) results in many unnecessary deaths for patients with any condition.

The NHS has produced an 'end-of-life care' website (NHS, 2020) which contains information about what end of life care involves, when it starts and the decisions people may want to think about, including financial issues and how and where people may want to be cared for, for example:

- care at home
- care in a care home
- care in hospital
- hospice care.

Residential and care homes

The Gold Standard Framework in care homes programme (GSFCH) was implemented in over 400 care homes in the UK (Thomas, 2007). The programme currently includes care homes that incorporate nursing care but the implementation programme will eventually include care homes that are also residential. The

GSFCH Programme has the same aims and key tasks as the GSF in Primary Care with the underlying philosophy of the programme being to enable residents to live well until they die. The focus is on quality of life as well as quality of dying.

The programme also aims to make it more possible for the resident to die in the place of their choice, which for most would mean remaining in the care home. However, no assumptions can be made as care must be appropriate for the patient's situation which may entail hospital-based care at some point of obvious medical need.

Planning ahead

The NHS is explicit about what the 'end of life' programme entails:

- Planning for the 'end-of-life' is explained as sometimes being called advance care planning and involves thinking and talking about wishes and feelings for how people are cared for in the final months of life. This can include treatments people do not want to have.
- Planning like this can help people while they are able to let others know their particular wishes and feelings. Informing family members about wishes could help them if they ever must make decisions about future care.

'End of life' care plans

These are commonly used and have, in effect, replaced the controversial LCP. The problem remains the same though: patients are put on a pathway which determines what care will and crucially, will not, be provided. This can simply be a route whereby food, fluids and medication are withdrawn so that death inexorably follows. It is also vital to be aware that some medications which may be administered at this time can also depress respiration, especially in the presence of dehydration (Cole and Duddington, 2021a).

Prognosis of dying in 'end of life' care

Prognosis as both a science and an art should be understood as notoriously difficult. Wise doctors and nurses accept this fact. Yet they also understand that there may be more ease in giving a prognosis when a patient has a cancer diagnosis. It is more difficult to issue a prognosis when being predicted as far in advance as a year, within the projected premise of 'end of life'. 'Approaching death' is a questionable concept, particularly for patients who are not terminally ill.

Evaluation of the Gold Standard Framework Strategy

Initial evaluation showed that the GSF's anticipatory approach to care has positive effects on pain and symptom control and that improved planning, particularly with regards to medication that might be needed, out of hours, has enabled some hospital admissions to be averted (King et al., 2005). The GSF has been endorsed by the NHS End-of-Life Care Programme.

The government's End-of-Life Care Strategy (2008) confirms the GSF as a major tool for improving care at the end of life. The GSF is not a prescriptive model but a framework that can be adapted according to local needs and resources. It enables teams to build on the good practice already present and provide coordinated care with a more patient-centred focus (Department of Health and Social Care, 2008).

The GSF is thought to provide a framework for a planned system of care in consultation with the patient and family. It promotes better coordination and collaboration between healthcare professionals. The tool helps to optimise out-of-hours care and is hoped to prevent crises and inappropriate hospital admissions.

'Inappropriate' is, however, a subjective word. Health professionals may not all agree on an opinion of 'inappropriate treatment' and may consider such a decision as 'defeatist'.

Reduced hospital admission a worthy goal?

Who then decides when an admission to hospital is inappropriate? Is the age of the patient associated with such a possibly discriminatory judgement? Reduction of emergency visits to hospital sounds a worthy aim as part of this 'strategy', but an emergency is just that and no amount of planning to prevent admission to hospital for elderly people can change this fact. Old people are not a homogenous group with similar health needs or prospects. Life cannot be so neatly controlled by a tidy label of 'end of life' care strategies. Who knows when a patient will die? How many patients have confounded an agreed prognosis, sometimes by years? True arrival at 'end of life' is a special circumstance with important patient and relative concerns that may not be easily incorporated into a care pathway or framework.

Implementation of the LCP, while having the apparently, good intention of setting 'end of life' care standards for imminently dying patients, had, on too many occasions, led to a withdrawal or reduction of care, a 'tick-box' mentality and actions which would appear to hasten the death of the patient (Centre for Policy on Ageing, 2014).

Advance directives

There are increasing calls for a national database of people's 'living wills', instantly accessible by all healthcare practitioners, both in primary care and hospitals and to be accessed also by paramedics and A&E doctors. This sounds very efficient; however, it should be considered unethical for someone to have an advance directive without being given an understanding of the MCA (2005) which defines 'treatment' as 'any diagnostic or other procedure'. This definition could have serious implications for those with a new condition needing investigation. Clinically-assisted nutrition and hydration (CANH) are now considered as medical treatment, according to the MCA. People, however, have the right to know about this change to past accepted treatment practice and often do change their mind about previous wishes.

Death at home

Dying at home may be an understandable wish. This is not achieved in many cases for multiple reasons, including a lack of caregivers, insufficient resources and unpreparedness of the patient and/or the family.

It is likely that many patients would prefer to die at home with family and friends but there could be problems with unexpected complications which require hospital interventions, such as a distressing haemorrhage, breathlessness, or pain, all of which require skilled interventions that could not be provided in a domiciliary setting.

Fixed decisions

Policies of 'care consistency' at 'end of life' may mean non-individualised care approaches. If home care is wanted and possible, this needs to be discussed further with the patient and family, early, enlisting relevant agencies. Flexible approaches are the way forward, not rigid pathways.

Templates for advance decision-making

There are many different templates for advance directives in circulation, the most popular of which is the Recommended Summary Plan for Emergency Care and Treatment (ReSPECT) process which was drawn up in 2016 by the Resuscitation Council UK (RCUK) and is now used by 150 hospital trusts.

The ReSPECT process was developed with healthcare professionals, members of the public and design experts at the Helix Centre at Imperial College London, to support professionals, patients and/or their families having carefully constructed realistic and person-centred conversations (RCUK, 2020).

The ReSPECT process creates personalised recommendations for a person's clinical care and treatment in any future emergency in which they are unable to make or express choices. Recommendations are created through conversations between a person, their families and their health and care professionals to understand what matters to them and what is realistic in terms of their care and treatment.

Patient preferences and clinical recommendations are recorded on a non-legally binding form which can be reviewed and adapted if circumstances change. The ReSPECT process can be used for anyone but will have increasing relevance for people who have complex health needs, people who are likely to be nearing the end of their lives and people who are at risk of sudden deterioration or cardiac arrest. Some people will want to record their care and treatment preferences for other reasons.

The ReSPECT process:

- Starts with a conversation between a person and a healthcare professional.
- Creates a summary of personalised recommendations for a person's clinical care in a future emergency in which they do not have capacity to make or express choices.
- Will be used to document conversations and recommendations made for care and treatment in an emergency.

The ReSPECT form

The form is a clinical record of agreed recommendations. It is not a legally binding document. The RCUK (2022) has updated and improved the ReSPECT form (version 3, available via the RCUK website). The version 3 form may be used with the person and either a health or social care professional, legal welfare proxy/lasting power of attorney (LPA) or family member involved in a ReSPECT conversation. As patients are often not able to make decisions about their priorities of care or treatment in an emergency, it is important to discuss what they would want to happen in advance.

Of particular concern is the section where clinical interventions or non-interventions will be documented under headings:

- prioritise extending life
- balance extending life with comfort and valued outcomes
- prioritise comfort.

'Comfort' as a term in this situation needs to be fully explained so that patients are aware of possible implications for them in the future. Many patients will be guided by the clinical section where clinical interventions or non-interventions are discussed, including about CPR. An obvious risk is that the layperson will defer to clinical opinion about realistic interventions, including potential non-admission to hospital (where new or existing problems would reasonably require hospitalisation).

Cardio pulmonary resuscitation (CPR)

ReSPECT is already widely used by health and social care organisations across England and in some parts of Scotland to support healthcare professionals and patients having important conversations in advance about their realistic emergency care choices. This includes discussion on whether CPR should be attempted in a future emergency. Such decisions made by mentally competent people need to be respected, bearing in mind that not all CPR incidents are doomed to fail.

Risks of the ReSPECT process

The Chair of the Medical Ethics Alliance illustrates the risks associated with the ReSPECT form.

It is, though, a form of advance directive and
subject to the limitations of advance directives
especially if it is long standing and the
patient's views have changed.
It puts before the patient the options
"Prioritise sustaining life, even at the expense
of some comfort", and
"Prioritise comfort, even at the expense of sustaining life"
In fact, often the best treatment may
lie between these two extremes
but there is a risk that it may
be seen as one or the other.
It is completed and interpreted
by the doctor.

There is a tick box at the bottom of the form concerning
cardio-pulmonary resuscitation which includes
"Not recommended".
In the case of where a patient lacks capacity should
they suffer dementia for example, a health
attorney should be consulted.
Next of kin does not have legal standing.
Where there is learning disability, autism, or psychosis
a health attorney or court appointed
guardian may be needed.
The mortality may be increased where these
conditions arise as shown by
the 2019 Learning Disabilities Mortality Review

(Cole, 2022)

Personalised templates relating to 'end of life' care

An example of helping patients is seen in the following statement, relating to 'end-of-life' choice documentation (Cole and Duddington, 2021a):

1. I am a Roman Catholic and in all decisions about my health care the teachings of the Catholic Church on end-of-life decisions must be observed.
2. I do not consider food and water to be medical treatment but instead consider them to be fundamental necessities of life. Therefore, I wish to be provided with food and water, including medically assisted nutrition and hydration.
3. I am absolutely opposed to euthanasia and expressly forbid any treatment or failure to treat – which might constitute euthanasia.
4. I do not wish any notice which says that I am not to be resuscitated to be placed on my bed or in any other place. Instead, I wish all decisions of this kind to be made in response to specific, medical situations.

For patients' appointed advocates, there is a prepared statement should they disagree with an end-of-life care proposal (see Chapter 5).

Giving time to patients

Just as pastors are concerned for their flocks, so too are nurses concerned for their patients' benefit. Patients' 'best interests', as a term, can be subjective. Caring is a complex process. It is also our greatest duty and opportunity, one that should evoke humility and not an overreliance on chemical agents to manage 'problems' rather than patients' real needs for palliation of any symptoms that may be present. In the practical circumstances, however, where staff caring for patients may feel under pressure and experience themselves as having little time, it is often difficult to provide the one thing – time, for the patient, which makes him or her feel cared for.

Holistic care needs assessments

Restoring wholeness is a legitimate goal of nursing and so the term 'holistic', from the Greek *Holos* meaning 'whole' or 'complete', is a very appropriate way to describe what we aim to do. Individualised assessments may be a better way of caring for people who wish to discuss 'end of life' care – as an individual with particular needs. This may provide needed time for patients, rather than risking the dangers of what can seem to be immutable, prescriptive pathways or frameworks.

The Nursing Code of Professional Conduct (NMC, 2018) states that nurses must make the care of the patient their first concern in line with the expectation of holistic care. A failure to relieve patient symptoms or address fears by referrals to the appropriate members of the multidisciplinary team for their specific expertise, does not comply with individualised, holistic care.

Subjective labels such as 'end of life' applied to fit and healthy older people may deny them the treatment and care that they require. The COVID-19 pandemic has highlighted the risk of discriminatory attitudes and denial of treatment for elderly people (see Chapter 11).

A holistic needs assessment (HNA)

An HNA is a simple questionnaire which aims to:

- identify a patient's concerns
- start a conversation about needs
- develop a Personalised Care and Support Plan
- share the right information, at the right times
- signpost to relevant services.

Assessment of needs meetings

Such assessments can help people focus on any of their needs together with their nurse. The following example originates from the Macmillan cancer charity (2021) but can be used for patients needing palliative care, with or without cancer (see Chapter 15).

The HNA usually has three parts:

1. **A questionnaire for patients**

   This allows patients to rate their concerns by giving them a score out of 10. These can be answered on paper (with an HNA concerns checklist) or electronically (an electronic HNA). It usually does not take long for patients to complete the assessment under the following four headings: *Physical, Emotional, Practical, Financial, Spiritual.*

2. **A conversation to discuss the answers.**

   This is an opportunity to talk about the patient's needs and concerns listed as above. The person may like to bring a family member, a friend or carer to the meeting if they find it helpful. The conversation usually lasts around 20 minutes.

3. **Creation of a personalised care and support plan (PCSP).**

   The nurse and patient together can create a PCSP which can help address a person's concerns and is achieved with the following interventions:

1. holistic needs assessments
2. end-of-treatment summaries
3. primary cancer care (or other condition) reviews
4. health and well-being information and support.

A PCSP can include information to help people self-manage, along with contact details of any helpful organisations or services.

A PCSP can help people, particularly those living with cancer to take an active and empowered role in the way their care is planned and delivered, with interventions and care tailored around the things that matter most to them. This is achieved through a series of supportive conversations in which the patient, or someone who knows them well, actively participates to explore the management of their own health and well-being in the context of their life and family situation.

The benefits of a PCSP

A PCSP can help to:

• facilitate conversations with patients
• identify their needs (with holistic needs assessments)
• share the right information, at the right times
• signpost to local support services.

Patients are given a copy of their care plan to keep with them for review with their nurse as required.

Patients' wishes and feelings

Practitioners should always maintain a degree of healthy scepticism where pathways or frameworks are used, or ideas are put to patients which focus on wishes and feelings alone rather than what treatment options remain and with due regard for individualised patient need. This is demonstrated by the disaster, in very many cases, of the LCP, where so often, no discussion occurred with people as to their wishes. Where discussion did occur, there were words such as 'comfort care' which would be promised but which was, in fact, quite the opposite for so many in terms of blanket medication, often, typically strong sedatives, opioids, without provision of hydration.

Conclusion

Once whichever framework or template is in place, some older patients may not be admitted to hospital where appropriate. Medical emergencies are no respecter of the age of patients and such events should be addressed in line with the need of any patient, which is to receive appropriate, beneficial care.

Pressure on elderly people for non-treatment?

Elderly patients, either in robust health or with increasing frailty or with a stable chronic illness, should not automatically become labelled as being in the near 'dying' or 'end of life' phase, nor should they be considered eligible for a care pathway or framework for dying patients without even a clear prognosis. This can easily become a form of pressure on elderly people to be persuaded to agree to avoidance of hospital admission at all costs. This approach is not medically ethical or realistic. This is not an evidence-based strategy or fair to elderly, fit patients. Patients warrant a culture of life and hope, not death. The public expect their doctors to be there to help when help is needed whether in the community, care home, or hospital setting, particularly in medical emergencies. These are no respecter of age and should be managed in a non-discriminatory, ethical manner for the benefit of each patient, regardless of age.

Patient labelling

Patients labelled as nearing 'the end-of-life' warrant the best care and treatment whether in an emergency or non-emergency situation. Patients with a poor prognosis need to be afforded a conversation in a sensitive manner about their situation. They need to understand the possible risks and benefits of treatment at their stage of the prognosis. Family members and the patient will understand the respect given by these reasonable, sensitive conversations with their health professionals.

Ensuring holistic care

Pope St John Paul II writes that the parable of the Good Samaritan,

> *… not only spurs one to help the sick, but also to do all one can to reintegrate them into society. For Christ, in fact, healing is also this reintegration: just as sickness excludes the human person from the community, so healing must bring him to rediscover his place in the family, in the Church and in society. In addressing the two aspects of sickness – disease and illness – the Good Samaritan removes the social stigma and poverty that entrap the victim.*

(Pope St John Paul II, 2000)

'Holistic care' must not be an easy term to use as a claim that it is offered to patients. Assessment and care must be undertaken with patience, effective communication and creative thinking to ensure no element of holistic need is missed. Health professionals may have to challenge the culture where optimum benefit for patients is at risk. This may be at the expense of the health professional's personal comfort to fulfil their role of advocate and to obey the dictates of conscience.

Ethical and moral development is needed by all human beings, despite the inherent faculty of conscience. Education of healthcare professionals in these areas is essential to further refine the collective understanding of what it means to be a trusted health professional for the most vulnerable in need of patient advocacy.

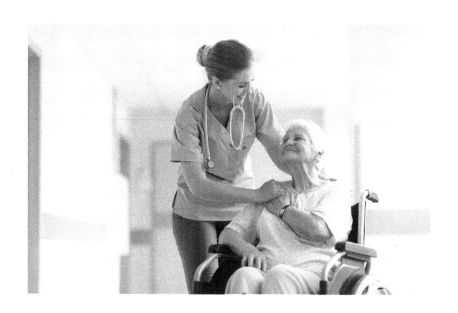

Chapter 5

The Mental Capacity Act 2005 and ethical principles for healthcare staff

---

The King will reply, "Truly I tell you, whatever you did for one of the least of these brothers and sisters of mine, you did for me".

(Matthew 25: 40)

Introduction

The Mental Capacity Act (MCA) 2005 is a set of laws that were passed by Parliament, which are designed to protect and give power to vulnerable people who lack the mental capacity to make their own decisions. It came into force in England and Wales in 2007. While not perfect, the laws are significant in safeguarding the lives of people who may lack mental capacity. There are areas of concern about this Act in relation to the need to promote patient benefit due to the changes brought in by the Act, regarding the definition of treatment defined as: any diagnostic or other procedure MCA, 2005, (section 64.1).

Who lacks mental capacity?

There is a two-stage test to work out if someone lacks mental capacity.

- **Stage one:** Does the person have an impairment of, or a disturbance in the functioning of, their mind or brain? This could include dementia, learning disabilities, mental illness, brain damage, etc.
- **Stage two:** Does the impairment or disturbance mean that the person is unable to make a specific decision when they need to? A person is unable to decide if they cannot:
  o understand information about the decision to be made
  o retain that information in their mind

o use or weigh that information as part of the decision-making process

o communicate their decision.

The MCA is underpinned by five key principles

1. Every adult has the right to make his or her own decisions and everyone should be assumed to be capable of doing this unless proved otherwise.
2. Everyone should be given all the support they need to make their own decisions before they are judged incapable of doing this.
3. People should have the right to make 'eccentric' or 'unwise' decisions – it is their capacity to make decisions, not the decisions themselves, that may be in question.
4. Anything done for or on behalf of people without capacity must be in their best interests.
5. Anything done for or on behalf of people without capacity should restrict their rights and freedoms as little as possible.

The fourth and fifth principles apply only when a person has been assessed to not have mental capacity for the decision in question. While it is not a principle of the Act, it is key to remember that mental capacity is time and decision specific.

'End of life' choices

Who can reasonably judge, considerably ahead of time, when 'end-of-life' is the true status of a person? From October 2007, under the MCA, admission to a hospital for almost any reason entails patients being asked whether they have or would like information about documents formalising their 'end of life' choices. These are commonly used, and have in effect, replaced the controversial LCP. There are obvious risks for patients who may have requested no treatment at the end-of-life, as according to the MCA, assisted food and fluid is now considered as 'medical treatment'. The Good Samaritan practitioner will ensure that this is understood by patients to prevent them becoming victims of potential fraud and deceit in relation to this change in medical practice where, hitherto, such 'treatment' was considered as humane care.

Advance directives

The MCA encourages the initiative known as 'living wills' – a concept advocated within the Act and believed to promise patients a say in their care, even after severe brain damage. People are encouraged by advance refusals to make forward plans, for a time when they may lose capacity and choose ahead of time to forego treatment. In an advance refusal or living will, under the MCA, a patient may request that life-preserving treatment be withdrawn if they become too ill to communicate. Death for those who have asked for treatment withdrawal would mean the removal of clinically assisted nutrition and hydration (CANH). This was a scandalous method of abusive neglect by omission, in so many cases, as part of the discredited LCP practices of often unnecessary opioids, sedation and dehydration.

False promises of advance directives

The MCA sets out rules about advance decisions to refuse medical treatment and creates new safeguards controlling many types of research involving people who lack capacity. Apart from the fact we cannot know how the patient feels or whether they might recover, there is the problem that we all change our minds. Such patients may be vulnerable to the decisions that they may have made some time before in an advance directive, which may later be used against them, reflecting a lack of justice for patients. They may be reliant on others who may be unwilling to offer a chance for any treatment (as part of expected beneficence) to aid in their survival or at least to assure remaining life quality.

Risks of advance directives

We need to examine the potential for any eugenic ethos (malevolence) under law, while the imperative for Christians in healthcare is to ensure patients' education and true understanding of such decisions.

Moreover, the potential of vulnerable patients becoming research subjects under the Act, when incapacitated, would appear to be a breach of the ethical principle of justice for patients. Ethical dilemmas, for those nurses wishing to act as patient advocates rather than agents of the state, can be envisioned.

The MCA was developed from the original Mental Health Act (1983/2007) which was concerned with financial affairs where mental capacity was impaired. The MCA adds to the original lasting power of attorney for financial matters to now include possible health needs.

Treatment

The MCA defines 'treatment' as: 'any diagnostic or other procedure' (MCA, 2005, section 64:1). This is quite a far-reaching definition with potentially unforeseen and unwanted consequences when people may have always believed that clinically assisted nutrition and hydration (CANH) is not 'treatment' and that diagnostic investigation for new health problems should not be denied where appropriate.

Defeatist healthcare, with consequences for conscientious objection, is all too easily the result of such a legal definition of treatment. Denying diagnostic investigations to patients in obvious need, irrespective of age, prognosis or original diagnosis, would be rightly considered as negligence.

Mental capacity and patients' rights

Contrary to a popular myth about the supposed aims of living wills, these did not spring from a patient's rights movement concerned about overzealous and unwanted treatment being 'forced' on terminally ill patients. Rather, the 'living will' was invented by the 'right to die' movement as a step towards legalisation of euthanasia (Grimstad, 2007).

Ethical issues

- Should professionals refuse to manage patients with advance directives?

- Should nursing homes have the right not to admit those patients with a living will?
- Should nurses and doctors address the precepts of the MCA with all patients, regardless of their long-held values and beliefs?

Patient understanding of living wills/advanced directives/refusals

Advance refusals simply presuppose more control over future care than is realistic. People making their own 'end of life' care plan (as part of the MCA) may not be aware of its implications. Do patients understand treatment complexity? Symptoms of treatable conditions at the end of life can be relieved. Even a patient's past verbal remarks can be considered for future decision-making by others under the MCA.

Therefore, the MCA may threaten death by treatment omission and widens the possibility of treatment withdrawal for many incapacitated patients. Prohibition can be exercised on simple treatments such as insulin, antibiotics (which can help with tissue pain due to infection) and CANH.

Enduring power of attorney and lasting powers of attorney

Any enduring power of attorney (EPA) made before the MCA came into force on 1 October 2007, remains valid.

- Under the previous law, an EPA was restricted to making decisions over property and affairs, which includes financial affairs and accessing the person's information.
- A lasting power of attorney (LPA) now has extended powers of attorney in relation to health. They can be made at any time when the person making it has the mental capacity to do so, provided they are aged 18 or over.
- Both an EPA and LPA must be registered. An LPA can be registered at any time, but a personal welfare LPA will only be effective once the person has lost the capacity to make their own decisions.

What Is a lasting power of attorney (LPA)?

Under UK law, an LPA can be made and be registered. The attorney represents the person who may be unable to make end of life decisions. An LPA is a legal document that allows a chosen person to make decisions for another who has appointed the health attorney. An LPA allows people to plan for when they no longer have capacity to make their own decisions and to make sure that these decisions are handled by a trusted person. The health attorney may, one day, be required to act as a Good Samaritan.

People who have appointed family members with an LPA must have their advocacy role respected. When acting under an LPA, an attorney (the appointed person, appointee) must make sure that the MCA's statutory principles are followed and check whether the person has the capacity to make that decision for themselves – if they do, a personal welfare LPA cannot be used and the person must make their own decision.

Attorney

The adult attorney does not have to be a lawyer or someone with specialist knowledge. It could be a partner, a family member, a friend, or a professional. This attorney has the legal power to make certain decisions on behalf of appointers and continues to make decisions for them after they have lost the capacity to make the decisions for themselves. Questionnaires for setting up an LPA can be accessed via a solicitor, but checking completed content is recommended by an independent healthcare professional to ensure full understanding of all involved as to the meaning of 'treatment'.

What decisions can a healthcare attorney make?

A healthcare attorney can only make decisions for another who is unable to make these decisions themselves. They can also decide about:

- finances
- property
- future healthcare
- future personal care and welfare
- daily routine (for example, eating and what to wear)
- routine medical care – when and where this should happen
- moving into a care home
- lifesaving or life-sustaining treatment.

The exact decisions that attorneys can take for someone else depends on what is documented in the signed, lasting power of attorney.

What the healthcare attorney can do

The healthcare attorney can be given power to refuse certain treatments for the person. For example:

- cardiac resuscitation after a heart attack
- blood transfusions
- medication
- electroconvulsive therapy (even if the person is sectioned and the responsible clinician or approved clinician prescribes this treatment).

What the healthcare attorney cannot do

The healthcare attorney will not be able to act in a way or decide, for example, outside of the law:

- consent to a deprivation of liberty being imposed without a court order
- make a decision that conflicts with a decision under guardianship which a guardian has the power to make, such as where to live
- make a decision that goes against any treatment refusals set out in the advance decision (if made after the appointment of the attorney). (This can, and should, be an area of debate.)

The doctor's motives

The MCA states that the doctors should not use the Act to be motivated by a desire to bring about the patient's death. This is a questionable point, as no doctor, it is hoped, would be motivated in such a way. It can be argued that this stated prohibition implies some inherent dangers in the Act for vulnerable patients.

Assisted food and fluid – 'medical treatment'

Due to the MCA now considering CANH to be medical treatment, there is an obvious danger of its discontinuation or its non-initiation in cases where patients may not be dying. It is argued that the MCA enshrines in statute law the decision made in the case of young Tony Bland, whose life was ended by withdrawal of his CANH, although his brain damage was not severe enough for him to have needed ventilator support (see Chapter 8).

Within the independent review of the LCP; More Care Less Pathway (DH, 2013), the chapter about '*Hydration and Nutrition*' states that if a patient wishes to eat and drink, then they should be supported to do so (1.64); failure to support oral hydration and nutrition when still possible and desired should be regarded as professional misconduct (1.64). Some patients may not be able to manage oral hydration. The Good Samaritan will ensure that the patient is appropriately cared for to prevent prolonged dehydration for which the most appropriate CANH route should be arranged. Hoping that the patient will die before the effects of starvation and hydration occur is an abusive approach to patients.

Care for the elderly

The MCA (2005) has relevance to everyone, with its emphasis on advance decisions, but particularly to elderly patients, who are known to commonly require costly investigation and treatments. Healthcare demand for costly interventions for the elderly often does not match supply in some impoverished NHS Trusts and many older people are sensitive to feeling a potential burden for the State and even their family members. The current focus about the 'right to die', which tends to dominate public debate, is a relentless, simplistic response to end of life care issues which endangers those who feel a burden and have some dependence or disability.

Elderly care assessment

A comprehensive assessment of care needs for an elderly person admitted for treatment and care will attend to diagnosis, treatment, health promotion and rehabilitation where required. Required home adaptation, support for family members/carers and personal and/ or palliative care will also be a focus where required. It is important to respect a patient's desires and be able to examine and to judge their preferences together with them, checking their understanding without compromise of long-accepted moral principles.

Ethical care for the elderly

The experience of the intrinsically flawed and ultimately discredited LCP should be salutary where 'end of life' labelling is expressed in pathways or frameworks that may 'straitjacket' patients into inappropriate 'care'. Emergencies and unexpected illness cannot be tidily managed with an overall aim of keeping old people out of hospital. Where treatment is needed it should be received, as for a younger person, and care outside of hospital may not be ethical or practical. The Good Samaritan nurse will ensure that old people are not disadvantaged in the future with plans made that they do not fully understand.

Treatment vs care

The choice between treatment and care is used by some to suggest a false dichotomy between the medical and social models of care. Both are required for people with complex needs. The five governing principles (outlined at the beginning of this chapter) that underpin the MCA serve as the basis for the detailed, complex piece of legislation which is supported by the MCA Code of Practice (2007).

The MCA Code of Practice (2007)

This is a statutory framework to empower and protect vulnerable people who are not able to make their own decisions or have no living will. The Act's Code of Practice can give guidance about the legislation and creates a new offence of neglect or ill-treatment. Most parts of the MCA apply to people aged 16 and over.

Independent Mental Capacity Advocates (IMCA). (General Regulations, 2006)

These regulations provide practical guidance on how the MCA is applied across various settings on a day-to-day basis for health professionals and other staff involved in the care or treatment of people who may lack capacity, as well as for unpaid carers and relatives of people who lack capacity. The MCA establishes a system for providing an Independent Mental Capacity Advocate (IMCA) for particularly vulnerable people without family or friends.

Safeguards for people without family or friends

The role of the IMCA is to support and represent the person in the decision-making process. Essentially, they make sure that the MCA is being followed. The MCA identifies this need when a person has no one other than paid staff with whom it would be appropriate to consult.

An IMCA must be over 18 years old and can be instructed for people in the following circumstances:

1. The person is aged 16 years or over.
2. A decision needs to be made about either a long-term change in accommodation or   serious medical treatment.
3. The person lacks capacity to make that decision.

4. There is no one independent of services, such as a family member or friend.

The MCA Code of Practice, (10.74–10.78), provides more information about how the decisions about IMCAs can be made. For example, if someone has limited family contact or if family members live some distance away, an IMCA can be instructed.

The MCA Code sets out the IMCA's role and functions. These are grouped into four key areas:

- gathering information
- evaluating information
- making representations
- challenging decisions.

Who is 'appropriate to consult' for people with no one to help them?

People without capacity who do not have friends or family to support them will be appointed an IMCA to represent them in any decision about

- serious medical treatment
- NHS or local authority accommodation
- adult protection: making some important decisions.

These appointees can only work with an individual once they have been instructed by an appropriate person/body

- For serious medical treatment decisions – the appropriate person will be a medical practitioner who has responsibility for the person's treatment.
- For accommodation decisions and care reviews – the appropriate body is likely to be the local authority responsible for the arrangements.
- For adult protection cases – this will be the local authority, coordinating the adult protection proceedings.

1. **Serious medical treatment**

    This is defined by the MCA as treatment which involves:
    - giving new treatment
    - stopping treatment that has already started
    - withholding treatment that could be offered in circumstances where:
        - if a single treatment is proposed, there is a fine balance between the likely benefits and the burdens to the patient and the risks involved
        - a decision between a choice of treatments is delicately balanced
        - the treatment proposed is likely to have profound consequences for the patient.

2. **Accommodation**

    Local authorities and NHS bodies can instruct an IMCA to support and represent a person who lacks capacity when:
    - they have arranged accommodation for that person
    - they aim to review the arrangements (as part of a care plan or otherwise)
    - there are no family or friends who it would be appropriate to consult.

3. **Adult protection**

    Local authorities and NHS bodies need to consider in each case whether they will instruct an IMCA for these decisions. An IMCA may also be provided to people for other decisions concerning care reviews or adult protection.

    In adult protection cases, an IMCA may be instructed even where family members or others are available to be consulted.

    When local authorities are using adult protection procedures, they can instruct an IMCA for either the person who is alleged to have been abused or neglected or a person who is alleged to have abused another person. The local authority must be thinking about or already have taken protective measures for the person. In adult protection cases, access to IMCAs is not restricted to people who do not have someone to represent them who is independent of services. People who lack capacity who have family and friends can still have an IMCA to support them in the adult protection procedures.

The nurse, as part of the care team, needs to be aware, as the Good Samaritan, of the importance of advocacy in identifying the need for an IMCA.

The new Court of Protection

This replaces the old court of the same name, which only dealt with decisions about the property and financial affairs of people lacking capacity to manage their own affairs. As well as property and affairs, the new court deals with both serious decisions affecting healthcare and personal welfare matters. These were previously dealt with by the High Court under its inherent jurisdiction.

The new Court of Protection is a superior court of record and is able to establish precedent (it can set examples for future cases) and build up expertise in all issues related to lack of capacity. It has the same powers, rights, privileges, and authority as the High Court. When reaching any decision, the court must apply all the statutory principles of the Act. In particular, it must make a decision in the best interests of the person who lacks capacity to make the specific decision. There will usually be a fee for applications to the court.

Details of the fees charged by the court, and the circumstances in which the fees may be waived or remitted, are available from the Office of the Public Guardian.

The MCA and ethical principles for healthcare staff
Ethical principles

It is argued and commonly accepted, that a principles-based common morality needs to be understood among professionals which can be interculturally and internationally accepted. A set of ethical principles can help in avoiding the two polar dangers: moral relativism and moral imperialism (Gillon, 2003).

Moral relativism

This finds that there is no objective way to establish that a particular morality is the correct morality and concludes that there is no reason to believe in one single, true morality. This it can be argued, is a deeply dangerous ideology to faith and morals. In the last homily he gave before becoming Pope Benedict XVI, Cardinal Joseph Ratzinger described modern life as ruled by a "dictatorship of relativism". He argued that this concept does not recognize anything as definitive and whose ultimate goal consists solely of satisfying the desires of one's own ego. Such a belief has been refuted by some others who argue for an intellectual and social life free of the desire for an infantilizing authority (Perl, 2007).

Moral imperialism

This is imposition of a set of moral values, either through force or through cultural criticism, onto a culture which does not share those values. The charge of moral imperialism is levelled against theorists and commentators who feel entitled to force a system of morality onto another culture or to criticise moral codes different from their own (Jenkins, 2011).

There are several principles for guiding ethical practice

Ethical principles are applicable across all fields of care and are particularly important in relation to research. The commonly discussed ethical principles include sanctity of life, confidentiality, fidelity, beneficence, non-malevolence, autonomy, justice and veracity.

Ethical principles about sanctity of life are debated in relation to abortion, assisted suicide and euthanasia. The sanctity of life ethic is increasingly challenged today where the quality-of-life ethic, according to modern bioethicists, is gaining prominence.

The sanctity of life

In his influential article titled *The Morality of Abortion*, the Protestant theologian Paul Ramsey (1968), claimed that 'from an authentic religious point of view' any sanctity or dignity of the life of human beings derives from God and not from biological processes or from any social or political order. While maintaining that a 'life's sanctity consists not in its worth to anybody', Ramsey rejected the idea that any human being's value could become dependent on contingent processes of valuing. Speaking positively, Ramsey's defence of the divine origin of humans' sacredness is a defence of the inalienability of human dignity and the inalienable right to life. This ethical stand on the sanctity of human life is increasingly in opposition to those who view life quality as superior to life's sanctity.

Quality of life is an important concept as is the sanctity of life moral principle. The latter principle is paramount while the former concept can be subjective and ill understood by those who perceive others' quality of life, as poor but very much prized by those individuals, despite the views of others.

A model for ethics in practice

Beauchamp and Childress (1994), set out four general ethical principles, an approach which can aim to serve as a model for ethics in practice:

1. **Beneficence or caring and promoting the welfare of patients**

    Beneficence is the most important principle particularly for those involved in clinical research. It is unethical to involve patients and research participants in any research if no benefit is expected either to the research subject or to society. The researcher should always place more emphasis on the safety of the research participant than any other factor. These ideals emphasise the necessity to benefit the patient and not to do harm. The aim of benefitting the patient applies as much to research activities as it does to clinical care (Gelling, 1999).

2. **Non-maleficence or the obligation to avoid the causation of harm, 'to do no harm'**

    A physical harm may be easily identified and, therefore, avoided, or minimised. Emotional, social and economic factors may be less obvious and the participant may be harmed without the researcher being aware. The risks should never outweigh the benefits and the researcher should be aware that there are potential risks with all research.

3. **Justice or equitable treatment, distributing benefits, risks and costs fairly**

    Researchers who plan to use a vulnerable participant population should justify this decision. This is usually done by applying for ethical approval. All potential research participants in the healthcare setting are vulnerable by nature of their compromised health status (Gelling, 1999).

4. **Patient autonomy or self-determination, respecting the decision-making capacity of persons**

    This ethical principle can be classified in three parts.
    i.   Autonomy of thought – this includes a wide range of intellectual activities that are described as thinking for oneself.
    ii. Autonomy of will – this involves the freedom of the individual to do something based on one's own deliberations.
    iii. Autonomy of action – when the decision has been made, individuals making the decision should be able to act as they wish.

Research ethics

The above ethical principles together with those of confidentiality, fidelity and veracity, apply to all patients and particularly participants in research. A researcher or practitioner who complies with these principles will practice to a high ethical standard.

Confidentiality

This is an important principle in the relationship of health professional and patient, underpinned by the professional, ethical codes. To establish the ethical principle of confidentiality, two conditions must exist: one person must undertake not to disclose information considered to be secret; another person must disclose to the first-person information that he or she considers to be secret (Gillon, 1985).

If the first person does not divulge the information, confidentiality is maintained. There may be rare instances when the health professional or researcher gains information which might be detrimental if kept confidential. Such instances would require careful management, while considering the other ethical principles.

Fidelity

For establishing a trusting relationship, the researcher must make sure that the research participant knows about the risks. The provision of this information should occur during the process of gaining informed consent. Hospital patients will often agree to anything a nurse or medical researcher suggests. A potential participant may view an invitation to take part as a recommendation rather than a request (Hewlett, 1996). The trust that research participants place in researchers, obliges researchers to be faithful to their commitment for the trust that research participants place in them, it obliges researchers to be faithful (Gelling, 1999).

Veracity

The fact that the potential participants may be deterred from becoming part of research due to all the potential effects being realised, should not deter researchers from their duty of telling the truth about the proposed research. A researcher who is not completely open and truthful may withhold information from the participant or raise false hopes about the potential benefits of the study intervention. Veracity is closely linked with the principle of respect for autonomy (Gillon, 1994). The autonomy of potential participants is infringed if they are deceived because information is withheld that may contribute to their decision-making principle of respect for autonomy (Gillon, 1994). People generally believe that others (particularly health professionals) will not be deceitful.

Research participants and the Mental Capacity Act (2005)

Leo Alexander, a psychiatrist and neurologist, wrote the Nuremberg Code in 1947, following World War II and the associated war crime trials of German physicians involved in unethical research on prisoners during that war. On 20 August 1947, the judges delivered their verdict against Karl Brandt and twenty-two others.

The German Kodex, which included such principles as informed consent and absence of coercion; properly formulated, scientific experimentation; and beneficence towards experiment participants, was thought to have been mainly based on the Hippocratic Oath. This was interpreted as endorsing the experimental approach to medicine while protecting the patient.

The Nuremberg code is generally regarded as the first document to set out ethical regulations in human experimentation based on informed consent. This code established moral, ethical and legal principles for experiments on humans. The goal has always been, and always should be, to conduct ethical clinical trials and protect human subjects.

Patient mental capacity for research

Throughout the MCA Code of Practice, 'a person's capacity (or lack of capacity) refers specifically to their capacity to make a particular decision at the time it needs to be made'.

'It is important that research involving people who lack capacity can be carried out and that it is carried out properly. Without it, we would not improve our knowledge of what causes a person to lack or lose capacity and the diagnosis, treatment and care of people who lack capacity' (MCA Code of Practice, 2007).

The MCA applies to all research that is intrusive. 'Intrusive' means research that would be unlawful if it involved a person who had capacity but had not consented to take part (MCA Code of Practice, 2007).

The research component of the MCA does not currently appear to be a focus of expected and rightful, public and professional concern in relation to clinical trials (e.g., testing new drugs). The 'appropriate body' – an organisation that can approve research projects – can only approve a research project if the research is linked to an impairing condition that affects the person who lacks capacity or the treatment of that condition (MCA Code of Practice, 2007).

Safeguards

The research components of the MCA are clearly concerning, despite the apparent 'safeguards' which are well known to be breached in other areas of practice, such as assisted suicide and abortion:

1. Any proposed research involving the person without capacity must either benefit them personally or cause them as little risk and intrusion as possible.
2. Carers or nominated third parties must be consulted and a research ethics committee must discuss the proposal as well.
3. If the person shows any reluctance to take part, the research must be stopped immediately.

Safeguards are notoriously liable to be considered as merely barriers to be overcome, as seen since the Abortion Act of 1967 with all the supposed safeguards. Abortion today is commonly 'on demand 'and we see assisted suicide in Europe with widened scope for permitting it.

The principles of the Nuremberg Code/Kodex and the Helsinki Declaration, among others, should be taught and understood by all involved in carrying out research who need to be mindful of their expectation of patient advocacy.

Patient autonomy vs patient advocacy and conscience rights

The former Lord Chancellor, Charles Falconer, set out the determination of the government to use draconian penalties to enforce living wills in *The Mental Capacity Act – Code of Practice* (Department for Constitutional Affairs, 2007). Lord Falconer's message in 2006 to the medical profession told doctors and nurses that new laws will require them to end lives rather than save them,

Those who decline to enforce this Act (MCA, 2005), in relation to treatment withdrawal (which, in their professional opinion, would disregard the 'duty of care'), will risk going on trial for assault. They may well face jail, or, alternatively, big compensation claims in the courts if they refuse to allow patients to die, who have made living wills, which are considered to be 'applicable and valid'.

(Falconer, 2006)

The threat of jail can influence medical judgement. There are many areas of ambiguity in these matters and the threat of jail, certainly could push medical decision-making towards a decision for death. The need for relationship building and effective communication with patients to ascertain their needs seems to be not important according to these simplistic, threatened 'penalties' advocated by Lord Falconer.

Conscientious objection no guarantee for patient safety

The guidelines issued with the MCA inform clinicians that if they have religious or moral objections to carrying out the instructions of a living will, the doctor or nurse may declare themselves conscientious objectors, but in that case, they must refer the patient onto another who will follow the instructions to allow the patient to die. This makes conscientious objecting professionals complicit in their deaths.

The inevitable ethical issues which will arise in practice, require the understanding and preparation of all practitioners considering the wide-ranging effects of this Act, not least the anticipated pressure felt by some patients to draw up a' living will' without understanding and who may already feel 'a burden' and a possible 'drain' on 'scarce' resources.

Nurses must be aware of and respect the belief systems of their patients and their families. Patients who have made a living will, requesting all treatment to cease in the event of incapacity, warrant full explanation to ensure proper understanding of the consequences of their request. Their advance refusals may well have been made in total ignorance of the potentially unpleasant, consequences of their decisions.

The Rights Revolution

It is evident that the Rights Revolution has reformed the shape and the law of healthcare provision since the 1960s. Developments have confirmed the need for increased patient involvement and empowerment. Lay patient groups, including self-help organisations, have had considerable effects on the administration and improvement of healthcare.

It can be argued that the Human Rights Act (1998) and the Data Protection Act (1998) have contributed to some 'consumers' of healthcare becoming ever more 'demanding' and willing to write to complain about their care, whether these are resolved by healthcare providers or the courts. This can be viewed as a positive development when learning about the NHS care scandals.

Patient empowerment

The terms 'patient empowerment' and a 'patient-centred approach to care' are on the political healthcare agenda in addition to 'patient choice'. The government remains committed to supporting these concepts despite the inherent difficulties. There are certain barriers to the implementation of patient empowerment, such as traditional medical views of the doctor knowing best although the concept of patient choice is more apparent today. Nevertheless, the government aims to avoid traditional medical paternalism, in line with a time of 'modernisation' and encourages patients to see themselves as equal partners with healthcare professionals.

Medical crises

Medical events cannot be predicted in detail, making most prior instructions difficult to adapt, irrelevant or even misleading. Furthermore, many proxies either do not know patients' wishes or do not pursue those wishes effectively. Thus, unexpected problems arise often to defeat 'living wills.' Because these can offer only limited benefit, advance care planning should emphasise not only the completion of refusals but the emotional preparation of patients and families for future crises.

Patients must be helped and educated to understand the implications of what they may want to sign up to in any advanced plan for care. The MCA (2005) will have relevance to everyone, with its emphasis on advance decisions, particularly to elderly patients, who are known to commonly require costly investigation and treatments.

The MCA includes the obligation for the provision of basic or essential care

This has been documented as the inclusion of 'the offer' of food and water by mouth. However, many patients with serious mental incapacity may not have the ability or strength to ask for or accept a drink and may not be able to swallow properly. Professionals need to be aware that this is unfair to those patients who may not be able to accept oral food and water and it may well be dangerous to try. We need to be conscious of the balancing force of obligations to help those who cannot help themselves. Merely 'offering' oral nutrition and hydration is unacceptable. 'Failure to support oral hydration and nutrition when still possible and desired should be regarded as professional misconduct' (DH, 2013). Therefore, nurses, as part of the multidisciplinary team, with the expectation of the role of advocate, in line with their duty of care, have a responsibility to act on their concerns about patients' inability to take both oral sustenance and hydration, and discuss suitable routes to provide this for safety and survival issues.

The right to die

It is argued that the 'right to die' enthusiasts, have had much success in trying to convince both medical personnel and the public that choice in dying is the ultimate principle. However, trying to micromanage death by such measures as withdrawal of basic treatment, terminal sedation, lethal overdoses and dehydration, profoundly changes the medical system, even for people who may recover, or who may live with disabilities (Valko, 2007). (See the suggested advocate prepared statement guidance form that follows).

Patient advocacy in action

As patient advocates, nurses must be prepared to explain alternative courses of action. Patients must be encouraged to think carefully about dealing with 'end of life' decisions. They should consider the option which gives the attorney authority to give or refuse consent to life-sustaining treatment and it is vital for people to make their informed wishes clear about end-of-life care.

Where patients are unable to communicate their wishes (even though they may be able to understand efforts to communicate with them), the nurse will need to discuss with family members the best course of action in line with the patient's benefit, not harm. However, family members and/or others may strongly believe that the patient should not receive treatment to survive, in what they perceive as in the patient's 'best interests.' The nurse will need to be alert to the possible financial motives which may accompany such decision-making.

<u>Advocates' Prepared Statement in the event of non-agreement – with an End of life Pathway Proposal</u>

1. I (Advocate.....................), as the legally- authorised Patient's Advocate of N (name/ connection, i.e., relative, friend. Parishioner ('The Patient') ....am obliged to record my non-agreement with the proposal End-of-Life Pathway ('Pathway').

2. The Patient has clearly directed in his/her signal **Medical Decisions Patient Document** (MDPD) statement, dated................and accompanying General Power of Attorney (made pursuant to the Powers of Attorney Act 1971, section 10) ('The Documents') (with certified, signed copies thereof lodged with all the Patient's healthcare providers and/or advisers) that all essential nutrition and hydration be given to him/her so as to protect his/her life.

3. The Patient further directs that death should not be hastened nor life be shortened and that an APNEA TEST should not be done at all (Joffe et al., 2010).

4. The Patient desires to receive appropriate and active care so that even when it appears that death is close, The Patient is provided with ordinary nursing and medical care, including pain relief which will not be likely to affect their alertness. The alternative to a syringe driver will be discussed, due to the incidence of misuse of these by the Liverpool Care Pathway (LCP).

5. The Patient in advance, refuses any form of palliative care which may entail an overdose of diamorphine and/or any other form of deep-level sedation that may have, as its consequence, the hastening of the patient's death.
   Seeking a second opinion is an accepted right of NHS patients (GMC, 2022).

6. The Patient wholly rejects any form of so-called 'assisted dying' (assisted suicide) even if, in any and all circumstances, the laws of the United Kingdom are adversely changed to allow it.

7. The religious faith and deeply held convictions of the Patient (as specified in the Documents) demonstrate his/her sincere wish for compliance and cooperation of the medical authority in line with his/her advocate's submissions on behalf of The Patient, allied to the legal protections governing End of life decisions for the welfare of The Patient. Religion and belief are included among the nine protected characteristics of the Equality Act (2010).

8. The Patient has registered an 'opt-out' (NHS certificate dated ....as part of ('The Documents') for organ, tissue and blood donation. No organs/tissue should be taken for transplantation or for any other purpose (The opt-out NHS certificate is noted in the <u>General Power of Attorney at page....... paragraph..........</u>).

9. The Patient directs that nothing should be done which will directly and intentionally impose death; nor should anything be omitted when such omission would directly and intentionally impose death on The Patient. Where possible, there should be a meeting between The Patient and relatives/the Advocate. In the event of patient incapacity, consent from relatives/the Advocate should be representative of The Patient's wishes.

10. The relatives or Advocate, ideally, should be the responsible patient representative on the question of Advance Refusal of an End-of-life pathway. Such a Pathway should not be given to The Patient without his/her fully informed consent and/or the said informed consent of The Patient's Advocate.

11. These instructions are binding, not only upon The Patient's Advocate(s) but also upon the health care professionals/facilities having responsibilities for The Patient's life and health.

12. Having regard to the aforementioned paragraphs 9-11, the Advocate requires that The Patient be removed from the Pathway forthwith and that written evidence ('Statement') should be promptly presented to the Advocate stating that this has been done.

13. The aforementioned Statement will (additionally) be sent to the various secretaries of the doctors engaged in care of The Patient as with appended, a video recording of the Advocate reading the Statement.

14. The Advocate relies upon the legal right to have any future meetings with the Patient's medical team recorded and minuted.

15. The Advocate submits that it is good case law as declared by Baroness Hale of Richmond in 2013 that the desires and wishes of The Patient and his/her appointed Advocate are listened to and their representations acted upon as made in The Patient's welfare and best interests.

16. Both the Advocate and The Patient maintain that the Pathway is predicated upon expediting a patient's death which is contrary to the provisions of the Mental Capacity Act 2005. It is opined that the Modus Operandi ('MO') of the Pathway(s) is to facilitate involuntary euthanasia/homicide which is (for now) a criminal offence.

17. Such an MO mitigates against the declared good practice which is set down in the Neuberger Report: *More Care, Less Pathway* (DH, 2013).

The above articulates that:

'There should be a duty on all staff to ensure that patients who are able to eat and drink should be supported to do so [unless they choose not to']. 'Failure to support oral hydration and nutrition when still possible and desired should be regarded as professional misconduct' (1.64).

Should there be a failure to observe the above guidelines, it will be incumbent upon the Advocate to contact the Chief Executive/Operating Officer of the hospital concerned, together with the provision of a formal report relating any alleged misconduct on the part of the doctors and/or support staff of the medical team so concerned, to the General Medical Council (GMC).

18. It will also be necessary for the Advocate to commence an action for protection of The Patient before the Court of Protection (High Court) and obtain legal advice and assistance in due process from a lawyer specializing in clinical/medical negligence as well as attendant human rights' law.

19. Other Considerations:

a) Contact the Consulate/Embassy of The Patient's [The Patient], a citizen of that State (e.g., UK, USA, Pakistan et al) is at risk of serious harm – that unless there is State/Consular intervention, then [The Patient] will die.

b) For out-of-hours emergency court applications: (+44) 020 7947 6000. Court Fees (likely to be in the hundreds of pounds not thousands)

Please note that the Court of protection may not automatically rule in the Patient's favour and that further costs might be incurred if it becomes necessary to proceed to the Appellate Division of the High Court on appeal.

NB. Nutrition and Hydration needs are separate entities and should be regarded and addressed as such. Subcutaneous (s/c) fluids are remarkably efficient, without adverse side effects. Nutrition can be administered where required via well-established iv (PICC) lines.

Resource: Help for relatives of loved ones who are being denied fluids: www.dehydrationlifeline.org

Communication needs

Nurses and physicians should provide guidance to patients in their past or present decision-making, despite the inevitable uncertainties.

They should share responsibility for those decisions; and, above all, should support patients and families through their problems and fears. Decisions made that can be considered as 'eccentric' will require the education of the patient and family with honesty, fairness, care and compassion.

MCA motives

Professionals and the public must be aware of and sensitive to the potentially fatal consequences in the apparent motives of sections of the MCA (2005):

1. The cost-saving implications for the NHS.
2. The advance refusals of treatment will clearly apply to those who may not be in the dying phase.
3. The research permitted on subjects without mental capacity.
4. The consideration of assisted food and fluid as 'medical treatment'.

Best interests

The MCA makes 'best interests' the criterion for clinical decision making. This criterion has been described as a 'construct which can be considered as eminently corruptible and, in any event, based on uncertainties in diagnosis and prognosis. Yet it would become determinative in matters of life and death. The MCA did not define 'best interests' but only how to approach making a 'best interests' decision' (Cole, 2019).

What means of protection are available for people who lack capacity to make decisions for themselves?

Chapter 14 of the Mental Capacity Act Code of Conduct gives guidance in pages 242-243 (Department for Constitutional Affairs, 2007):

Always report suspicions of abuse of a person who lacks capacity to the relevant agency in relation to:

- Concerns about an appointee
- Concerns about an attorney or deputy

- Concerns about a possible criminal offence
- Concerns about ill treatment or willful neglect

The Act introduces new criminal offences of ill treatment or wilful neglect of a person who lacks capacity to make relevant decisions (MCA Section 44).

If someone is not being looked after properly, contact social services

In serious cases contact the police.

Concerns about care standards

- In cases of concern about the standard of care in a care home or an adult placement scheme or about the care provided by a home care worker, contact social services.
- It may also be appropriate to contact the Commission for Social Care inspection (in England) or the Care and Social Services Inspectorate for Wales.

Concerns about healthcare or Treatment

- If someone is concerned about the care or treatment given to the person in any NHS setting (such as an NHS hospital or clinic) contact the managers of the service.

Conclusion

Patient empowerment

The government aims to avoid traditional medical paternalism, in line with 'modernisation' and encourages patients to be equal partners with healthcare professionals, to be 'stakeholders' in their own treatment in line with the concepts of the *NHS Plan* (DH, 2000a). The government remains committed to inclusion of 'choice', 'patient empowerment' and a 'patient-centred' approach, despite the inherent difficulties. However, some healthcare professionals prefer the professional safety of dominant relationships with patients. There are certain barriers to the implementation of patient empowerment, not least because time afforded to all patients appears to be a vanishing commodity (see Chapters 9–11).

Many people including health professionals, believe that a review of the MCA is due in line with the above concerns. The Good Samaritan practitioner will be vigilant to exercise the role of patient advocate where patients lack mental capacity and must understand that this capacity may fluctuate and refer people to appropriate services where required. This includes liaising with the IMCA, particularly for those with no family. This safeguarding particularly applies where research is being considered.

Patient protection

The protections of the MCA need careful analysis. Some are structured to protect patients from abuse. However, some protection against their own possibly 'eccentric decisions' as described in the Act (in line with an Advanced refusal), is lacking. Such decisions must be respected according to the Act and appear to be encouraged.

Patients need to understand the complex term 'treatment' and the potential reasons for emergency treatment. Patients should know that acute urinary retention, as one example, requires emergency treatment for safety and comfort

Back door euthanasia

Some doctors have openly admitted that where the law expects that they collude in bringing about patients' deaths due to the MCA Advance refusals, forcing them to let their patients die, they will risk jail over 'back door euthanasia'

(Doughty, 2007)

Patients or their advocates, may not be able to dictate treatment but are entitled to refuse a 'pathway' approach to care, akin to the LCP (see Chapter 10). This is the type of 'care' that is known to be unacceptable to them at the end of their life or beforehand.

The forms that are available for this declaration have been documented within this chapter and Chapter 4.

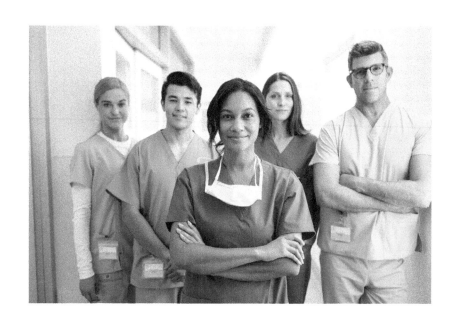

Chapter 6
Organisational culture

Creating the right corporate culture is essential for shaping a business' identity and most importantly, nurtures and engages your workforce.

(Sodexo, 2021)

Introduction

Organisational culture is important to patients, carers and healthcare professionals and is not a new concept. The literature on the subject is well established. The terms 'patient empowerment' and a 'patient-centred' approach are on the political healthcare agenda in addition to 'patient choice'.

"There are too many places for people to hide. The integrity of the organisation remains vulnerable to threat" (Casey, 2023). This statement relates to yet another investigation into the Metropolitan Police culture and standards of behaviour by Baroness Louise Casey. It could be applied to any other vast organisation where leadership and management in many areas is complacent, defensive and disengaged from its mission.

Leadership

It has been argued that firstly, leadership is a real and vastly consequential phenomenon, perhaps the single most important issue in the human sciences. Second, leadership is about the performance of teams, groups, and organizations. Good leadership promotes effective team and group performance, which in turn enhances the well-being of the incumbents; bad leadership degrades the quality of life for everyone associated with it. Third, personality predicts leadership—who we are is how we lead—and this information can be used to select future leaders or improve the performance of current incumbents (Hogan and Kaiser, 2005). The same authors argue that in the current post-modern business world, organizations are facing several challenges, which raise many questions on the inability of the traditional leadership styles to deal with issues and compete in today's business environment. Thus, now organizations need leaders instead of administrators. Leaders, who have strong motivation, can actually extend an organization's life or give a new life to it (Hogan and Kaiser, 2005).

In the leadership literature, leadership is treated as a fundamental claim; so, leaders influence priorities and goal setting through motivating people, and also through enabling, inspiring, and creating a conducive psychological atmosphere (Bass, 1990).

Transformational vs Transactional leadership

A Transformational leadership style is described as being recognized universally as a concept requiring higher moral development and may be directive or participative. This style Bass (1999) argues, contrasts with the transactional leader who practises contingent reinforcement of followers. It has been observed that an important research question has only been partially answered as to why transformational leadership is more effective than transactional leadership in a wide variety of business, military, industrial, hospital, and educational circumstances (Bass, 1999).

Leadership and learning

The literature has explored commonalities between a transformational style of leadership and learning mainly because leaders have significant influence, and they also have the ability to play a crucial role in enhancing organizational learning. Many research articles have been published so far, which deal with organizational learning and leadership. It is argued that the only sustainable source of competitive advantage is continuous learning because the environment is rapidly changing, and it increases organizational performance (Mohamed and Otman, 2021).

Continuous learning and professional development is mandatory in nursing for ongoing critical reflection and for ensuring competent practice as related to the code of conduct for standards of practice and behaviour.

The culture of an organisation is pivotal for the ethical care of people in need and for promoting staff welfare. This equally applies to Higher Education institutes where important critical enquiry must be respected, particularly where healthcare is the focus of research proposals.

Issues of today

Currently, there is constant discussion in the media and elsewhere on issues such as patient autonomy, 'death with dignity', withdrawal of treatment, terminal sedation, assisted suicide, 'living wills', 'futile treatment' and the more recent legislation on presumed consent to organ donation. All these developments herald inevitable challenges to nursing practice and those opposed to changes which they cannot agree with and are vulnerable to pressure to comply in practice.

The long-held right to conscientious objection is compromised or even eliminated if some 'modern' bioethicists are taken seriously by medicine and nursing. Bullying of staff within the NHS is sadly well known, so students and practitioners need to be aware of their rights.

Organisational justice

Organisational justice refers to the extent to which employees perceive workplace procedures, interactions and outcomes to be fair in nature (Baldwin, 2006). In nursing, Kuokkanen et al., (2014) found that organisational justice correlated with empowerment and that organisational justice increased the extent to which nurses felt empowered in their role, as well as their commitment to their job and motivation to work. Ponnu and Chuah (2010) found that organisational justice or lack of it, contributed to nurses' intentions to leave their role, as well as their job satisfaction and commitment to their organisation.

It has been proposed that organisational justice has three main components: distributive, procedural and interactional justice (Altahayneh et al., 2014).

1. Distributive justice – defined as an individual's perceived fairness of resource allocation.
2. Procedural justice – an individual's perception of fairness, based upon organisational policies and the processes by which these policies are put into action.
3. Interactional justice – the perceived fairness of individuals with regards to organisational interpersonal communications, that is, how a person perceives the quality of an interaction with another person during the implementation of formal policies.

A significant negative correlation has been concluded between perceived organisational justice and turnover intention, suggesting that lower levels of perceived organisational justice increase the likelihood of a nurse leaving their role (Tourani et al., 2016).

Justice and management responsibility

A recent study by Bakeer et al. (2021) made the following recommendations:

- Nurse managers should provide extra attention to strategies that promote organisational justice among nurses. In particular, it may be worthwhile focusing on aspects that improve procedural justice, for example, providing clear explanations of organisational policies, rules and regulations.
- Ensure nurse managers are aware of the concept of organisational justice, its principles and how it is applied to nursing.
- Consider evaluating nurses' current levels of organisational positive behaviours described as 'citizenship' behaviours to provide nurse managers with ideas to encourage or promote these behaviours using validated assessment tools (Bakeer et al., 2021).

Unethical leaders

Recent research from Maastricht University has confirmed that ethical leadership can reduce the prevalence of corrupt behaviour in an organisation. Researchers found that greater levels of ethical leadership are associated with lower levels of corrupt behaviours in subordinates. In contrast, unethical behaviours of leaders are more likely to encourage corrupt behaviours (Manara and van Gils et al., 2020).

The research concluded that ethical leaders are good role models, stimulate ethical conduct and use reward and punishment to decrease unethical behaviour, such as corruption, a specific form of unethical behaviour characterised by a misuse of power. Ethical leaders create a context where people intuitively refrain from choosing unethical behaviour.

Clinical governance

The murderous activities of the infamous Dr Harold Shipman, who worked in isolation from other doctors in his one-man GP practice, is a salutary lesson in the need for vigilance for required standards of ethical care. The seemingly constant NHS healthcare scandals can reflect a lack of clinical governance in action.

Clinical governance is a system through which NHS organisations are accountable for continuously improving the quality of their services and safeguarding high standards of care by creating an environment in which excellence in clinical care will flourish (Scally and Donaldson, 1998).

The concept of clinical governance is, or should be, accepted by all organisations which are engaged in healthcare and by all health team members. Clinical governance is an umbrella term which covers activities that help sustain and improve high standards of patient care.

The seven pillars of clinical governance are:

- clinical effectiveness and research
- audit
- risk management
- education and training
- patient and public involvement
- information and IT
- staff management.

Moral behaviour

This can be defined as a sense of concern for others, responsible behaviour, relating to keeping one's promises, a commitment to altruism and helping a stranger in need (Ketafian, 1989). A moral problem is a broad concept, encompassing certain categories: moral uncertainty, moral dilemma, moral distress and another concept can be added, that of 'moral outrage' (Pike, 1991).

The experience of moral distress can be distinguished from the experience of moral dilemmas. In moral distress, a nurse knows the morally right course of action to take, but institutional structure and conflicts with other co-workers create obstacles. A nurse who fails to act in the face of obstacles also may experience reactive distress in addition to the initial distress (Jameton, 1994). Such a situation contributes to the need for formalised clinical supervision (support) for nurses throughout health and social care settings.

Peer support

Students contribute to and cooperate with each other in a clinic setting informally (Roberts, 2008) and peer support is important for learning. In a qualitative study, it was determined:

- that the students utilised peer support in their clinical practices,
- that peer support encouraged them to help each other to cope with their shortages in clinical practices,
- that the students found the answers to their questions more easily and that they considered peer support valuable in this respect (Roberts, 2008).

These findings can equally be applied to qualified nurses who can access the additional provision of clinical supervision (support) which can be invaluable for improving critical thinking, learning and performance (see Chapter 7).

Nursing defences against anxiety

A child and adult psychoanalyst, Isobel Menzies, wrote a seminal paper on the structure of a hospital nursing service, titled: *A case-study in the functioning of social systems as a defence against anxiety.* Although the study refers to 'the hospital', it in fact discusses a group of hospitals. In the paper, Menzies made the original proposition that work in healthcare and social care organisations entails significant anxieties for staff and that defences against this anxiety are part of organisational life. Menzies notes that as the research proceeded, she came to attach increasing importance to understanding the nature of the anxiety and the reasons for its intensity (Menzies, 1960). For Menzies, the anxiety is connected to primitive anxieties aroused in the nurse by contact with seriously ill patients.

Emotional containment

Alongside anxiety, Menzies notes another crucial theoretical concept, the relationship between emotion and its 'containment'; that is, the ways in which emotion is experienced or avoided, managed, or denied, kept in, or passed on, so that its effects are either mitigated or amplified. The capacity to think, on the part of individuals or groups, is related to the capacity for containment of anxiety. Menzies also suggests that this, to-be-expected anxiety is amplified by the techniques used to contain and modify it. The main message of her paper is the elaboration of how these defensive techniques are played out in the organisation of the nursing service. They are:

- splitting up of the nurse-patient relationship
- depersonalisation, categorisation and denial of the significance of the individual
- detachment and denial of feelings
- the attempt to eliminate decisions by ritual task-performance
- reducing the weight of responsibility in decision-making by checks and counterchecks
- collusive social redistribution of responsibility and irresponsibility
- purposeful obscurity in the formal distribution of responsibility

- the reduction of the impact of responsibility by delegation to superiors
- idealisation and underestimation of personal development possibilities
- avoidance of change.

(Menzies, 1960)

Menzies' conclusions give a powerful picture of dynamic processes at work within an institutionally defensive system. Her paper illustrates the complex defence system used by the nursing culture but does not address adequately what to do about it. She asserted that the paper had been misunderstood and had led people to believe that providing support groups for staff was the answer to anxiety-provoking work. Menzies was strongly against this idea of staff support groups. She thought that the issue of anxiety was overemphasised in relation to the other side of the process – containment. She felt that the organisation needed to be designed in a way that offered staff effective containment of their anxieties.

Clinical support for healthcare staff

Since this renowned study by Menzies, a formalised method of staff support, along with the promotion of psychological safety, has been introduced for nurses. This support method, termed 'clinical supervision' has the primary purpose of providing independent support for nursing staff. It was an innovation, as was clinical governance, initiated following the alarming number of known murders of patients committed by the British GP, Dr Harold Shipman in the 1980s and 1990s. It is believed that his crimes may have also occurred during the 1970s and that in total, the number of murders was close to 260. He murdered his patients by administering opioid drug overdoses to them in their own homes in Hyde, Cheshire.

There was clearly no measure in place for the oversight of Shipman's one-man GP practice. If there had been, he may have been resistant to such attempted oversight, thus provoking concern by those charged with such supervision. Such resistance would have allowed a red flag of concern to be raised during his clinical practice from 1974–1998. One patient advocate, from another Hyde GP practice, raised her clinical concerns about the number of untoward deaths of elderly people at the time but her attempts to have an investigation initiated were thwarted.

Continual killings?

In the book written about Dr Shipman's killings: *'Healthcare serial killings: was the case of Harold Shipman unthinkable?* the author states that he still feels it was,

> *unspeakably dreadful, just unspeakable, unthinkable and un-imaginable that he should be going about day after day pretending to be this wonderfully caring doctor and having with him in his bag his lethal weapon... which he would just take out in the most matter-of-fact way.*

(Hurwitz, 2013)

This narrative by Hurwitz relating to Dr Shipman's crimes could be applied to any of those healthcare professionals who were involved for many years in the starvation, sedation and dehydration of dying and non-dying patients as part of the discredited practices of the LCP. Those who maintain such practice is acceptable and go further to implement it, even to the present day, should refer to the following questions and comments about a possibly, future dystopian culture of healthcare.

The following questions and thoughts can be applied as much to doctors as to nurses. Imagine a world in which healthcare staff no longer subscribe to the principle of beneficence or do so erratically and unpredictably. Beneficence is so often watered down by respect for autonomy – that 'first among equals' of moral principles running counter to it (Gillon 2003) – that one wonders how determinative it may be of good healthcare (Downie and Macnaughton, 2007).

Imagine now that doctors no longer manifest the character traits and dispositions to act for the good of others or that they oscillate in doing so. What then? What would healthcare look like if its principal actors relied on quite different moral virtues, dispositions and motivational drives from those we associate with doctoring, if they were intermittently to crave patient harm? Variability of healthcare outcomes might make the consequences of such traits difficult to see (Spiegelhalter and Best, 2004; Aylin et al., 2003; Mohammed et al., 2001). Imagine now, a darker possibility, one in which such contrarian practitioner traits are systematically directed against the medical and healthcare interests of patients (Hurwitz, 2015).

Dr Shipman, during the 12 months before his arrest in 1998, was killing someone, on average, every 10 days (Hurwitz, 2015). Such questions about a looming 'care' culture cannot be dismissed as just fanciful. They can help us review our own philosophy of patient care and respect the concept of conscientious objection.

Healthcare organisations have a duty to the communities they serve for maintaining the quality and safety of patient care. Whatever structures, systems and processes of an organisation, it must be able to show evidence that standards are upheld in relation to its service users and staff.

Patients at risk of harm

Any nurse with concerns about practitioners who appear unfitted for their role, whether regarding known sympathies with eugenic or paedophilic ideology, incompetence or other behaviour such as known alcohol or drug abuse which puts patients at risk of physical or psychological abuse is accountable for reporting such concerns. Such colleagues cannot be protected by a 'cover – up' ethos which must be considered as indefensible in healthcare.

Staff collaboration

Patient safety relies, among other factors, on teamwork, communication and collaboration between professionals. These factors are essential for patients with multiple comorbidities who rely on treatment from different teams and specialists and a coordinated approach.

Despite this important need for staff collaboration on behalf of patients, the incidence of staff bullying can affect both staff and patients. It can poison an organisation's morale. It has been recognised as a problem in both medicine and nursing and organisations need to be professional in dealing with its origins and repercussions.

The NHS bullying problem

A staff survey conducted by the NHS shows that bullying and harassment remains an extensive problem in the health sector, with 24% of all NHS staff having reported that they have experienced some form of bullying. Other research has shown 29.9% of all NHS staff say they have suffered psychological stress due to bullying behaviours (NHS, 2016a).

Bullying defined

'Bullying may be characterised as offensive, intimidating, malicious or insulting behaviour, an abuse or misuse of power through means intended to undermine, humiliate, denigrate, or injure the recipient' (The Advisory, Conciliation and Arbitration Service (ACAS), 2022).

Bullying and harassment

Bullying or harassment may be conducted by an individual against an individual (perhaps by someone in a position of authority such as a manager or supervisor) or involve groups of people. It may be obvious, or it may be insidious. Whatever form it takes, it is unwarranted and unwelcome to the individual. Bullying can impact on an individual's psychological safety and severely disrupt the ability of teams to function and communicate effectively and to manage patients (GMC, 2014).

The Protection from Harassment Act (1997)

Harassment is conduct that causes alarm or distress on at least two occasions. The Act prohibits the pursuit of a 'course of conduct which amounts to harassment of another'. The goal is to make provision for protecting persons from harassment and similar conduct. The House of Lords in 2006, held that, in some circumstances, a bullied employee can win damages under the Protection from Harassment Act (1997 – Section 3). This is the case, although the Act was originally intended as an anti-stalking measure and notwithstanding that there was no negligence on the part of the employer. The National Bullying Helpline explains the route by which employers can be made liable to pay huge damages for harassment of an employee by fellow employees.

The Protection from Harassment Act (1997) makes it a criminal offence to commit an act of cyberbullying with the intent to harass another person or which the perpetrator knows, or reasonably ought to know, amounts to the harassment of another person. A person found guilty of this behaviour could face imprisonment of up to six months, receive a financial penalty or both.

Section 4 of the Act provides the potential for greater punishment to those found guilty of causing another person to believe, on two or more occasions, that violence will be used against them. A person found guilty of this offence could face up to five years imprisonment. The Act also gives courts powers to grant restraining orders against those found guilty of one of the above offences.

Management bullying

Research led by the University of Leicester (2016), analysed survey data, showing that 21% of mental health workers had been bullied and 8% discriminated against by their managers in the previous year. Of these, 86% had gone sick in the year before the survey for an average of 11 days in total. Over 13% of trainee doctors reported being victims of bullying and harassment in their training post, according to a yearly survey report from the GMC. Bullying and undermining has a serious impact on the quality of training and on patient safety. It should not be accepted as part of the healthcare culture (GMC, 2014).

The NHS silent epidemic

Roger Kline's report, *Bullying: the silent epidemic in the NHS* (2013), reported that a quarter of staff in the NHS felt they were bullied and the rate of reported bullying had doubled in just four years. Staff previously surveyed said less than half of cases of bullying, harassment, or abuse cases were reported and the proportion of cases being reported is falling, down from 54% in 2004 to 44% in 2013.

In December 2016, former Department of Health (DH) Minister, Ben Gummer, chaired a round table of NHS leaders and academic experts after which he asked the Social Partnership Forum (SPF) to develop a plan to tackle bullying in the NHS. On 7 December 2016, the *Tackling Bullying Call to Action* was launched. Leaders across the NHS are committed to making a difference by promoting supportive cultures where staff can flourish and problem behaviours such as bullying are tackled.

Leading this initiative, is the NHS Social Partnership Forum (SPF), which brings together DH ministers and officials, NHS employing organisations, NHS England, Health Education England, NHS Improvement, NHS Employers and trade unions. It has developed a better understanding of the most effective interventions to tackle bullying, by working with academics to explore the evidence and gathering experiences from within the NHS and beyond.

Positive confrontation

Abuse of power is not an unknown concept in any area of life, whether in the NHS, private, or voluntary sector. Some bullies have no power outside of the workplace and demand it at work. This problem can often originate from professional jealousy, due to the interplay of personal and professional insecurity. Sometimes, deeply held ethical views and perhaps religious conviction may be resented.

Often the perpetrators need as much help as the subjects of the bullying so that the toxic cultures they create can be minimised, if not eradicated. Those with power to change the culture may 'look the other way' as confrontation is felt to be too daunting, or they are ill-prepared as managers. Bullies can thrive on the belief that confrontation to address their behaviour is too difficult for those accountable for recognising and managing a toxic work culture. Confrontation does not necessarily connote with negativity; it can be a positive behaviour which can be learnt.

Whistleblowing: the legal and ethical issues

The expectation of the role of the nurse as patient advocate can be sometimes linked to whistleblowing. It has been argued that patient advocacy is not for the faint-hearted, but whistleblowing can be a traumatic experience for the whistle blower.

Whistleblowing has been described as a stigmatised and hidden activity that carries considerable ramifications for all concerned. In the health sector, when episodes of poor practice or service provision are identified, it is frequently nurses who are the whistleblowers. Despite this, there is remarkably limited literature that explores nurses' experiences of whistleblowing (Jackson et al., 2010).

Legal protection for whistleblowers

Practitioners need all support possible during and after the event of whistleblowing. They often feel unable to return to a previously loved job, despite the promised legal protection.

The Whistleblowing Act (2012)

The person who blows the whistle does not personally have to be affected by the dangerous practice or illegal activity at work. The Act does not require the whistle blower to prove the malpractice; it is sufficient that they just raise the concern. Any dismissal will automatically be considered as unfair if it is wholly or mainly for making a 'protected disclosure'.

Whistleblowing: the ethical issues

The following is an excerpt from Steven Wilmot's 2001 paper, titled: *Nurses and whistleblowing: the ethical issues*:

> Whistleblowing presents practical and ethical dilemmas for nurses and needs to be seen as part of a spectrum of increasingly confrontative actions against miscreant organisations by their employees. The ethics of whistleblowing can only be understood in relation to its moral purpose, whether that is to achieve a good outcome (a consequentialist view) or fulfil a duty (a deontological view). The consequentialist perspective is unable on its own to resolve problems arising from the balance of good and harm resulting from the act of whistleblowing (where considerable harm might be caused) or of responsibility for that harm.
>
> A deontological approach provides an analysis of these problems but raises its own problem of conflicting duties for nurses. However, a strong argument can be made for the precedence of the nurse's duty to the patient over duty to the employer. Although both duties to the patient and the employer are based on an implicit or an explicit promise, the promise to a person (the patient) must take precedence over the promise to an organisation.
>
> It can even be argued that duty to the employer may in fact justify whistleblowing by nurses in some circumstances. However, the consequences of whistleblowing are forced upon nurses in a different way by the fact that the danger of reprisals acts as a deterrent to whistleblowers, however justified their actions may be.
>
> (Wilmot, 2001)

The Protected Disclosures Act (2014) updated by the Protected Disclosures (Amendment) Act 2022

The Act provides enhanced protection for whistle blowers. It provides a statutory framework for the protection of workers who raise concerns about relevant wrongdoing in their workplace from dismissal, penalisation or other sanctions by their employers. To qualify for protection, you must have a "reasonable belief" that a wrongdoing has occurred or is likely to occur. It is not necessary for the wrongdoing to have occurred but that you believe it to be possible. The Act ensures that safeguards exist should reprisals be taken against workers and provides for a "stepped" disclosure regime in which a number of distinct channels (internal, regulatory and external) are available.

The Act requires every public body to establish and maintain procedures for dealing with protected disclosures and to provide written information relating to these procedures to workers. A case can be taken to an employment tribunal if a worker has been treated unfairly having blown the whistle.

Further information can be accessed from the whistleblowing charity, 'Protect', the Advisory, Conciliation and Arbitration Service (Acas), Citizens' Advice, or the relevant trade union.

The Act makes clear that a worker who makes a disclosure must reasonably believe two things:

1. They are acting in the public interest. This means that personal grievances and complaints are not usually covered by whistleblowing law.
2. They must reasonably believe that the disclosure tends to show past, present, or likely future wrongdoing falling into one or more of the following categories:
    - criminal offences (this may include, for example, types of financial impropriety such as fraud)
    - failure to comply with an obligation set out in law
    - miscarriages of justice
    - endangering of someone's health and safety
    - damage to the environment
    - covering up wrongdoing in the above categories.
       (Department for Business Innovation and Skills, 2015)

Support for whistle blowers

The Freedom to Speak Up Review (2015), chaired by Robert Francis, found that there is still a 'serious issue' around the treatment of whistle blowers. It calls for a change in culture within the NHS to ensure all staff feel safe to speak up and that raising concerns becomes a normal part of their routine. Francis also recommends training for students about raising concerns which should be 'embedded' within undergraduate and postgraduate courses. This should be implemented by regulators, including the NMC and workforce planning body, Health Education England (Francis, 2013).

Internal and external staff support

Stressful as it can be, there are support systems to help staff who decide to whistle blow and should be known by the relevant employee.

1. The NMC guidance on 'raising concerns' (NMC, 2013) should be used with whistleblowing policies issued by the employer.
2. Employees should know the local clinical governance and risk management procedures, providing information on the need for early reporting of incidents or near-misses.
3. Employees should understand and follow safeguarding policies.
4. Educational emphasis on accountability and encouragement to raise concerns can help identify and prevent more problems, to protect the public.
5. Appropriate systems for raising concerns must be in place and all staff should be able to access them.
6. Stress management techniques are essential for employees engaged in the process of whistleblowing.
7. The chief executive officer (CEO), professional bodies and trade unions should be considered as good means of support, should other managerial support fail.

The 'Protect' Charity

The 'Protect' charity has operated for over 25 years and has supported more than 40,000 people. The first whistleblowing support organisation in the UK, it has been helping people raise concerns through their advice line since 1993 and played a key role in campaigning for the whistleblowing law in the UK, the Public Interest Disclosure Act (1998).

This independent UK whistleblowing charity provides free, confidential advice to employees. It aims to protect workers' rights, organisations' reputations and wider society, by encouraging safe and responsible whistleblowing. The charity believes that whistleblowing ultimately protects clients, beneficiaries, staff and the organisation itself.

How can I best express my caring responsibility?

It is suggested that it is not duty that is primarily to be the guide to recurrent moral problems but situated questions of responsibility and agency, such as how can I best express my caring responsibility? When is it justified for me to be held responsible? How can I best deal with vulnerability, dependency and suffering? (Sevenhuijsen, 2000b).

Support and encouragement for protection of conscience is vital for oneself, students and colleagues to challenge situations where risk or even harm can threaten our vulnerable patients, to whom we always must remember our duty of care, taking forward an ethical agenda.

Staffing levels, a safety risk?

The RCN has spoken of a perfect storm of factors leading to a record 50,000 nursing vacancies nationwide (RCN, 2021a). One of these factors is a vicious circle of increasing workloads deterring new recruits. It can be argued that nursing services remain largely invisible to other providers, to administrators and policy makers and to theorists in fields such as bioethics and health economics.

Lack of adequate staffing can contribute to patient safety risk or missed care. The RCN has acknowledged that it may be challenging for nurses to log their concerns about staffing and safety, but it is important to follow the organisation's incident reporting procedures.

The Health and Safety Executive

The Health and Safety Executive (HSE) describes an incident as:

- a 'near miss' (an event not causing harm but has the potential to cause injury or ill health, including dangerous occurrences) or

- undesired circumstances (a set of conditions or circumstances that have the potential to cause injury or ill health, for example, lack of appropriately trained nursing staff to safely move and handle patients).

Raising concerns – a model letter (RCN, 2021b)

The RCN is aware that staffing inadequacy may be beyond the employer's control, but a letter is a quick and easy way of documenting concerns. The RCN created two model letters, one for RNs and one for care assistants during the COVID-19 pandemic.

RCN model letter for registered nurses raising concerns:

Dear [send to your line manager and their manager or director of nursing],

As a registered nurse I have an obligation under the Nursing and Midwifery Council code to raise and escalate any concerns about issues that will impact patient care or safety.

As my employer, under health and safety legislation, you have a duty of care towards your staff and the patients they care for and should take all reasonable steps to address these concerns. With both these points in mind, I am writing to raise these concerns.

[Add detail as appropriate. You might want to mention specifically when there weren't enough nursing staff to deliver safe care; staff-patient ratios; staffing levels and skill mix; patient numbers and acuity, leadership, or management; adverse events; and other ways you have tried to raise this concern].

As a registered nurse, I act, at all times, to deliver safe and effective care to patients and uphold the highest professional standards. I have done all I can, but care is currently being compromised. Given the nature of my concerns, I am formally asking you to intervene in the interest of safe care.

I intend to share a copy of this letter with my professional body and trade union, the Royal College of Nursing.

Yours Sincerely,

[Insert name]

The RCN UK Nursing Support Workers Committee (formerly the RCN UK Health Practitioner Committee) represents the thousands of health care assistants, health care support workers, assistant practitioners, nursing associates and trainee nursing associates.

RCN model letter for care support workers raising concerns:

Dear [send to line manager],

As an employee I have a duty to report any concerns I have about the health and safety of my workplace and issues affecting the safety of our patients.

As my employer, under health and safety legislation, you have a duty of care towards your staff and the patients they care for and should take all reasonable steps to address these concerns.

With both of these points in mind, I am writing to raise the following concerns. [Add detail as appropriate. You may wish to mention: On (X shift on X Day) there were not enough nursing staff to deliver safe care; staff-patient ratio; staffing levels and the skill mix; number of patients and their acuity; availability of appropriate PPE; clear leadership or management; adverse events; and other ways you have tried to raise this concern].

As an [insert role title], I act at all times to deliver safe and effective care to patients and uphold high standards. I have done all I can, but care is currently being compromised.

Given the nature of my concerns, I am formally asking you to intervene in the interests of safe care.

I intend to share a copy of this letter with my trade union, the Royal College of Nursing.

Yours Sincerely,

[Insert name]

What if the staffing situation does not improve?

Having submitted the letter and nothing improves, the suggested next step is to formally raise concerns. If issues remain unresolved, the RCN suggests that the nurse should follow their advice at rcn.org.uk/raising concerns or call the RCN.

The NHS 'market' ethos

There appears to have been a change in the organisation of the NHS, where management skills have often been celebrated more than clinical skills.

Under the Thatcher era, the NHS underwent major changes that, in addition to the competence-based approach to professionalism, included the introduction of general management, competitive tendering, privatisation of ancillary services and the introduction of internal markets.

'Extreme efficiency'

It has been argued that the long-standing tension that exists between the ideals and reality of nursing practice in relation to the biophysical model of nursing and the increased demands of emotional labour, may also reflect the concept of disengagement. This was identified by Ritzer, who suggests that the fast-food restaurant represents the rationalisation of society in the quest for extreme efficiency (Ritzer, 1993).

Such an argument also considers that a side effect of globalisation is cultural homogeneity and the emergence of 'McDonaldisation' (Herdman, 2004). It is arguable that the irresistible effect of 'McDonaldisation' offers an efficient method for satisfying many of our needs, services that can be easily quantified and calculated, including predictability and control. The result is greater productivity, dehumanisation and homogenisation.

Post-emotional society

Meštrović (1997) extends the thesis of McDonaldisation to the emotions, arguing that McDonaldised emotions are rationally manufactured, a 'happy meal' of emotions consumed by the masses. Meštrović believes that emotions are absent from most sociological theorising and that contemporary Western societies are entering a new developmental era in which synthetic, quasi-emotions become the basis for widespread manipulation by self, others and the culture industry (Meštrović, 1997).

A new form of totalitarianism

Meštrović proposes that a neo-Orwellian process of emotional manipulation is affecting the Western world and that a consequence includes the fact that 'any policy or event, no matter how repulsive it might be, by old fashioned inner-directed standards, will be acceptable as long as it is packaged properly' (Meštrović, 1997). This, he argues, is a new form of totalitarianism, likened to that proposed in the book *One Dimensional Man* (Marcuse, 1964/1991).

It is difficult to oppose the 'nice face' of this new form of totalitarianism. Differences are apparent; heightened rationality cannot resist the trend of post-emotional control as it targets the emotions rather than the intellect. It is now argued, however, that due to the competition between fractionalised groups, opposition does not lead to action (Herdman, 2004).

Reisman (1997) describes a post-emotional society as one in which people do not react to events and crises in the same way as in the past. Instead, people are blasé and uninvolved, despite being able to intellectualise events as important.

Academic institutional power vs critical enquiry, knowledge and beliefs

A new academic journal is to be published in which academics may write under pseudonyms, for fear of retribution. The truly alarming motive for the founding of this new publication, known as *Journal of Controversial Ideas*, is simply to avoid persecution by the universities that employ contributors to this new journal. Universities will not always favour free discussion; the resort to pseudonyms by some authors, convicts universities of betrayal (Gartside, 2019). This reflects a 'closed shop' academic culture which persecutes anyone who ventures outside the fashionable consensus.

The historical duty of universities for critical enquiry, means supporting proposals which are new in the field, and relate to the important subject of conscientious objection. My research proposal wanted to know how do nurses manage orders they cannot fulfil and was titled: Can the code of conduct help nurses to act as the patient's advocate? This needed consideration rather than viewing such credible, critical enquiry as too controversial, university lecturers' academic integrity should trump the fear of funding withdrawal by government over supposed controversial proposals. My study proposal, as just described, was focused on conscientious objection, but was declined by the university tutors at a late stage. It was clearly related to the government-approved and ultimately discredited LCP, which was at the height of its implementation at the time.

Perhaps universities' dependence on funding by government can trump the expectation of promotion of objective, critical enquiry. Critical questioning of the LCP's aims, and outcomes was emerging well before the independent review of 2013, which revealed the betrayal of many patients and families in practice and recommended the LCP's discontinuation.

Safe proposals

The power of some universities can be recognised today as unhealthy. Tutors who do not fulfil their remit as educators will be held to account for their lack of moral fibre by protecting their status and so-called 'reputation' by selecting 'safe' research proposals.

University-based student coercion

The rather pejorative terms 'woke' and 'snowflake' commonly applied to young people today, and commonly to students, can be applied equally to some of their supervisors who have been seen to act with impunity against their students and sometimes even their own peers. They have sometimes been denied their right to freedom of expression, having been 'de-platformed' in recent high-profile cases.

Academic rigour is clearly under threat within some UK universities. Some staff members no doubt feel the same pressure as healthcare staff feel when their vocation to practise in an ethical and intelligent way is under threat. The historical, cosy complacency and protection afforded to staff by universities' institutional, unassailable power needs to change and is changing.

Critical enquiry warrants respect

The philosophies of universities need to incorporate the concept of 'conscience', which must apply in all fields. Without the due respect for diversity of thoughtful enquiry and freedom of expression, any institution becomes a focus of ridicule and contempt. It has been argued that: it is self-centred and narcissistic to be able to see things only through the prism of how it makes you feel – it is how toddlers engage with the world. Time for the adults to speak up (Knight, 2020a).

It is fortunate that over time, and more clearly since the pandemic, students have at last learned that their unacceptable educational experiences as consumers cannot continue. They warrant a value for money, credible educational experience and must do all in their power with government to achieve this.

University thought and word policing

In November 2019, the Cardiff University Student Union (CUSU) adopted an official 'pro-choice' stance. The union established that all official societies must be pro-abortion and that terminology used in literature will be strictly controlled. For example, the term 'unborn baby' is not allowed. Instead, the less emotive term 'foetus' will be used in case women are upset by any suggestion that an unborn child is human. Humanity is to be obscured by terminology (Treloar, 2020b).

Denial of freedom of speech

Catholic students were then told they cannot take part in official societies at Cardiff University. The university chaplain, Father Sebastian Jones, said that no Catholic could remain a member of an organisation that upholds the promotion of and material support for the procurement of abortions. He added: 'For a Catholic to participate in such an organisation would risk them incurring excommunication'.

While the Student Union said it recognised its responsibility to uphold freedom of speech and to allow students to take a stance on sensitive issues, it is not easy to reconcile what the Students' Union motion stated with their response to subsequent questioning. The motion that was passed at its annual general meeting (AGM) in which the following is unequivocal, though contradictory, makes it impossible for a Catholic, in conscience, to be an officer of the union. Catholic students have been excluded by an intolerant and aggressive secularism as follows:

- CUSU will publicly announce their stance as pro-choice and clearly state on the CUSU 'Pregnancy Support' webpage and any other applicable webpages such as in the 'Policy' webpage.
- Changing the pregnancy and abortion-related terminology throughout the Student Union to make it unbiased and medically accurate. For example, on the CUSU 'Pregnancy Support' webpage, referring to a foetus at 13 weeks instead of a 'baby'.
- The VP [Vice President] of Welfare and Campaigns will be responsible for ensuring that the Student Union campaigns and strategies support the pro-choice stance to provide an equal, safe and inclusive environment for students.

(Treloar, 2020b)

Dangerous cancel culture

The French philosopher, Bernard-Henri Levy, offers his opinion on 'cancel culture' as: 'I'll tell you what cancel culture is, it's a school of imbecility churning out ever more imbeciles. And it is profoundly dangerous. Cancel culture goes against the very contract of life: it is the opposite of life and living (and philosophy)' (Levy, 2021).

Protection of legitimate views

Tougher measures, however, to strengthen free speech and academic freedom at universities in England are planned by the government to stamp out unlawful 'silencing' on campuses. The plans include the appointment of a new Free Speech and Academic Freedom Champion. This is a crucial step in making sure legitimate views can be held and expressed on campuses across the country.

More authority means more accountability

A lack of awareness of poor or even unethical practice is not an option for chief executive officers of NHS Trusts or university vice chancellors. These post holders must be accountable and transparent due to the greater authority invested in them on behalf of patients, staff and students, respectively.

Employees should never fear involving the CEO where other means employed for patient advocacy have failed at lower managerial levels. Relatives, too, are often unaware of the accountability expected of the hospital CEO whether in the NHS, private, or voluntary sector.

University sector power without responsibility

Accessing a university vice chancellor's office, has been described by one unfairly treated student as trying to approach an impregnable fortress, to be permanently shielded from students.

A journalist, who wants to protect the name of a student who suffered cancellation of a PhD study by a university for spurious reasons, has reported that "Universities can cancel your degree for wrongthink – and there's no real right to appeal" (Samuel, 2023). This case is not an isolated one.

The Office of the Independent Adjudicator (OIA) in this case, had rubber stamped the regulations and conclusions of the university, rather than maintaining its supposed responsibility as a robust and cheap safeguard in the form of scrutiny. The Government claims it is going to fix this kind of problem by passing the Higher Education (Freedom of Speech) Bill. But even by this new law, if a student wanted a judicial review, it seems that a university would only be concerned for its reputation by having picked on a student with bottomless financial resources, with a willingness to have their name trashed. Otherwise, they can operate with impunity. A human rights barrister, Paul Diamond has said:" [This] is not an operating safeguard system". It is not a pretty picture of our university sector either (Samuel, 2023).

The NHS Patient Advice and Liaison Service (PALS)

Another NHS innovation was the introduction of the Patient Advice and Liaison Service. This service provides an opportunity for patients or relatives, both in hospital and the community, to voice their experiences, whether good or poor. The service also offers confidential advice, support and information on health-related matters and provides a point of contact for patients, their families and carers. The PALS office can give information about the NHS, as well as support groups and services outside the NHS. The PALS also helps to improve the NHS by listening to concerns and suggestions.

The Good Samaritan healthcare professional will be aware of patients' right to the complaints process in line with patient advocacy, within NHS hospitals and community healthcare settings. Any complainants, whether from patients or relatives, need to be informed of the existence of the relevant organisations that are there to support hoped-for resolution or restitution.

Should the department not resolve a situation, the person will be informed of the NHS complaints procedure, including how to get independent help if a complaint is desired. Thereby, the complainant has explored the internal source for support, which is essential in any external furtherance of a complaint, such as to the Parliamentary and Health Service Ombudsman (PHSO).

The Parliamentary and Health Service Ombudsman (PHSO)

Complaints about the NHS in England and UK government departments can be referred to the PHSO, but a complaint must be made to the original organisation in the first instance. The PHSO has a complaint checker tool on the website homepage which can then link to the correct complaint form. Private healthcare can be investigated only where NHS treatment has been provided.

What to expect from the Ombudsman?

The PHSO will accept a complaint where an organisation has not acted properly or fairly or has given a poor service and not put things right. If the PHSO decides that the organisation got things wrong and had a negative effect on the person, recommendations can be made about what it should do about this.

What can be recommended by the Health Ombudsman

The PHSO can ask an organisation to take action to put things right for the complainant (or somebody else affected). This could mean getting the organisation to acknowledge its mistakes, apologise, or recompense for any financial outlay required because of what happened.

An organisation can be asked to look again at a decision it has made, but only if it is clear that it made mistakes, acted unfairly, or did not follow its process when making the decision.

The PHSO can ask an organisation to improve its services to avoid the same things happening again. This can include asking an organisation to review its policies or procedures, guidance, or standards (PHSO, 2021).

Final decisions on unresolved complaints

The PHSO makes the final decisions on unresolved complaints about the NHS in England and UK government departments and other UK public organisations. Almost 80% of cases investigated by the PHSO service in a year annually are about the NHS and the rest are about UK government departments and other organisations.

Case summaries are published on the PHSO's website and can be searched by entering key words such as cancer, diagnosis and death, as well as by organisation, for example the name of a hospital trust and by location (PHSO, 2016).

Poor care for the elderly

The PHSO reported on 10 investigations into complaints made to its office about the standard of care provided to older people by the NHS. This report titled *Care and Compassion*, was published in 2011 and included stories from the results of investigations concluded in 2009 and 2010 which are not easy to read. These stories illuminate the gulf between the principles and values of the NHS Constitution and the reality experienced of being an older person in the care of the NHS in England. The report raised critical issues which emphasised that patients should receive the highest quality of care, which the service is expected to deliver (PHSO, 2011).

Poor and neglectful care

A representative of the King's Fund has written as follows about the PHSO's report in relation to multifactorial problems resulting in poor and neglectful care:

> *The Ombudsman is not known for emotive language,*
> *but she says her "harrowing" findings, reveal "an attitude*
> *which fails to recognise the humanity and individuality*
> *of the people concerned and to respond to them with*
> *sensitivity, compassion and professionalism".*

(Cornwell, 2011)

If we have learned anything in the past decade about providing safe, high-quality care, it is that it requires sustained, continuous effort and focus over a period of years: it cannot be fixed overnight.

The report is a clarion call to think much more deeply about how and why vulnerable people suffer at the hands of the people there to look after them. The failings in the PHSO's report point to something more than callous attitudes on the part of a few 'bad apples'. The stories are about personal and institutional failure. Reliable quality cannot be achieved by single individuals acting alone.

At senior level, board and executive team members should be active, talking to patients, visitors and staff and seeing for themselves what goes on in wards, waiting areas and clinics. In the best organisations, senior leaders demonstrate by word and deed that quality of care is non-negotiable and take an active interest in what is required to deliver it.

Staff need active, sustained supervision and support. In the high-volume, high-pressure, complex environment of modern health care, it is very difficult to remain sensitive and caring towards every single patient all the time, but it is possible with an agreed ethos of good care throughout the organisation.

Requests of dying patients

We ask ourselves how it is possible that anyone, let alone a nurse, could ignore a dying person's request for water? What we should also ask is whether it is humanly possible for anyone to look after very sick, very frail, possibly incontinent, possibly confused patients without excellent induction, training, supervision and support (Cornwell, 2011).

Conclusion

> *Openness is not the end;*
> *it is the beginning*
>
> (Heffernan, 2012)

The culture of an organisation, whether in a hospital, higher education Institute, or community care settings, can make or break the experience for patients and staff. Educators of both nurses and doctors must strive to promote the roles of patient advocate, patient educator and evidence-based practitioner regardless of what may be considered 'taboo' topics, or academic ideological orientation.

Higher Education institute staff must accept the historical responsibility for allowing critical enquiry, particularly where it relates to patient care. Research studies on the concept of patient advocacy are vital. Politically correct-minded academics must never consider this important concept and responsibility as 'too controversial'.

A required new vision for NHS improvement and leadership

The NHS new vision is for team leaders at every level of the NHS to develop improvement and leadership capabilities among their staff and themselves (NHS, 2016b). This will help protect and improve services for patients in the short term and for the next 20 years.

A college of health service management and managerial registration?

There is also to be the biggest review of NHS management in 40 years. The creation of a college of health service management is long overdue; it would set standards for managers and provide relevant education and training as well as professional qualifications in the same way that the royal colleges do for the medical profession. A logical next step might be professional registration (Cooper, 2021).

Pay and conditions

Most nurses enter nursing with a clear vision of helping patients and remuneration has always been understood historically as no barrier to nursing entrants. Over time, financial rewards improve, together with career progression and this has always been accepted by nurses.

Managers should champion the needs of nurses to be able to care for their patients effectively. They could start by urgently considering the issue of recruitment and retention, the 12-hour shifts, and the need for suitable accommodation (historically this was always locally available for nurses and students, where required) to minimize long travelling times at the beginning and end of their shifts.

Aleksandr Solzhenitsyn summarised the importance of a spiritual orientation to life:

> *The strength or weakness of a society depends*
> *more on the level of its spiritual life than*
> *on its level of industrialization... A tree with a*
> *rotten core cannot stand.*

(The Imaginative Conservative, 2011)

Lessons to be learned?

Parents affected by the tragedy of the Lucy Letby case, the paediatric nurse, recently sentenced to a whole life order for the murders of seven babies and the attempted murder of six others, will find no comfort from this often-repeated phrase following healthcare scandals. Past lessons clearly to be learned, often appear to be forgotten or even willfully ignored. Time and again to disregard the credible judgement and suspicions of clinicians and to punish them for acting as whistleblowers and Good Samaritans appears as moral cowardice, irrespective of the considered case complexity.

Lessons must be learned. Concerned healthcare workers and patient relatives may decide that approaching the police if their concerns are not listened to by managers and other staff, may be their only recourse for protecting vulnerable patients of whatever age, who they honestly believe to be in danger of a murderous practitioner at large. One future, positive development for healthcare organisations could be what the BMA is now calling for, regulation for non-clinical healthcare managers as exists for clinical staff. Proven systemic failures may precede corporate manslaughter charges.

The need for educated staff at all levels in healthcare must be respected and acted upon to achieve the goal of Good Samaritan patient care. Making change must be a personal mission of all, in line with the duty of care to patients and staff. This is, however, a responsibility also of those in whom most authority is invested to influence a positive and safe culture for the organisation.

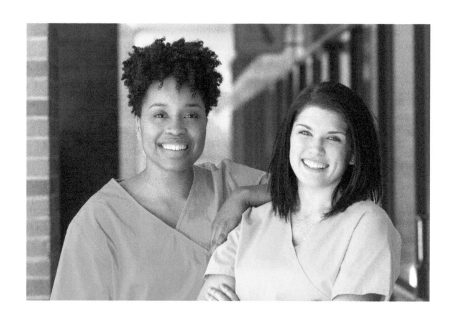

Chapter 7
Conscientious objection, courage and staff support

Be strong and very courageous. Do not be
terrified, nor be dismayed, for the Lord, your
God is with you wherever you go.

(Joshua 1:9)

Introduction

The elements in the title of this chapter require equal exploration. They help in understanding the position of ethical health professionals, of any religious denomination or none, who are working within ethically-difficult situations.

The extent to which nurses have the freedom to decline assignments that they oppose on ethical grounds is arguable in some of today's healthcare settings. New laws may not allow for conscientious objection. The moral dilemma for the ethical practitioner is apparent, as complicity in evil is always a risk in such situations though not always perceived as such by some others.

The appeal of the Florence Nightingale legend relied on its ability to combine virtue, self-sacrifice and physical endurance, all played out in a hostile foreign environment. This description of the qualities required of a nurse such as Florence Nightingale, could be applied equally to ethical practitioners of today. They may also have to play out such qualities in a difficult work environment where conscientious objection is required.

The concepts of legality and morality today, should be understood as mutually exclusive. What is deemed as legal is not always moral. This is seen in the unethical laws and guidance that feature in the past and continue into the present day.

Conscience

> *There is no true peace without fairness, truth,*
> *justice and solidarity.*

(Pope St John Paul II, 1999)

The following clauses (372–375) from the Catholic Catechism examine moral conscience:

What is the moral conscience?

Moral conscience, present in the heart of the person, is a judgement of reason which at the appropriate moment enjoins him to do good and to avoid evil. Thanks to moral conscience, the human person perceives the moral quality of an act to be done or which has already been done, permitting him to assume responsibility for the act. When attentive to moral conscience, the prudent person can hear the voice of God who speaks to him or her.

What does the dignity of the human person imply for the moral conscience?

The dignity of a human person requires the uprightness of a moral conscience (which is to say that it be in accord with what is just and good according to reason and the law of God). Because of this personal dignity, no one may be forced to act contrary to conscience: nor within the limits of the common good, be prevented from acting according to it, especially in religious matters.

How is a moral conscience formed to be upright and truthful?

An upright and true moral conscience is formed by education and by assimilating the Word of God and the teaching of the Church. It is supported by the gifts of the Holy Spirit and helped by the advice of wise people. Prayer and an examination of conscience can also greatly assist one's moral formation.

What norms must conscience always follow?

There are three general norms:

1. One may never do evil so that good may result from it.
2. The so-called *Golden Rule*, 'Whatever you wish that men would do to you, do so to them' (Matthew 7:12).
3. Charity always proceeds by way of respect for one's neighbour and his conscience, even though this does not mean accepting as good something that is objectively evil.

The following clauses (377-378) from the Catholic Catechism examine the Virtues:

What is a virtue?

A virtue is habitual and firm disposition to do the good. 'The goal of a virtuous life is to become like God' (Saint Gregory of Nyssa). There are human virtues and theological virtues.

What are the human virtues?

The human virtues are habitual and stable perfections of the intellect and will that govern our actions, order our passions and guide our conduct according to reason and faith. They are acquired and strengthened by the repetition of morally good acts and they are purified and elevated by divine grace (Compendium of the Catechism of the Catholic Church, 2005).

Virtues

Aristotle follows Socrates and Plato in taking the virtues to be central to a well-lived life. Like Plato, he regarded the proposed nine ethical virtues (*wisdom; prudence; justice; fortitude; courage; liberality; magnificence; magnanimity and temperance*) as complex rational, emotional and social skills. But Aristotle rejected Plato's idea that to be completely virtuous, one must acquire an understanding of what goodness is through a training in the sciences, mathematics and philosophy.

Aristotle believed that to live well, we need a proper appreciation of the way in which such goods as friendship, pleasure, virtue, honour and wealth fit together as a whole. To apply that general understanding to particular cases, we must acquire, through proper upbringing and habits, the ability to see, on each occasion, which course of action is best supported by reason (Stanford Encyclopaedia of Philosophy, 2018a).

A change in thinking about ethics

Elizabeth Anscombe, a British analytical philosopher published a paper in 1958, titled *Modern Moral Philosophy*. This changed the way other philosophical theories were viewed. She emphasised the importance of the emotions and understanding of moral psychology. Among the theories she criticised for their reliance on universally applicable principles, were J.S. Mill's utilitarianism (*Greatest Happiness Principle*) and Kant's deontology (*Categorical Imperative*) which both claimed to be applicable to all moral situations.

Anscombe's recommendations that virtue requires a more central position in our understanding of morality have been taken seriously by some philosophers. The consequence of such theories and beliefs is what is described as virtue ethics.

Virtue ethics and the 'good nurse'

'Virtue ethics' is a term used for theories that give a focus to the role of character and virtue in moral philosophy. Rather than either doing something out of duty (deontology theory) or acting to bring about good consequences (utilitarianism), people will simply act in virtuous ways. This can be viewed in healthcare as a consistent approach to living a virtuous life.

Virtue ethics as a term, is used often enough for a simple shared meaning to be assumed. A virtue ethics for nursing is concerned with the character of individual nurses. It seeks ways to enable nurses to develop character traits appropriate for actions that enhance patient well-being and qualities which enable us to act in accordance with our 'higher selves'.

Principles for cooperation in evil

Moral philosophy classically considers cooperation with evil in two ways: *formal or material.*

- Formal cooperation involves directly willing the evil at hand and thus is always wrong.
- Material cooperation does not involve directly willing evil but providing some form of material support and it can be remote or proximate depending on how close it is to the act (Schneider, 2020).

In either case the ethical practitioner will need strategies for avoidance of evil acts according to their conscience. There are several questions we need to ask ourselves when facing unethical situations at work:

- How do health professionals manage orders that are against their conscience?
- How do health professionals reconcile their relationship with God and moral integrity?
- Are we ready to refuse an immoral assignment or are we prepared to do anything?
- What choices make us complicit with evil?
- How can we avoid being complicit in evil?

Deliberate cooperation is always morally wrong. Even attending, planning, or preparing and supporting the immoral action is wrong. No one wishes to put at risk their means of livelihood but making an ethical stand is a declaration of good will to patients. The Good Samaritan can determine good, mutually courteous and respectful relations with colleagues. Having equal determination to avoid immoral acts is essential.

There is a greater awareness of the importance of respect for human rights today, and the rights of health professionals for exercising conscience cannot be an exception. This requires avenues of support.

The UK Equality Act (2010)

This Act lists the nine protected characteristics – one of which is religion or belief.

The right to conscientious objection

Other means to support an ethical stand for health professionals, include conscience, which is a clear guide to moral behaviour. A duty of care to patients is expected of health professionals and is enshrined in codes of professional conduct. Codes of conduct, when honoured, can act as a protection for both the patient and the practitioner. Where conscientious objection is not accommodated in certain fields of care, then we need to be prepared for the challenge to exercise this right.

The code and communicating to managers

The code of conduct can act as a moral compass. Formal and early documentation of ethical concerns can clarify one's position clearly for line managers, while individuals' access to sources of professional, personal and spiritual support is vital.

Harm

The injunction, 'to above all, do no harm' (*Primum non nocere*), has been an axiom central to clinical pharmacology and to the education of health professionals for many years. The injunction remains a clear and powerful reminder that every medical and pharmacological decision carries the potential for harm (Smith, 2005).

Harm can occur by commission or omission in life. Harm in healthcare can occur with a subtle interplay of factors which may be powerful, organisational, professional or personal. Those who attempt to protect patients from harm may suffer professionally, personally and emotionally and even financially should the result mean having to leave a much-loved job. It is not far-fetched to expect the Good Samaritan practitioner to be punished for attempts to act as the patient advocate, which may require whistleblowing, despite this being an expectation of the code of conduct. The role of patient advocate is important for all patients, particularly those who are sadly without any support and dependent only on the good will of members of their care team.

Health developments

Ethical challenges for health professionals are characterised by the demands of legal, professional and government developments and 'modern' bioethicist opinions. All of which can demand compliance with an encroaching culture that can be opposed to moral and ethical practice, requiring practitioner conscientious objection. This may be compounded by the need for whistleblowing, with all the potential associated negative consequences for those wishing to act as the Good Samaritan. Such developments can be a cause of attrition from the nursing profession, which has never been in more need of skilled, committed nurses.

Health professionals need to have their right to conscientious objection respected and not be limited or curtailed by managers or 'modern' bioethical opinion (see Chapter 16). The killing of nine million babies in the UK (mainly for social reasons), since the Abortion Act of 1967, has resulted in many healthcare practitioners being unable to work in their favoured specialty of obstetrics and gynaecology due to their conscience rights being perceived as a 'problem'. Many committed pro-life clinicians and nurses believe it to be a pointless exercise to apply for posts in these work settings. They have, therefore, been effectively eliminated from the specialty for over 50 years in the UK.

Helpless practitioners

In some environments it is difficult, sometimes paralysing due to fear, to speak up and represent a patient's rights and interests. Certain environments may lead to the feeling of helplessness. Nurses need to prevent this by being able to identify hostile and dangerous environments.

Nurses concerned about the threat to life of patients in their care environments, must recognise such threats and attempt to guard themselves against becoming helpless practitioners.

Affirming conscience

Uncaring actions directed at people due to their vulnerability, lack of economic viability, or even a perceived lack of humanity, are actions against conscience. The strength required to act as the patient's advocate is equal to the strength required to exercise the right to conscientious objection. The two concepts are inextricably linked.

Strengthening conscience

Oppression of and disregard for those considered as the least among us requires a response strategy for the strengthening and affirming of conscience. Christianity asks us to monitor our lives and to give up easy options if they stand in the way of achieving some spiritual good. An example of this could mean, for example, leaving a job where conscience cannot approve a healthcare culture where treatment is often inappropriately considered as 'futile' and patients are given inappropriate, unethical 'end of life' care.

Sensitive conscience

Cultivating a sensitive conscience is a pre-requisite for nurses to ensure provision of compassionate care. There are several potential dangers to patients, such as the encroaching culture of treatment 'futility', the continued LCP's lethal practices (though recommended for discarding) and the definition of 'treatment' by the MCA (2005). This defines treatment as 'any diagnostic or other procedure' a definition with far reaching consequences.

Laws and guidelines affecting conscience rights:

- The MCA considers assisted food and fluid to be 'medical treatment'.
- The foreseen dangers of the Presumed Consent to Organ Donation Act (2020) (see Chapter 12).
- Specific medical guidance, e.g., British Medical Association (BMA) guidance on CANH (BMA, 2018) (see Chapter 8).

- The repeated push by lobbyists for a change in UK law for assisted suicide (see Chapter 13).

Conscientious objection in practice

All those with a conscientious objection have varying religious, philosophical or political reasons for their beliefs. Conscientious objection requires sensitivity to the need to act as the Good Samaritan, concerned about the patient's benefit, not their harm, in any area of treatment and care. This applies whether staff work in direct or indirect contact with patients from the level of CEO to that of healthcare assistant staff.

The code of conduct for nurses (NMC, 2018) makes provision for conscientious objection in practice. However, there is currently a statutory right of conscientious objection for nurses, midwives and nursing associates in only two documented areas in nursing: abortion and in-vitro fertilisation.

Conscientious objection to participation in treatment allows nurses and midwives in Scotland, England and Wales, along with nursing associates in England, to refuse to participate in the process of treatment which results in the termination of a pregnancy because they have a conscientious objection, except where it is necessary to save the life or prevent grave, permanent injury to the physical or mental health of a pregnant woman:

The Abortion Act (1967) – (Scotland, England and Wales) Section 4.

4 (1) Subject to subsection (2) of this section, no person shall be under any duty, whether by contract or by any statutory or other legal requirement, to participate in any treatment authorised by this Act to which he has a conscientious objection: Provided that in any legal proceedings the burden of proof of conscientious objection shall rest on the person claiming to rely on it.

4 (2) Nothing in subsection (1) of this section shall affect any duty to participate in treatment which is necessary to

save the life or to prevent grave, permanent injury to the physical or mental health of a pregnant woman.

Section 38 of the Human and Fertilisation and Embryology Act (1990)

This provision allows nurses, midwives and nursing associates the right to refuse to participate in technological procedures to achieve conception and pregnancy (which involves disposal of unwanted embryos) because they have a conscientious objection. This applies to healthcare professionals working in the UK.

Part 7 of The Abortion (Northern Ireland) Regulations 2020

This provision allows nurses and midwives in Northern Ireland to refuse to participate in the process of treatment which results in the termination of a pregnancy because they have a conscientious objection, except where it is necessary to save the life, or to prevent grave permanent injury to the physical or mental health, of a pregnant woman.

The right to conscientious objection for healthcare professionals can be a threatened and actual casualty in secular cultures, as exemplified by the case of the two Glasgow midwives (Doogan and Wood v Greater Glasgow and Clyde Health Board, 2014).

The case of the Glasgow midwives

Despite the Equality Act (2010), which protects employees from discrimination on the grounds of religion or belief, two senior UK Catholic midwives who were asked to supervise abortion lost their case on conscientious objection at the UK Supreme Court (Doogan and Wood v Greater Glasgow and Clyde Health Board, 2014).

The Supreme Court in London, the UK's highest court, concluded in 2014 that these two Catholic midwives did not have the right to avoid supervising other staff involved in abortion procedures. The Supreme Court ruled that Mary Doogan and Connie Wood should have to support staff who are caring for women having terminations. This ruling meant the case was 'lost' yet, draws into sharp focus the problem of conscientious objection for many healthcare professionals who must be aware of their rights to expression of beliefs under the Equality Act (2010).

The scope of section 4 of the Abortion Act in the case of the Glasgow midwives

There were three possible interpretations put forward to the Supreme Court:

- The Royal College of Midwives, who were acting as an intervener, suggested a very narrow view, namely that 'treatment authorised by the Act' is limited to the treatment which actually causes the termination of a pregnancy, i.e., the administration of drugs which induce premature labour, and does not extend to the care of a woman during labour, or to the delivery of the foetus, placenta and membrane, or to anything that happens after that.
- Mrs Wood and Ms Doogan suggested a wide view, namely that section 4 confers the right to object to any involvement with patients in connection with the termination of pregnancy to which an individual has a personal conscientious objection. In their case, they were uncomfortable with receiving and dealing with the initial telephone call booking a patient into the labour ward for an abortion, the admission of the patient, assigning a midwife to look after the patient and supervising staff who were looking after the patient, both before and after the procedure, as well as any direct involvement in the abortion procedure itself.
- The Health Board argued for a halfway house, whereby 'treatment authorised by the Act' begins with the administration of drugs and ends with the delivery of the foetus, placenta and membrane. So, section 4 would not cover making bookings or other administrative, supervisory, or managerial tasks.

The court largely agreed with the Health Board's proposition, but slightly extended it to include all the usual care and support given during the delivery of the baby.

Following this case, Lady Hale recommended that: 'Employers should make reasonable adjustments to the requirements of the job in order to cater for religious beliefs, either under the Human Rights Act or under the Equality Act' (Hale, 2014). This recommendation appears lacking in the final judgement in the case of the two Catholic midwives refusing to supervise abortion.

The Nursing Code of Professional Conduct: standards of practice and behaviour refers to the right of conscientious objection:

> 4.4 Tell colleagues, your manager and the person receiving care if you have a conscientious objection to a particular procedure and arrange for a suitably qualified colleague to take over responsibility for that person's care.
>
> (NMC, 2018)

How can doctors and nurses be expected to be an accomplice to something that is against their conscience? Some people may be unaware of how ethical dilemmas cause soul searching in their colleagues. We do not intend to encourage others in wrongdoing but can sensitively inform them that we know that they would not want to dismiss our beliefs. For us to transfer what we know to be unethical to another degrades us both, 'we are not a cog in a wheel, using others to do our dirty work' (Watt, 2022).

Conscientious objection, cowardice, or bravery?

The following is argued, controversially, by a 'modern' bioethicist: 'Shakespeare wrote that "Conscience is but a word, that cowards use, devised at first to keep the strong in awe"' (Savulescu, 2006).

The concept of conscientious objection does not offer a charter for cowards.

People over the centuries in times of Christian persecution knew they would suffer for their faith and would never surrender, even on pain of death, as with the English martyrs during the Reformation. One martyr, St Edmund Arrowsmith, on the scaffold at the time of his martyrdom, said: 'Nothing grieves me much as the England which I pray God soon to convert' (Atherton and Peyton, 2013).

Savulescu continues,

Conscience, indeed, can be an excuse for vice or invoked to avoid doing one's duty. When the duty is a true duty, conscientious objection is wrong and immoral. When there is a grave duty, it should be illegal. A doctor's conscience has little place in the delivery of modern medical care. What should be provided to patients is defined by the law and consideration of the just distribution of finite medical resources, which requires a reasonable conception of the patient's good and the patient's informed desires. If people are not prepared to offer legally permitted, efficient and beneficial care to a patient because it conflicts with their values, they should not be doctors. Doctors should not offer partial medical services or partially discharge their obligations to care for their patients.

(Savulescu, 2006)

The 'services' he included, relate to termination of pregnancy, including those at late term. Savulescu argues, as a 'modern' bioethicist, that as doctors have historically decided which treatments are appropriate for patients, conscientious objection equates with paternalism.

Conscience vs secularism

Blunting or elimination of conscience can be a means of coping with a hostile culture or caused by experience of bullying. The results are morally and psychologically damaging for nurses and ultimately for their patients. The conflict between a sensitive conscience and a militantly secular culture can be difficult to resolve. Nevertheless, rights of conscience need to be cherished by nurses who accept the importance of conscientious objection and should be respected by fellow professionals and secular bioethicists who have probably never cared for a patient in the clinical area.

Christian persecution

If they persecuted me, they shall persecute you, also.

(John 15:18–25)

St John Henry Newman, writing a letter to the Duke of Norfolk about conscience, points out that conscience is the internal witness of the existence and the will of God, but that nowadays when people speak of the rights of conscience, they have no thoughts of God at all, but simply mean the freedom to act as they feel like doing (St John Henry Newman, 1875).

A belief that Christian persecution exists only in far off lands is not realistic today. In the 'civilised' world of the West, Christian men and women who take their religion seriously are subjected to bigotry when being considered for a judicial appointment and Christian university societies are denied the right to have Christians lead them.

In a forthright address to the inaugural Catholic Medical Association conference for healthcare students in 2014, the Archbishop of Westminster, Cardinal Vincent Nichols, said:

> *As evangelists in the world of healthcare, you encounter incredibly complex ethical questions. You need to give strong and courageous witness to the inviolable and intrinsic worth of every human life from conception to natural end. You will, and already do, face determined and sometimes aggressive opposition. Never let this deter you from engaging in debates about euthanasia, abortion, fertility, the just provision of care for all, irrespective of financial means, age, or illness.*

(Nichols, 2014)

World Medical Association and conscientious objection

The right to conscientious objection is often deprecated and even its elimination is now being championed by certain 'modern' bioethicists and 'respected' bodies, such as the World Medical Association (WMA). Draft proposals in 2021 were being debated for the association's International Code of Medical Ethics which could have resulted in the right to conscientious objection for doctors being curtailed or removed. The opposition to this plan caused the WMA to review their radical and unjust proposed plan.

The WMA was essentially planning to deny conscientious objection and force doctors to become executioners. Changes to the International Code of Medical Ethics would be significant because they will be incorporated into the Geneva Declaration that is binding on all states. In the draft of the paragraph dedicated to conscientious objection, it was restricted so much that it was practically non-existent. Among other things, it required the objecting doctor to refer a patient to another non-objecting doctor. How can the WMA force physicians to participate in actions that are unacceptable to their conscience? This is what the reviewed World Medical Association International Code of Medical Ethics now states regarding conscientious objection:

29. This Code represents the physician's ethical duties. However, on some issues there are profound moral dilemmas concerning which physicians and patients may hold deeply considered but conflicting conscientious beliefs.

The physician has an ethical obligation to minimise disruption to patient care. Physician conscientious objection to provision of any lawful medical interventions may only be exercised if the individual patient is not harmed or discriminated against and if the patient's health is not endangered.

The physician must immediately and respectfully inform the patient of this objection and of the patient's right to consult another qualified physician and provide sufficient information to enable the patient to initiate such a consultation in a timely manner

(WMA, 2023).

After considerable debate, a compromise agreement was reached that does not require doctors to refer in case of a conscientious objection.

This agreement was achieved after lengthy discussion and contributions from British and American Catholic and Jewish physicians.

The United Nations and the right to conscientious objection

The Universal Declaration of Human Rights – Article 18 states: 'Everyone has the right to freedom of thought, conscience and religion...'

Human rights

> *Rescue those who are being taken away to death.*
>
> (Proverbs 24:11)

Human rights, including the rights of the child, must be interpreted in the light of the Charter of the United Nations (UN), which was set up following World War II, to highlight to all nations the barbarity of the anti-life Nazi ideology, tragically revealed during that war. Today, it may be argued that the unborn baby is increasingly considered as an enemy within the womb to be brutally discarded.

Pregnancy, is not a disease, it is argued that 'it is a relationship from which we all benefited as foetuses'. Care of children is expected of parents but for those in particularly difficult circumstances, societal norms should expect prenatal care to be available to them (Watt, 2016).

The Charter of the United Nations (2016)

The charter has committed member states under Article 55 (Chapter 9) to promote the 'universal respect for and observance of human rights and fundamental freedoms for all, without distinction as to race, sex, language, religion, political or other opinion, national or social origin, property, birth, or other status'. The right to life of the unborn appears to be omitted in this commitment.

The humanity of the unborn?

A former American footballer, Benjamin Watson, who won the Super Bowl in 2005 with the New England Patriots is a vocal defender of the unborn. He now works for the US pro-life organisation, Human Coalition.

Watson has condemned society's dismissal of the worth of the unborn. He argues that,

> *The preborn have to prove they won't inconvenience us. If the preborn are deemed too burdensome, too genetically different, or just too untimely and un-welcome, they can be killed... But this approach seriously misunderstands what it means to be a human being. Nobody should have to pass a test to deserve to exist.*

(Society for the Protection of Unborn Children, 2021)

The United Nations and the right to life of the unborn?

The international instruments on human rights are ambiguous on the issue of whether the unborn child is protected or not. An analysis of the International Instruments on Human Rights shows that there is no explicit protection of the right to life of the unborn child. The regional commissions, the Courts of Human Rights and some national courts have refused to declare categorically that the unborn child is a subject of the right to life. Consequently, the protection of the right to life and other inherent rights of the unborn child is left to the free decision of the states.

The principles proclaimed in the Charter of the UN, including recognition of the inherent dignity and of the equal and inalienable rights of all members of the human family, are the foundation of freedom, justice and peace in the world. Even though in reality, the unborn child has a legal personality in the laws of many states, because the child is a subject of some rights which the law recognises, the fact remains that it is only from birth that the unborn child acquires legal personality. Thus, the legislations of many states stipulate that legal capacity begins with birth (Ibegbu, 2000).

The UN Convention on the Rights of the Child (1989)

The convention states: 'the child, by reason of his physical and mental immaturity, needs special safeguards and care, including appropriate legal protection, before as well as after birth' (Convention on the Rights of the Child, 1989). Those most in need of protection today, of their right to life, appear to be the defenceless unborn, the most vulnerable in society. The right to life is the building block for future generations whose rights are generated from having been allowed to survive in the womb.

The United Nations Human Rights Committee

This committee, by 2019, drafted a memo which stated, very controversially, that abortion and physician-assisted suicide should be universal human rights. The memo, or 'general comment', on the International Covenant on Civil and Political Rights calls for abortion to be decriminalised everywhere. Nations and states should 'not introduce new barriers and should remove existing barriers [to abortion]... including barriers caused as a result of the exercise of conscientious objection by individual medical providers.

Therefore, the UN Human Rights Committee has openly discarded the protection of the unborn, despite the 2016 Charter for the UN, regarding its declaration on 'human rights and fundamental freedoms for all' and the long-held right to conscientious objection for health professionals.

Thou shall not kill

Christianity and other world religions have the well-established commandment against killing. The law against killing is written in the conscience of every human person. Consequently, every human person is conscious of it. Thus, the constitutions of many states stipulate that every human person has a right to life and not only that human life is sacred, but it is also inviolable. No one, therefore, has the right to take away human life; instead, we have the duty to care for it, to protect it and to defend it. Only God is the owner and Master of human life.

According to figures from the World Health Organisation (WHO), between 40 and 56 million abortions are performed every year. The cruelty and violence of the deaths are cloaked under the slogan of reproductive health rights and 'the right to choose'. However, increasing reports of coercive control in relation to abortion and detrimental post-abortion effects on women, both psychological and physical, can no longer be ignored or suppressed.

The United Nations promotion of the 'right' to abortion

Archbishop Bernardito Auza, the Holy See's Permanent Observer to the UN, has spoken out forcefully against the so-called 'right to abortion' that is currently being promoted at the UN, particularly by its European members. Speaking to the UN's Commission on Population and Development, Archbishop Auza stated:

> *Suggesting that reproductive health includes a right to abortion… defies moral and legal standards within domestic legislations and divides efforts to address the real needs of mothers and children, especially those yet unborn.*
> *Formulating and positioning population issues in terms of individual "sexual and reproductive rights" is to change the focus from that which should be the proper concern of governments and international agencies. Governments and society ought to promote social policies that have the family as their principal object, assisting it by providing adequate resources and efficient means of support, both for bringing up children and looking after the elderly, to strengthen relations between generations and avoid distancing the elderly from the family unit.*

(Grogan, 2017)

Abortion decriminalisation

Pharmaceutical abortion (Mifepristone or RU486) now accounts for over half of all abortions (Jones et al., 2022). There are current moves by the pro-choice movement to decriminalise abortion in England and Wales. The Abortion Act of 1967 is now considerably extended in terms of the grounds for abortion, effectively allowing abortion on demand for social reasons.

A physician trained in law, Dr Philip Howard, argues against this move and examined the important, related issues: Now most abortions (97–98%) are performed on the grounds that continuance of the pregnancy is thought to entail a greater risk to the mental health of the mother than having an abortion. However, there is very considerable doubt that pregnancy adversely impacts mental health. In future we could see changes to abortion law in England and Wales to decriminalise abortion, which would:

- *allow abortion for any reason at all, up to 24 weeks of pregnancy*
- *make it lawful for anyone, medically qualified or not, to supply pills or instruments for an abortion*
- *make it much easier for abusive men to coerce women into having an abortion.*

Decriminalisation of abortion would mean that it is no longer a criminal offence. It would remain a medical or surgical procedure provided essentially for social reasons. The implications of full decriminalisation to birth would be considerable and would lead to an increase in abortions. Decriminalisation of abortion means that it would be regarded as a social issue, though performed as a medical procedure. Therefore, doctors and midwives could be sued for not performing foeticide or abortion competently and the rights of doctors and midwives to conscientious objection would be seriously undermined as abortion and foeticide would no longer be crimes at all. If prenatal foeticide becomes permissible for "failed" surgery or other interventions, what logically, would prevent

*perinatal euthanasia for failed intrauterine surgery, or indeed
for perinatal disability discovered at birth? What would this
mean for disability discrimination and attitudes towards those
who are disabled if they could have been destroyed shortly
before (or after) birth for their disability? What, if
any limit or threshold would be placed on foeticide
or active post-natal euthanasia?
The issue of foeticide will inevitably raise the question
of the rights of the unborn and the neonate. If foeticide
is legal, immediately before birth, why not euthanasia
immediately after delivery? What is the moral distinction
if any, between immediate pre- and post-natal existence?
What legal or moral change happens at birth? The possibility
of a requirement for abortion or foeticide would impact
on the development of prenatal therapies and the development of
foetal medicine. There would be moral confusion over the meaning
of the rights of the pre-born or immediately post-natal child.
The decriminalisation of abortion is likely to remove
the right of conscientious objection as it would become
a social rather than a medical issue except where there was
a claim for the misuse or supply of abortifacients
in clinical negligence.*

(Howard, 2018)

Foetal pain

While abortion is a moral issue with ongoing debate about the rights
of the mother versus the child, ethical issues are expanding due to
emerging physiological evidence about embryonic development in
relation to foetal pain experienced in utero.

A recent study finding (that may compound the emotional suffering
of women post-abortion) relates to surgical abortion (although becoming
less common than medical abortion) and the issue of foetal pain, which
should be reconsidered as being a phenomenon as early as at 12 weeks'
gestation. The study authors state that to their knowledge, they are not
aware of any procedures where invasive foetal intervention proceeds
without anaesthesia or analgesia, except for abortion (Derbyshire and

Bockmann, 2019). In a recent paper published by the authors, titled *Reconsidering Foetal pain*, they state their belief that,

> *Foetal pain does not have to be equivalent to a mature adult human experience to matter morally and so foetal pain might be considered as part of a humane approach to abortion.*
> *The possibility of the foetus experiencing more pain through efforts to abolish pain seems highly unlikely, even fanciful.*

(Derbyshire and Bockmann, 2019)

The prevailing understanding is that all clinicians or surgeons working with foetal patients advocate the use of foetal anaesthesia and analgesia as standard practice. To the authors' knowledge, in reconsidering foetal pain, this is not the practice during surgical abortion. While further studies might be welcome to address the optimal procedures necessary to improve outcomes, there is consensus that the use of foetal anaesthesia and analgesia improves maternal and foetal cardiovascular stability, provides the necessary immobility of the foetus and prevents a dangerous foetal physiologic reaction or 'stress response' to the surgery (Rollins and Rosen, 2014; Van de Velde and De Buck, 2012).

Non-maleficence

For therapeutic procedures, therefore, such pain can be ethically offset. The principle of non-maleficence implies that we should first do no harm. Current neuroscientific evidence undermines the necessity of the cortex for pain experience. Even if the cortex is deemed necessary for pain experience, there is now good evidence that thalamic projections into the subplate, which emerge around 12 weeks' gestation, are functional and equivalent to thalamocortical projections that emerge around 24 weeks' gestation.

Compassion for animal vs human embryos

Human rights campaigner and member of the House of Lords, David Alton has highlighted the double standards of the Animal

Welfare (Sentience) Bill (DEFRA, 2021) currently being considered by the House of Lords.

There are glaring double standards in UK law. The Animals (Scientific Procedures) Act (1986, Amended regulations, 2012) stipulates rightly that animal foetuses must be killed in humane ways, but no parallel legal provision exists for human foetuses. Unborn children in the UK are left without such protections. When Lord David Alton inquired whether some of the bill's safeguards might be extended to unborn homo sapiens, he was told that the bill had been cast in such a way as to prevent this.

No requirement to give pain relief to babies during an abortion

Babies undergoing abortion at 20 weeks' gestation 'via surgical dilatation and evacuation' are not provided with pain relief. This procedure is described by the Royal College of Obstetricians and Gynaecologists (2010) as 'where the foetus is removed in foeticide, where potassium chloride is injected into the heart to cause immediate cardiac arrest'. It has been highlighted that potassium chloride is 'excruciatingly painful if administered without proper anaesthesia' (Human Rights Watch, 2006).

Foetal pain inquiry

Lord David Alton took part in an inquiry in 2020 into foetal pain, organised by 18 parliamentarians from both Houses. They found that recent studies strongly suggest that unborn children may feel pain much earlier than previously thought. In an article published in the Journal of Medical Ethics, researchers say there is now 'good evidence' that the brain and nervous system, which start developing at 12 weeks' gestation, permit the unborn baby to feel pain (Derbyshire and Bockmann, 2019). Lord Alton describes one of the researchers as a 'pro-choice' British pain expert who used to think there was no chance that unborn babies could feel pain before 24 weeks. He too is now erring on the side of caution (Alton, 2021).

Thus, current neuroscientific evidence supports the possibility of foetal pain before the 'consensus' cut-off of 24 weeks. Such emergent evidence should be seriously considered, notwithstanding the moral prohibition on abortion, for most people who have a faith and for those who do not.

'We celebrate when charity is offered to animals... but allow abortion up to birth for human beings with disabilities' (Alton, 2021). Lord Alton also explains how a double standard towards animals and humans could be due to poor public understanding of unborn life, exacerbated by the pressure and censorship often faced by open discussions on these issues. 'Those who criticise such laws risk being de-platformed or pushed into political no-man's-land. This silencing of debate has led from illogic to ignorance' (Alton, 2021).

Some British people do not believe that human beings are alive until birth

A 2013 YouGov Poll found that a shocking 17% of British people do not believe that human beings are alive until birth. 'Perhaps, given the brutal reality of abortion, they do not wish to consider the implications of the opposite being true. And government policy seems to imply the same' (Alton, 2021).

Animal vs child welfare

Lord Alton went on to discuss the hypocrisy of many people's approaches to the rights of animals in comparison to unborn children:

I have met people who claim to be great champions of animal rights and yet are vehemently in favour of abortion – including some who are trying to amend the law to allow abortion in all circumstances right up to birth. We rightly celebrate when charity is offered to animals who suffer from a particular injury or disability, yet we allow abortion up to birth for human beings with any kind of disability, including cleft lip, cleft palate, or club foot – to say nothing of Down's syndrome.

(Alton, 2021)

Ethics of vaccines' components

There are obvious ethical issues in relation to vaccine development and other drugs using foetal cells. Giving or using such products requires conscience examination and even where involvement in such practice may be refused by practitioners with conscientious objection, full patient understanding and informed consent is required in view of both the ethical issues and potential side effects. Nurses who administer medication must be aware of the possible side effects and ethical makeup of the drug components. Any concern about these must be respected and nurses and care staff must not be forced to administer or receive products, e.g., foetal cell lines as utilised in vaccines against the COVID-19 pandemic. This would be contrary to the conscience of ethically minded practitioners.

Embryo experimentation

It would seem likely that the decriminalisation of abortion would reduce the rights and confuse the legal identity of the embryo and unborn child. If the embryo was no longer considered a human person, experimentation on embryos is likely to be extended. The human embryo would have less legal protection than a laboratory animal as it would be regarded as no longer human. It would be easy for the in vitro embryo to be used as an experimental entity for genetic research, studies on embryonic development, pharmacological research and drug testing.

(Howard, 2018)

The concept of 'choice' in abortion

The concept of the so-called 'right to choose' is heavily undermined by the associated coercion of women which is known to be linked to domestic abuse. This often results in abortion. The concept of choice, it can be argued, is a fallacy in many such situations.

Nurses need to be aware that women often change their mind during the medical abortions by drugs which are so much more prevalent today. The need for abortion pills to be taken at home was legally accepted as a temporary measure as part of the emergency powers of the Coronavirus Act (2020). The ongoing risks by continuing use of these drugs for the unborn and their mothers' mental and physical health, including the obvious dangers of coercive control as part of domestic abuse, cannot be underestimated.

Women's 'choice' – fact or fiction?

Should a woman change her mind after taking Mifepristone and seek help, receiving progesterone in a timely manner, within 72 hours after taking the first abortion pill, allows an overall 68% chance that the baby will survive (Kearney, 2019).

The role of the nurse as the patient advocate is obvious in these life-endangering situations. Women who have had their pregnancy saved have much gratitude for the Good Samaritan help received. To quote one young woman whose child sadly died, despite provision of progesterone: 'Your kindness will never be forgotten and the help you gave us, gave our baby a chance. Thank you from the bottom of my heart. If anything, my faith in humanity was restored' (Kearney, 2021).

The abortion industry launched an ultimately, unsuccessful complaint to the GMC about this and other successful 'rescue' missions. 'Women's choice', it seems, can only apply when it is deemed possible by certain 'powerful' bodies.

The 'powerful' bodies in this case came to learn that there was no case found against Dr Kearney, a true Good Samaritan. Similar practitioners will be able to continue to offer safe and ethical help to women, where possible, who change their minds about proceeding with a medical abortion.

Abortion effects on women's mental health

Evidence gathered from studies concludes that foetal loss seems to expose women to a higher risk for mental disorders than childbirth and shows that abortion can be considered a more relevant risk factor for mental disorder than miscarriage (Bellieni and Buonocore, 2013). The findings of an earlier, more specific study of young women post-abortion suggest that it may be associated with increased risks of mental health problems (Fergusson et al.,

2006). The emerging research about the alarmingly negative effect on women's mental health post-abortion can no longer be ignored.

Applying Gillick competence and Fraser guidelines

The Fraser guidelines still apply to advice and treatment relating to contraception and sexual health. But Gillick competency is often used in a wider context to help assess whether a child has the maturity to make their own decisions and to understand the implications of those decisions.

School nurses have the power to dispense the morning-after pill, a powerful hormonal drug, to girls under 16 years of age, free of charge with no requirement for the girls' parents to be informed. This undermines parents in the struggle to protect their children. School nurses who refuse to become agents of the state, by acting against their conscience in this way, are placed in an impossible position, so are effectively excluded from such school posts.

A child protection organisation recommends encouraging children to tell their parents or carers about the decisions they are making. If they don't want to do this, you should explore why and, if appropriate, discuss ways you could help them inform their parents or carers. For example, you could talk to the young person's parents or carers on their behalf (NSPCC, 2020).

Do no harm?

The ongoing transformation in the methods and ethics of medicine raises profound moral questions for doctors, nurses, pharmacists and others who believe in the traditional virtues of Hippocratic medicine. This proscribed abortion and assisted suicide and compelled physicians to 'do no harm'. This imperative, to date, has generally been accommodated by society as has medical conscientious objection.

No doctor in the US is forced to perform abortions. Indeed, when New York mayor Michael Bloomberg sought to increase accessibility to abortion by requiring that all residents in obstetrics and gynaecology in New York's public hospitals receive training in pregnancy termination, the law specifically allowed doctors with religious or moral objections to opt out on grounds of conscience. The assisted suicide laws of Oregon and Washington, for example, permit doctors to refuse to participate in hastening patient deaths.

Medical disinterest emerging in higher training in abortion

In 2016, emerging evidence reported that only 1% of UK trainee obstetricians and gynaecologists were taking higher training in abortion (Goldbeck-Wood, 2016).

A spokesperson for 'Right to Life UK' said: 'The extremely low number of trainee obstetricians and gynaecologists who are taking higher training in abortion, likely reflects an innate human reluctance to end life' (Robinson, 2020).

Attempts to increase those numbers in recent years have come from the Royal College of Obstetricians and Gynaecologists (RCOG) and from Marie Stopes International. The RCOG released a report in 2019 stating its intention to teach and assess 'abortion skills' as part of its core curriculum.

> The RCOG's proposals fail to mention any conscientious objection provision for pro-life students who do not want to provide abortion skills. The college issued a 'Better for Women' report which states:
>
> 1. The General Medical Council (GMC) should review the Undergraduate medical curriculum to include the importance of abortion care to students.
>
> The RCOG will teach abortion skills as a part of its core curriculum and assess those skills through examination.
>
> (RCOG, 2019).

Such aims compound the past and present elimination of Catholics, Christians and other pro-life people from this speciality. Such a position is indefensible in our supposed liberal age of tolerance, fairness and purported respect for inclusivity and diversity.

Practitioner choice?

All doctors who practise medicine in the UK must be registered with the GMC, if the proposals are adopted, and pro-life medical students could be forced to sit through the knowledge and undefined 'abortion skills' training or risk losing their membership of their medical body.

Student indoctrination

Marie Stopes International is attempting to encourage nursing students into providing abortions as it faces potential shortages in trained medical professionals willing to do abortions. The abortion giant is working with Health Education England and a range of UK universities as it seeks to promote its new abortion clinic placement programme to these students. Marie Stopes International's new placement scheme is nothing but an attempt to indoctrinate young students: 'Future healthcare professionals' training should be directed at offering the best possible care to all humans, including unborn babies' (Robinson, 2020).

This is another area where the nurse's right to conscientious objection will, no doubt, be sorely tested.

Overturn of Roe v Wade

The consequences of abortion denial, as reported by Rocca et al., (2021), based on Turnaway Study data, found that 96% of women after five years no longer wished they had received an abortion. In Ethiopia, liberalising abortion law has vastly increased abortion incidence without an appreciable decrease in maternal or abortion mortality (Miller, 2022). Poland, which has a strict abortion law, has one of the lowest rates of maternal mortality in the world.

Billed as 'health care', abortion is an undeniably violent 'solution' to issues for which women deserve life-respecting solutions for themselves and the young lives they support. (Watt, 2022).

What are healthcare workers' rights under law?

The Equality Act 2010 legally protects people from discrimination in the workplace and in wider society. It replaced previous anti-discrimination laws, making the law easier to understand and strengthening protection in some situations. The Act lists nine protected characteristics, without a hierarchy:

- age
- disability
- gender reassignment
- marriage and civil partnership
- pregnancy and maternity
- race
- religion or belief
- sex/sexual orientation

Clearly, religion and belief are protected equally alongside the other characteristics. Therefore, it can be argued that: 'We have a right to call for respect of that belief. And we surely have a right to call any attempt to suppress or denigrate that belief a hate crime' (Rose, 2018).

Freedom of religion and of speech

At the same time, the rights to freedom of religion and of speech as set out in Articles 9 and 10 of the European Convention on Human Rights are protected by the Human Rights Act of 1998. It allows defence of people's rights in UK courts and compels public organisations – including the government, police and local councils – to treat everyone equally, with fairness, dignity and respect. Therefore, there is a protected right under English law to state and to defend our belief.

The Glasgow Midwives' failed case is salutary for all medical professionals who wish to exercise their right to conscientious objection. The midwives' case appears to be a precedent now set for different ethical scenarios. One example is the case of 'Y', a brain-injured man whose family wanted his 'treatment' to be discontinued. The 'treatment' consisted of CANH. This basic, humane intervention was judged to be no longer of benefit to him by the Supreme Court in 2018. Many patients with brain injury are not dying and may well recover in this time of increasing knowledge of the brain's capacity for recovery in many cases (see Chapter 8).

Courage and staff support

> *The simple step of a courageous individual is not to take part in the lie. One word of truth outweighs the world. In keeping silent about evil, in burying it so deep within us that no sign of it appears on the surface, we are implanting it and it will rise up a thousand-fold in the future.*

(Solzhenitsyn, 1973)

It is suggested that individuals will have 'modules' of courage rather than composite courage. Modules of courage enable a nurse to respond courageously to some, but not all, of the situations that inspire fear (Adams, 2006).

Courage in action

Recently media reports and research in the UK and Ireland have addressed poor practice in healthcare. In one situation an Irish inquiry team investigated an unacceptably high rate of postpartum hysterectomies at the Lourdes hospital in Ireland over a 25-year period. The team commented that they had difficulty understanding why so few had the courage, insight, or integrity to say, 'this is not right' (Harding-Clark, 2006).

Defeatism vs beneficence

Psychosocial aspects of caregiving have tended to command secondary status. Training that gives emphasis to professional detachment may have a detrimental impact later, on the interpersonal relationships between nurses and patients – and to the quality of care delivered. The nurse wishing to represent the patient's need for beneficence may experience a prevailing culture of treatment defeatism, exemplified by the unethical assumption of treatment futility for some patients for whom appropriate treatment is required. This culture is difficult to negotiate, so nurses need all the support available to them.

Clinical supervision (support)

Clinical supervision is an activity that brings skilled supervisors and practitioners together to reflect upon practice. It is a means of peer support and provides time for nurses or midwives to think about their knowledge and skills and how they may be developed to improve care. Nurses can be supported greatly with clinical supervision in their attempts at patient and staff advocacy or the exercise of conscientious objection.

Importance of formalised staff support in practice

The role of education in teaching nursing staff professional values and standards is so important in healthcare. Clinical supervision, although not uniformly offered to nurses today, can provide practitioners with a forum for open and honest dialogue about their experiences of delivering care. A psychologically safe environment is essential in which to discuss the everyday challenges, frustrations and pressures of the job – in which stories and feelings about patients and their care are shared, explored and validated. The clinical support facilitator may be sourced externally and may be from a related discipline. A system of clinical supervision is a vital method of staff support. It helps to remind busy staff that every patient is individual and unique; it provides support to nurses; encourages communication within the team; and it helps to improve team dynamics.

Strengthening courage in practice

It remains challenging to ensure widespread implementation of clinical supervision for nurses across healthcare organisations. There is an increasingly evident need for formalised support in nurses' busy practice settings, so it is important to provide and improve the quality of clinical supervision in healthcare. Effective clinical supervision can achieve skilled reflection in a critical way to allow the nurse more courage to act as the Good Samaritan where a culture of treatment 'futility' may be present as an inappropriate and unethical patient management approach.

The UK Conscientious Objection (Medical Activities) Bill (2018)

The Medical Activities Bill, introduced by Baroness O' Loan in 2018, was designed to afford necessary protection for the careers of medical practitioners on matters of life and death. The bill aims to strengthen the conscience rights of healthcare professionals who believe it would be wrong to be involved in three specific activities – abortion, activities under the Human Fertilisation and Embryology Act 1990 (such as embryo disposal or research) and the withdrawal of life-preserving treatment.

Lord Singh, speaking from a Sikh perspective, in support of the bill, stated: 'Majority opinion can, at times, be unthinking and we need to be wary of being pushed or pushing others to support debatable attitudes that at times affront ethical and moral principles' (Singh, 2018).

Conclusion

Persecution for one's beliefs can affect Christians and those of other faiths who also will experience opposition, for clinging to their ethical beliefs on behalf of their patients in need.

The Human Rights Act of 1998 allows the defence of people's rights in UK courts. It compels public organisations – including the government, police and local councils – to treat everyone equally, with fairness, dignity and respect. Under the Human Rights Act (1998), Article 9 protects freedom of religion and Articles 10 and 11 protect the linked rights of freedom of speech and freedom of association.

Together with the Equality Act 2010, there is a protected right under English law to defend Christian and others' belief systems, including conscientious objection in healthcare settings. Under the Equality Act 2010, it is illegal for employers to discriminate against employees or applicants for jobs because of their religion or belief; it is also illegal for public authorities, schools, businesses, etc., to discriminate against people or organisations because of their religion or belief.

The European Convention on Human Rights applies throughout the UK because of the Equality and Human Rights Commission (1998)

Employment Claims

Under the Equality Act 2010, claims relating to employment are brought in an Employment Tribunal. Other claims under the Equality Act or under the Human Rights Act are brought in the County Court.

Expectations of practitioners' moral judgements

There is no true peace without fairness, truth, justice and solidarity

(Pope St John Paul II, 1999)

Legal protection exists for those wishing to exercise the right to conscientious objection. Nurses are expected to provide individualised and compassionate, safe patient care in line with the code of professional conduct.

It is argued, by Weinstock (2014) that,
... just as democracies benefit from citizens thinking and deliberating about complex moral issues that arise in the general policy context, so healthcare institutions benefit from healthcare professionals feeling empowered to reflect about the laws, rules, codes of conduct and protocols that govern their professional practice... the work of doctors

*and nurses involves them in daily interaction... in which
moral judgement and agency is required. The work
(of health care professionals) would simply be impossible
were they not to feel that they possessed scope within
which to exercise such judgement. The recognition of
a right to conscientious exemption is one of the elements
through which they are enabled to develop the moral
agency required for their professional practice.*

Professionals warrant support in respecting their code and need to be sure how to access such support. This may be clinical, legal, emotional, psychological, spiritual or practical. Such support can strengthen required courage on occasions of ethical conflict which are associated with conscientious objection.

Practitioners need to understand that their right to conscientious objection, in line with their religious beliefs, does not involve complicity with acts against their conscience and their professional mission by being expected to act as agents of the state.

Acting against the code of conduct, the role of patient advocate and dictate of conscience are not options for ethical health professionals. Support, for them, however, is essential in fulfilling the required expectations of their vocation.

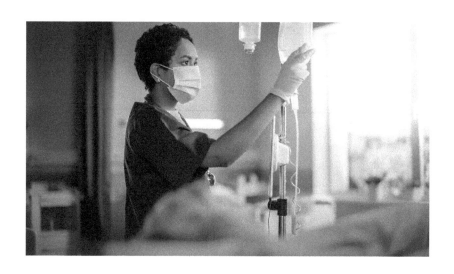

Chapter 8
Clinically-assisted nutrition and hydration: duty of care vs legal and professional guidance

---

For I was hungry, and you fed me. I was thirsty, and you gave me to drink.

(Matthew 25:31–46)

Introduction

This chapter explores the important responsibility of caring for vulnerable patients who are totally dependent on the provision of clinically-assisted nutrition and hydration (CANH) for their well-being and hoped-for recovery with a focus on the duty of care expectation of health professionals.

Recent legal and professional guidance, however, appears not to favour life chances for those with a brain impairment due to either injury or disease. The denial of CANH for many people was a practice approved, in a vast majority of cases, by the LCP. Many patients were placed on the pathway but were not in the dying phase with often a non-cancer, chronic condition. Such discredited practice appears now to be endorsed by the following two, relatively recent developments which both occurred in 2018:

1. The UK ruling of the Law Lords on the case of 'Y' (a brain-damaged man)
2. BMA guidance on CANH withdrawal for brain-injured people.

These two developments in 2018 relating to legal and professional guidance must be an inevitable cause of ethical conflict for committed pro-life health professionals. Denying CANH to patients with brain damage as agreed by the treating clinician and family members without a need for recourse to law, is compounded by BMA guidance (BMA, 2018) on withdrawing CANH.

What is CANH?

Views on medical treatment have changed, so that basic needs to support life, namely CANH, which were always accepted to be within the province of humane care are now considered as 'medical treatment'. This can now be stopped or not commenced in line with any advanced directive (documented or verbally made about 'treatment') and with the agreement of close family members for mentally incapacitated patients. Therefore, people who are contemplating an advanced directive (treatment refusal) need to be clear about what is meant by 'medical treatment' today.

Decisions about whether to start, continue, or stop CANH are made daily – but few decisions are more challenging for healthcare professionals. It is important to approach both clinically-assisted food and fluid as separate entities depending on the situation of dying and non-dying patients.

Many patients can benefit from various means of CANH in today's health settings where patients may be living longer, but have some swallowing difficulties following a stroke or simply with muscle weakness due to ageing or chronic health conditions. Many patients can learn to manage their own feeding regimes and many patients have good life extension and quality through these techniques. They can prevent repeated chest infections when even soft or pureed food or thickened fluids are unsafe. Some consider this form of feeding to be medical treatment. Others argue that it is basic, humane care for patients who are in obvious need of nutrition and hydration and are going to suffer and die without this assistance.

A deadly agenda for 'healthcare'

The Supreme Court in 2018 ruled that doctors with family agreement would be able to withdraw food and fluids from brain-damaged patients in a persistent vegetative state (PVS) or a minimally conscious state (MCS) without needing to apply to the Court of Protection.

Inflicting unnecessary symptoms on patients is not in keeping with moral, ethical principles, duty of care principles and codes of conduct, aimed at ensuring humane patient care. How can patients with conditions with unclear recovery potential be victim-blamed for surviving, inconveniently – by some family members and health professionals? These may have, at best, a defeatist attitude to rehabilitation and, at worst, a deadly agenda where finance may, of course, be a lurking factor.

What helps in our role with patients with brain damage?

Patients with brain damage, for whatever reason, may not be dying and will suffer and die because of discontinuation of life-sustaining 'medical treatment' as CANH is considered today. Understanding the concept of the duty of care and the code of conduct can help us in our role as the patient's advocate.

This is a perfect example of an occasion where ethical practitioners can work together to provide a protective guard for such vulnerable patients and refuse unethical direction. Practitioners need to remember that laws can be immoral and unjust and the patient has great need of advocacy for their chance of humane care, improvement and potential survival.

Evidenced-based care

Keeping up to date with the ongoing and improving developments in treatments for people with brain damage and the capacity for brain recovery in some patients is essential. This is part of our need for an evidence base to our practice in line with the expectation of codes of conduct.

Duty of care

In tort law, a duty of care is a legal obligation which is imposed on an individual, requiring adherence to a standard of reasonable care while performing any acts that could foreseeably harm others. It is the first element that must be established to proceed with an action in negligence. The long-held duty of care is defined simply as a legal obligation to: always act in the best interest of individuals and others, not to act or fail to act in a way that results in harm.

The Nursing Code of Conduct: standards of practice and behaviour for Nurses and Midwives states, 'Nurses need to remember the duty of care enshrined in their code of conduct: to act as the patient's advocate and be evidence-based in their practice' (NMC, 2018).

The code expects nurses to do no harm, conduct holistic needs assessments, be evidence-based in their practice and act as an advocate for the vulnerable. If a vulnerable adult is neglected or not given the medicines or food they require, then this is neglect, which is recognised in safeguarding as a form of abuse.

The code of conduct documents the standards (17.1 – 17.3) in relation to patient risk:

17. Raise concerns immediately if you believe a person is vulnerable or at risk and needs extra support and attention.

17.1. Take all reasonable steps to protect people who are vulnerable or at risk from harm, neglect, or abuse.

17.2 Share information if you believe someone may be at risk of harm, in line with the laws relating to the disclosure of information.

17.3 Have knowledge of and keep to the relevant laws and policies about protecting and caring for vulnerable people.

Treat people in a way that does not take advantage of their vulnerability or cause them upset or distress.

(NMC, 2018)

Acts of neglect by omission can include ignoring medical or physical care needs, failure to provide access to appropriate health, social care, or educational services and the withholding of the necessities of life, such as medication, adequate nutrition and heating.

Good Samaritan care

The Good Samaritan who goes out of his way to aid an injured man (Luke, 10:30–37) signifies Jesus Christ who is the physician of souls and bodies, 'the faithful witness' (Rev. 3:14) of the divine salvific presence in the world.

How can nurses make this message concrete today?
How to translate it into a readiness to accompany a suffering
person in the terminal stages of life in this world and to offer
this assistance in a way that respects and promotes
the intrinsic human dignity of persons who are ill, their
vocation to holiness and thus the highest worth of
their existence.

(Congregation for the Doctrine of the Faith, 2020a)

Hydration needs of vulnerable patients

Emotional and cultural factors influence decision-making about assisted nutrition and hydration. Lack of information and misperceptions of CANH can play a predominant role in the decision to begin or suspend nutritional or hydration support (Del Rio et al., 2021).

It has been extensively argued as to whether provision of food and water is to be regarded as a basic nursing measure (which is unquestionably part of humane care) or as medical treatment, provision of which is at the discretion of medical staff, according to the MCA (2005). Apart from the likelihood of major variations within categories such as congenitally brain-damaged infants, healthy people with traumatically acquired injuries and elderly people with dementia, it is unwise to consider all people from such widely differing groups as potential candidates for 'withdrawal' (McCullagh, 1996).

Withdrawal of clinically-assisted nutrition and hydration

This means of ordinary care can be withdrawn in extreme circumstances – an appropriate decision when death is clearly imminent. But fit patients with unconscious states should not qualify for removal of feeding and hydration. For dying and non-dying patients, safe monitoring by competent staff avoids such risks as fluid overload.

When did nutrition and hydration become 'medical treatment'?

Let food be thy medicine and medicine be thy food.

(Hippocrates)

Recent and past healthcare legislative developments and relevant cases in the UK increase the growing concern about how CANH is considered by some, and is deemed by the MCA, to be medical treatment. This concern is illustrated by the following:

- The case of 'Y' (2018), revealed that where family and clinicians were agreed, CANH for brain-damaged people could be discontinued without recourse to the court.
- BMA guidance on CANH (2018), directed doctors about denial of assisted nutrition and hydration, and coincided (interestingly) with the ruling on 'Y' the same year.
- The case of the Polish Catholic man (RS) in Plymouth (2020). Doctors stopped providing life support treatment to this middle-aged man, known to be 'RS' who had been at the centre of a legal dispute after falling into a coma. The family was divided on the decision.
- The Tony Bland case (1993). Judges considered 'assisted feeding was futile' although this was his only required form of life support.
- Vincent Lambert (2019, France) and Terri Schiavo (2005, USA). Both young people had their assisted nutrition and hydration stopped, following unsuccessful legal challenges by their parents, advocating for it to be continued (against the wishes of other existing and ex family members). These cases are discussed more fully later in this chapter.

A change in spiritual outlook?

There were no medical breakthroughs that initiated this new way of thinking about brain-injured people, but various factors can be attributed to this new attitude to brain-damaged people.

Firstly, it was a changing spiritual outlook, together with legal precedent and professional guidance and secondly, the introduction of futile treatment bioethical theories.

All these factors set yet another precedent for health professionals, who, once legal decisions are made that are not in favour of life, are expected to cease the humane feeding of such patients. Such decisions trouble the conscience of ethical healthcare staff who are placed in an impossible ethical position. The ethical stand taken by pro-life staff with conscientious objection against such future decisions will need support from each other, relevant managers and those charged with staff welfare and their pastoral care.

The Mental Capacity Act (2005)

'Treatment' under the MCA is defined as: 'any diagnostic or other procedure'. This definition can rein in the scope for those patients who may need investigation and treatment, regardless of their original diagnosis and predicted prognosis. The IMCA service within the MCA, nevertheless, is aimed at protecting vulnerable people by representing a person's wishes and feelings and challenging the decision-makers when the person has no one else to do this on their behalf.

If people have been assessed as lacking capacity, then any action taken, or any decision made for, or on behalf of them must be made for their true benefit. Some decisions made by the patient may be considered as 'eccentric' but must be respected according to the MCA. This implies a need for nurses to ensure patients are fully informed of a possibly negative impact on their health due to their decisions they may have made. The concept of 'best interests' is under review with a more favourable and more objective concept being proposed – that of 'benefit versus possible harm'.

The UK case of 'Y'

The Supreme Court ruling of July 2018 allows doctors and families to allow people in long-term persistent, non-responsive states to die without legal application. If both the family and the medical team agree, then a patient can, in essence, be starved and dehydrated to death, without there being any need for a legal check and balance. This has undeniably moved the goalposts for the vulnerable, closer to 'euthanasia by omission'.

The case of 'Y' involved a brain-damaged man in the UK whose family wanted his feeding stopped and agreed with the medical team to seek required court intervention. Previously, further to the Bland judgement of 1993, it had been recommended 'as a matter of good practice' that reference be made to the courts where doctors were contemplating withdrawal of CANH from a patient in a persistent vegetative state. Since the Bland judgement (1993) and the MCA (2005), such recourse to law has not been considered a strict duty.

The judgement on 'Y'

In the summer of 2018, concerning the case of 'Y', it was decided by the UK Supreme Court that decisions regarding CANH no longer had to be routinely referred to the court. This development puts decision-making about this important and ethical issue in the hands of doctors and family members. Such decisions will affect people who have suffered a brain injury, have dementia, have had a stroke, have Parkinson's disease, or are in a persistent vegetative state (PVS) (more positively known as persistent non-responsive states) or a Minimally conscious state (MCS).

All the listed categories of patients lack mental capacity to make decisions for themselves so that the ruling is concerned with the circumstances when CANH can be withheld or withdrawn, to end the life of the patient.

Exceptions

The two circumstances when CANH will be provided are:

- if there is a decision by an authorised health and welfare attorney or
- following a clinician-led 'best interest' process which supports the use of CANH.

One legally qualified physician, remarking on this judgement, noted that:

> *This will have considerable repercussions for: mentally incapacitated patients with profound neuro-disability, including persistent vegetative states, minimal consciousness states and severe head injuries as well as those with strokes.*

(Howard, 2018)

BMA guidance on CANH in England and Wales

All the listed categories of patients will lack mental capacity to make decisions for themselves, so that the guidance is concerned with the circumstances in which CANH can be withheld or withdrawn to end the life of the patient. It is not difficult to predict the dilemma for practitioners who do not agree with such guidance which can affect patients who are not imminently dying.

Patients in whom CANH is not considered clinically indicated

The court (An NHS trust and others (Respondents) v Y, 2018), the GMC (2010) and NICE (2018) have made clear that health professionals are not required to offer treatments that they consider to be clinically inappropriate, which may be because:

- it is not possible to provide it (e.g., it is not physically possible to insert a feeding tube, or the patient repeatedly pulls it out)
- the clinical risks associated with CANH are too great, e.g., patients for whom tube placement (usually PEG or RIG) is considered a high mortality risk
- there is an elevated risk of aspiration
- CANH would provide no clinical benefit in terms of extending the patient's life or providing symptom relief and would carry potential risks (e.g., in patients with end-stage dementia for whom the inability to take sufficient intake may indicate that they are approaching death).

Hydration is particularly important where prognosis is always uncertain, despite conditions being considered as 'end stage'.

What does the BMA mean by CANH being unable to achieve its clinical aim?

Any clinical aim worth its name needs to be compassionate above all else. Clinical aims are for providing essential services that promote health, prevent diseases and deliver healthcare services to individuals, families and communities.

The following was stated at the Supreme Court in the case of 'Y':

The BMA can see no principled or logical reason for requiring court review in relation to patients with persistent vegetative states (PVS) and minimally conscious states (MCS), but not for a patient with a different condition. Similarly, it (the BMA) can find no logical reason why one form of medical treatment (clinically-assisted nutrition and hydration), is treated differently from other forms of medical treatment such as artificial ventilation.

(An NHS trust and others (Respondents) v Y, 2018)

The BMA guidance for UK doctors states:

> Although there is a very strong presumption that it will be in a person's best interests to prolong life, for some patients, CANH will not be in their best interests, because it is not able to provide a quality of life that they would find acceptable – and in these circumstances, legally and ethically, it should not be provided.
>
> (BMA, 2018)

The BMA is assuming that vulnerable patients such as these would agree with being starved and dehydrated to death by those judging their quality of life as unacceptable. Their potential for recovery is not considered. This leaves many helpless people who are by no means imminently dying to a long, cruel death by dehydration and starvation. It is not difficult to predict the dilemma for those practitioners who do not agree with such guidance. It is not unknown for guidance to be overlooked where patients' benefits are compromised by it.

The BMA guidance removes safeguards that, for all its shortcomings, the practice of referral to the Court of Protection did provide. It appears that the BMA proposals will enable euthanasia 'by stealth'.

The case of 'RS'

A middle-aged Polish man known only as 'RS' in a coma following a heart attack in Plymouth, was at the centre of a divided family opinion on his care. On 15 December 2020, the Court of Protection ruled that keeping him on life support was not in his best interests, saying that he should be provided with palliative care to retain the greatest possible dignity until his death. The members of his family contesting the decision said that video footage proved RS was able to breathe unaided and had responded to stimuli. After their appeal to the European Court of Human Rights on his behalf, was rejected, the hospital proceeded to withdraw food and water.

The case drew widespread attention and criticism from Poland, with senior politicians, church figures and neuroscience expert witnesses being involved, to no avail. The opportunity to save him was tragically lost. This disturbing case can be considered as the beginning of further anti-life judgements by those in a position of authority and influence. The greater the authority invested; the more accountability is expected. Disregarding unjust laws and guidance is a human right of all.

Tony Bland

Tony Bland was injured at the age of 19 in the Hillsborough football stadium disaster in April 1989, which resulted in him being in a PVS for nearly four years. A PVS is often rather more hopefully and accurately termed a 'persistent non-responsive state'.

Crossing the Rubicon

Such judgements can be considered as 'crossing the Rubicon'. On 10 January 49 BC, General Julius Caesar crossed the Rubicon, a stream separating Rome from the province of Gaul. Crossing the Rubicon began a civil war that would end the Roman Republic.

Article 2 of the Convention on Human Rights (1998) states 'no one shall be intentionally deprived of his life'. An action or omission can have a clear intent to end the life of a patient. The five Law Lords agreed in 1993, that Tony Bland's nutrition and hydration could be removed and the doctors caring for him at Keighley Hospital in West Yorkshire would not be acting unlawfully by doing so.

The court, therefore, forced the 'crossing of the Rubicon' in the case of Tony Bland when it was deemed that food and fluid were medical treatments and could therefore be withdrawn. And it was deemed by one of the judges in the case that Tony Bland had no 'interests' let alone 'best interests' in his continuing unresponsive condition.

The five judges did state that this case did not create a precedent and that doctors, wanting to discontinue feeding in other cases should first seek a declaration from the court. This element of some degree of vulnerable patient protection in that judgement, appears to have been superseded by the judgement on 'Y'.

Patient protection?

Did the apparent 'futility' of Tony Bland's nutrition and hydration justify its termination? Patients have reported feeling terrible thirst and other effects when being denied hydration. The nurses' code of conduct (NMC, 2018) expects nurses to do no harm, conduct holistic needs assessments, be evidence-based in their practice and act as an advocate for the vulnerable. One of the five Law Lords, Lord Mustill, had admitted to: 'having felt profound misgivings about almost every aspect of the Bland case'. He said that nurses' long-held expectations of care will be turned upside down... and that 'the law is now left in a morally and intellectually misshapen state' (Airedale NHS Trust v Bland, 1993).

The legal situation

Legal prohibitions appear to have been ignored by the preceding cases listed because they are in contravention of Article 2 of the European Convention and of the Human Rights Act 1998, which states: 'No one shall be deprived of his life intentionally'. There are no caveats or exemptions which would meet what has been allowed in recent times in the UK (Knight, 2003).

The best treatment in such cases is likely to fall within the scope of the state's positive obligations under Article 2 of the European Convention on Human Rights.

It can be argued rightly that failure, even to advise clinicians of the importance of compliance with the principles set out in Articles 3, 6 and 8 of the European Convention on Human Rights renders guidance which promotes withdrawal of food and fluid as unlawful. Therefore, knowing this, staff should feel more empowered to exercise their rights to conscientious objection despite professional guidance on withholding food or fluid.

Chapter 10 makes clear how such legal cautions of the European Convention on Human Rights were apparently ignored.

Vincent Lambert (France)

Following a head injury in 2008, a 42-year-old nurse, was slowly being starved to death in France, in 2019 when the French high court ruled in favour of the doctors to discontinue his life-sustaining feeding support which had been provided since severe brain damage and quadriplegia after a motorcycle accident. His parents and two of his siblings fought a long legal battle against Vincent's wife, his other siblings and his doctors who all believed it was time for him to die. A lengthy court battle over his medical care led to his death by starvation and dehydration on 11 July 2019.

Vincent's parents, Pierre and Viviane Lambert said they were 'resigned' to his death after they exhausted all options to save his life.

Vincent's father, criticised the courts and doctors for killing his son, saying it is 'madness' to starve a disabled man to death. 'It's murder in disguise, it's euthanasia,' he told reporters outside Sebastopol Hospital in Reims, France. His mother, Viviane, expressed similar desperation in a letter to French president Emmanuel Macron in May 2019, writing,

> 'Mr. President, my son was sentenced to death… my son did not deserve to be hungry and dehydrated… Vincent's not in a coma, he's not sick, he's not connected. It's not a machine that keeps my son alive. He's breathing without assistance… Vincent is disabled but alive.'

Vincent's doctors and other medical specialists confirmed that he could breathe without the assistance of a respirator and he also responded to external stimuli. His condition was listed as stable prior to removal of basic intervention keeping him alive.

At the height of the controversy in 2015, Mr Lambert's parents released a video via a conservative Catholic website on YouTube which they said showed him reacting to family members.

Terri Schiavo (USA)

The case of Vincent Lambert drew the attention of international human rights advocates. Many see similarities to the fight over the life of Terri Schiavo, an American woman who died by slowly being starved to death after her life-sustaining feeding support was removed based on her husband's wishes. Schiavo's family also lost a long legal battle to provide medical care to their daughter (Bilger, 2019).

This is a more fear-provoking scenario than the typical 'death-with-dignity' campaign because it clearly moves beyond the tyranny of the depressed person acting against their own life Such developments see a state which exerts lethal power over a vulnerable person, a person who cannot even exercise their will at all, whose alleged verbal wishes in such a situation are believed and can be seen to trump the possibility of rehabilitation potential and progress.

Brain-injured patients are not always 'dying'

Many patients needing CANH today may not be dying at all. They may be otherwise fit, as cases testify, but are suffering from incapacity, perhaps due to brain injury. These patients can now be at risk of death due to withdrawal of life-sustaining food and fluids ('medical treatment') in line with legal and professional precedent: the MCA (2005), the cases of 'Y' (2018), Tony Bland (1993) and doctors' medical guidance (BMA, 2018). These developments portend ethical dilemmas for those practitioners with conscientious objection.

While the withdrawal of CANH has been advocated as a general proposition for patients with a variety of conditions, much less attention has been directed to the specific capacities and limitations of individual patients.

It is surprising that, while debate over whether individuals within groups with identified disabilities retain 'personhood', little attention has been given to the question as to whether any of the individuals from whom hydration and nutrition are to be withdrawn could possibly experience persistent thirst throughout the period from withdrawal of hydration until death. Thirst inflicted, registered and documented on animal subjects, in studies, should be heeded as important research.

'Personhood'

The Education and Research Officer of the Anscombe Bioethics Centre, a Catholic research institute based in Oxford, argues that:

> ... the question about benefitting from continued life is ultimately the wrong question to ask. Life is not a possession or a commodity that we sometimes benefit from and sometimes do not, in which case it no longer has value. On such a view, undue weight is placed on conscious experience and the pleasures that may entail. One may not "enjoy the benefits of life" without consciousness, but life itself is always an intrinsic benefit. True, such a benefit may be very limited, but treatment may only be withdrawn if its burdens outweigh the benefits, which must include continued life.

(Wee, 2019)

Thirst

According to McCullagh (1996), questions for the management of unconscious patients should include the following:

- What is known about brain functions required for thirst experience?

- How soundly is that knowledge based?
- How confidently can knowledge about thirst sensation derived from animal studies be transferred to the human situation?
- How likely are the brain lesions of patients considered for withdrawal of CANH to be compatible with retention of the capacity for thirst?
- How can this likelihood be assessed in individual patients?

It can be argued that the possibility of thirst experience seems to be set aside on the basis that lack of indications from patients' awareness of their surroundings, automatically equates with a lack of capacity for thirst. This is a gross and alarming assumption, since patients with 'locked in' syndromes with perceived incapacity to appreciate thirst are also unable to communicate. Evidence appears to be insubstantial about the lack of capacity for patients for experiencing thirst, if considered at all, following withdrawal of hydration (McCullagh, 1996).

Masking anticipated and unnecessary symptoms

Dehydration is a very cruel way to inflict death on anyone. The obvious significant effects over periods of starvation and dehydration (sometimes for weeks in the case of many patients placed on the LCP) meant that such patients receive doses of opioids to aim to mitigate the effects of starvation and dehydration, yet there is evidence that dehydration minimises the effects of those opioids. The cause for hydration and nutrition is overwhelming in terms of compassion (and common sense) to allow the patient some comfort.

Required questions about patient 'nil by mouth' orders

Withdrawal and non-commencement of assisted food and fluids happened for years as part of LCP practice without consideration of the impact on thirst sensation, as questions tended not to be asked. Required questions often not asked are:

- Why does the patient need a 'nil by mouth' (NBM) order? Some relatives are too afraid to question such orders and even some staff may accept this order without questioning it.
- Has the cause of swallowing difficulty been investigated/ ascertained?
- When did the patient last drink?
- How is the patient going to be adequately hydrated?

Prohibition of torture

The fight against torture is at the core of the Council of Europe's activities. Article 3 of the Convention of Human Rights (2009), under the heading 'Prohibition of Torture', states that: 'no one shall be subjected to torture or to inhuman or degrading treatment or punishment'. Unlike other convention clauses, it allows for no exceptions. When interpreting this article in its judgements, the European Court of Human Rights has stated that even in the most difficult circumstances, such as the fight against terrorism, the convention completely prohibits torture and inhuman or degrading treatment or punishment, irrespective of the conduct of the person concerned.

The European Court of Human Rights and Torture

This court has interpreted that for ill-treatment to fall within the scope of Article 3 of the Convention of Human Rights it must attain a minimum level of severity and it is necessary to assess the circumstances of the case, such as the duration of the treatment, its physical or mental effects and other factors such as the purpose for the ill-treatment.

Rights of condemned prisoners

Condemned prisoners are not expected to suffer in the process of execution in countries or states where the death penalty is legal. The ethics in such situations are now being carefully considered with clinicians exercising their right to conscientious objection not to be involved and their decision being respected.

Dehydration – comfort care/compassionate care?

When patients are thought to be dying that does not mean that fluids become futile.

(Finlay, 2008)

'Comfort care' can be a meaningless, hollow term without true comfort care aims, actions and outcomes for the benefit of patients. Several doctors who have experience of elderly, palliative and paediatric care, respectively, have commented on the importance of hydration as 'ordinary care' where appropriate, feasible and non-burdensome (Craig, 2002 and 2004; Finlay, 2008; Cole, 2015).

Concerns voiced about prolonging life, by use of clinically-assisted fluids should not take precedence over the aim for patients' benefit in terms of comfort and life quality. Patients who are relegated to receiving 'only comfort care' are known to feel terrible thirst and other effects, including restlessness and agitation when being denied hydration (see Chapter 15).

Discontinuing treatment

Pope St John Paul II addressed the participants in the international congress on 'life-sustaining treatments and vegetative state: scientific advances and ethical dilemmas' a year before he died in 2005, saying:
The evaluation of probabilities, founded on waning hopes for recovery when the vegetative state is prolonged beyond a year, cannot ethically justify the cessation or interruption of minimal care for the patient, including nutrition and hydration. Death by starvation or dehydration is, in fact, the only possible outcome, as a result of their withdrawal.

In this sense it ends up becoming, if done knowingly and willingly, true and proper euthanasia by omission.

(Pope St John Paul II, 2004a)

Guidelines vs conscience

The prospect of disagreeing with a decision made between the family and clinicians to stop feeding and hydrating a non-dying family member is daunting for staff whose conscience cannot comply with such an order.

The foreseen practice of starvation and dehydration of the non-dying will become contagious and is being reported as having occurred with impunity and even against the wishes of some members of the family as in some of the cases listed.

Despite the legal backing and professional approval for such orders imposed on patients and their carers, conscience cannot be blunted and stifled by the dictum of 'just following orders'. Staff support is vital in such circumstances. Non-acceptance of the concept of conscientious objection by employers is open to counterargument and claims in relation to recognised human rights in law. Can we really allow attrition of healthcare professionals at such a time of shortages who just want to care compassionately for their vulnerable patients?

Difficult orders

Such legal decisions and professional guidance will see nurses and doctors opposing this ruling as heroes and heroines, considering the potential cost and negative outcome for their careers. However, 'strength in numbers' is a useful maxim for like-minded health professionals wishing to abide by their codes of conduct, duty of care and conscience.

Relatives who made submissions to the LCP independent review (DH, 2013) were critical of the common occurrence of fluid and nutritional needs being disregarded, regardless of whether the patient was dying. The need for the education of healthcare professionals in relation to CANH that the LCP review panel recommended cannot be disregarded and supplanted by this BMA guidance of 2018 on CANH.

Nazi ideology – those unworthy of life

During the Third Reich, the *Untermensch* were considered unworthy of the right to life. What sort of liberty is it which provides a state with the power to judge who is worthy of life and who is unworthy of life?

New evidence on prolonged disorders of consciousness

At the same time as the UK case of 'Y' and the BMA issued guidance on CANH (both in 2018), a report was published in August 2018 from the American Academy of Neurology, updating their own guidelines for managing prolonged disorders of consciousness. It contains some startling conclusions that are highly relevant to the BMA guidance on CANH:

1. Four in ten people who are thought to be unconscious are actually aware.
2. One in five people with severe brain injury from trauma will recover to the point that they can live at home and care for themselves without help.

(Giacino et al, 2018)

Care goalposts moved

Doctors and campaigners have warned that the judgement on 'Y' has 'moved the goalposts' on end-of-life care closer to the 'slippery slope' of 'euthanasia by omission'. Could this mean that healthcare staff and organisations such as nursing homes and hospices with conscientious objections to the withdrawal of CANH would not be allowed to care for certain categories of patients with swallowing difficulties and cognitive impairment and could be forced into complicity in the deliberate ending of patients' lives.

The new BMA guidance on CANH (2018), which can be argued is detached from clinical and moral reality, will not stop health professionals' right to conscientious objection, which will be exercised in line with the expectations of professional codes and their own regard for ethical principles and duty of evidence-based care for vulnerable humanity. Patient advocates need each other, for strength in numbers to support and protect their patients.

Death by thirst

Dr Tony Cole, a retired paediatrician and chairman of the Medical Ethics Alliance, has been reported as saying that many of the most distressing cases in the evidence to the LCP review were of horrifying situations that can only be described as patients dying of thirst saying,

> *This is totally unacceptable! If the BMA guidelines [then in draft form] do not eliminate this danger, then they will also be discredited. As a doctor who has seen death from thirst twice, I can say it is something not easily forgotten.*

(Cole, 2015)

Compassion is expressed in true care for people who are or who are not dying and need life-sustaining, humane interventions. A positive, questioning, compassionate and educated approach is required, together with required knowledge of developments for brain-injured people to ensure opportunity for a patient's possible recovery.

Conclusion

It is suggested that an astute practitioner, confronted with what is said to be a 'bioethics norm', will probe further to seek the root of the norm, alert to spurious arguments (Murphy, 2004).

How can 'modern' (secular) bioethicists impose their views on issues such as conscientious objection and promote its obsolescence when nurses face moral problems every day in their practice due to their closer relationships with patients as well as the difficulties and distress they experience in their capacity as moral agents?

Duty of care

Cruelty is indefensible in healthcare. The health professions have a record of dutiful care to all patients, regardless of age or economic productivity. Care is perhaps the most basic element of a patient's treatment that a nurse can provide, yet it is the most essential. The impulse to care, together with the desire for nurses to put the interests of others' good before their own, can be a clear declaration of a nurse's own ethical position.

Nurse-patient advocacy does not normalise deviant practice. Nurses must be prepared to stand up and speak out for people in need. Advocacy for patients must transcend fear, professional obligations and relationships with colleagues as exemplified by the actions of the Good Samaritan.

'Them and us'

The Catholic Church's perspective is invaluable: 'sick and disabled people are not some separate categories of humanity; in fact, sickness and disability are part of the human condition and affect every individual, even when there is no direct experience of it' (Congregation for the Doctrine of the Faith, 2008).

It is important to move beyond the Enlightenment preoccupation whereby one's ability to know and master the world is a measure of one's humanity. We should also reject a neo-liberal conception of personhood that reduces the concept to an individual's productivity. Instead, we should look toward the way that human beings relate to each other to identify the essence of personhood (Symons, 2021). We are all part of the same human family.

Recommended training programmes

The review panel of the discredited LCP which had resulted in many terrible deaths, recommended that 'Specialist services, professional associations and the Royal Colleges should hold and evaluate: Education, Training and Audit programmes' (DH, 2013). This approach can ensure educated, compassionate practitioners who must care for patient's hydration needs.

The aim of this recommendation was to teach healthcare professionals how to discuss and decide with patients, relatives and carers, the management of hydration needs at the end of life (DH, 2013).

Wisdom

God takes no pleasure in the extinction of the living.

> *Death was not God's doing,*
> *He takes no pleasure in the extinction of the living.*
> *To be – for this, He created all:*
> *the world's created things have health in them,*
> *in them no fatal poison can be found,*
> *and Hades holds no power on earth:*
> *for virtue is undying.*
> *Yet God did make man imperishable,*
> *He made him in the image of His own nature:*
> *it was the devil's envy that brought death into the world,*
> *as those who are his partners will discover.*

(Book of Wisdom 1:13–15, 2:23–24)

The goal of acting as the Good Samaritan may be achieved by the nurse ensuring ethical misgivings are verbalised, both with colleagues and relatives as one would with own family members. There are many ways to act as the Good Samaritan in healthcare, e.g., patients under our care may be considering writing an advance directive and may be ignorant of how the concept of 'treatment' has so radically changed in medicine to consider assisted food and fluid as 'medical' treatment.

This chapter has focused on how we can accompany and protect a person who is or is not dying and who should not suffer the result of discontinuation of life-sustaining assisted food and fluid, always to be considered as care which is humane. Treatment denial may occur simply due to what may be a temporary or extended period of physical incapacity. Rehabilitative treatment is not without success today for many patients.

> *Nurses wishing to respect their conscience, the duty*
> *of care and act as the patient's advocate can take heart*
> *by remembering the words of Jesus:*
> *Whatever you did to the least of these, you did to*
> *Me and whatever you neglected to do for the least*
> *of these, you neglected to do it for Me.*

(Matthew 25:31–46)

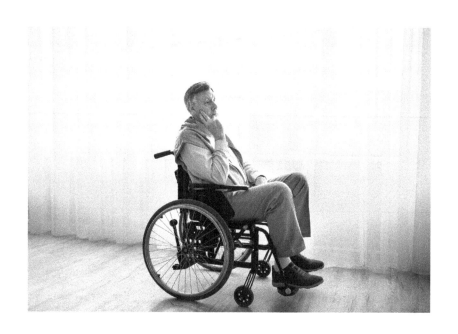

Chapter 9
NHS healthcare scandals – A: Failure to care

Thou shalt love thy neighbour as thyself.

(Matthew 22:37–39)

Introduction

The NHS healthcare scandals reveal the tragic results of the mismanagement of patients, in many care areas and over considerable periods of time. The affected patients, together with their families were rendered totally powerless against a system of neglect in so-called 'care' settings.

The compounding factor to relatives' suffering is the inability of the relevant hospital trusts to acknowledge the 'pain, trauma and deep harm' which had been experienced by the people involved (Hawkins, 2021). People repeatedly acknowledge that things can go wrong in healthcare, but transparency and acknowledgement, apology and some form of restitution by those accountable can be a contributory factor in healing of the pain and damage caused.

Healthcare scandals have served to bring the role of the nurse as the patient advocate into sharp focus. The role of the Good Samaritan health professional, however, is not an expectation only of those working in clinical practice.

Vulnerable adults

In 2009, a DH report about safeguarding vulnerable adults, highlighted how the assumption that, 'As a matter of course, NHS care must be safe, blinkers people to the obvious' (DH, 2009).

Despite the professionalisation of nursing and the increasing autonomy of nurses in their roles, the need for nurse-patient advocacy has never been more obvious when examining the NHS healthcare scandals. These are coming to public attention and national scrutiny, often after years of being unchallenged or not investigated by both healthcare professionals and NHS management. Those professionals who attempted to act as whistleblowers did so generally unsuccessfully and at great cost to themselves in terms of being ostracised and bullied.

The long overdue exposure of the NHS care scandals uncovered either poor patient care and treatment standards or neglect and abuse, all of which lessens trust of the public. It appears that the culture of healthcare settings where unethical practices occurred in action, or by omission, involved acceptance by many staff. The uncovered NHS scandals are, sadly, blots on the UK healthcare landscape.

Scandals

NHS scandals involved long term, inappropriate and generally unchallenged opioid overdose prescription together with unwarranted sedation at many 'care' institutions over many years. The care failings of the Mid Staffordshire NHS Trust, the lack of care for the learning disabled, the lack of parental rights' recognition, the midwifery disasters and the discredited LCP (see Chapter 10) all add to the litany of NHS tragedies.

Parental rights

British parents have increasingly had to fight to achieve their children's right to treatment or rehabilitation. This is advocacy by parents for a culture of life and hope for their vulnerable children, against the apparently increasing, defeatist healthcare culture. The recent UK cases in the media spotlight have resulted in other (European) healthcare settings being eager to provide dedicated, rehabilitative care for such children.

Cases of medical staff who have forbidden parents from taking their children out of the UK for more pro-life, positive attempts at rehabilitation or newer treatments elsewhere, reveals the worst type of paternalistic approaches to treatment and care. This can result in a lack of parental trust in both the hospital management and healthcare team.

A conspiracy of silence?

A common denominator of these sad, scandalous incidents appeared to be a general conspiracy of silence by many staff at all levels. Is this caused by fear, indoctrination, bullying, lack of support, agreement of practices, or apathy? In most cases, in seeking restitution, it is the public who are most demanding of justice for their loved ones.

Despite the quest for (and success in) nursing professionalisation and the acquired autonomy of nurses, harm has been experienced by patients where criminality was eventually exposed yet punishment by law not achieved. Other practitioners who have caused harm and even death have never been exposed and brought to justice. Due to such actions revealed in the NHS scandals, many families remain in unresolved grief due to the often-delayed realisation of what happened to their loved one and the awareness of an overall lack of justice.

Power imbalance

Many families believe that they cannot achieve justice due to their experience of immense power exerted by 'the system'. The intransigence of some practitioners has been described by other staff and informed relatives as 'driven by a culture of death', maintaining a conspiracy of silence as evidenced by many adherents of the discredited non-individualised 'cult' of the LCP. The LCP practices were incentivised by financial reward for NHS Trusts due to the pathway's 'quality' status in line with the Commissioning for Quality and Innovation (CQUIN) framework by NHS England.

Resources and attitude factors involved in poor care

Several Healthcare Commission investigations have shown in detail how senior managers have failed in their most basic duties as regards patient safety, with disastrous consequences. In each of these cases, patient safety was found to have been crowded out by other priorities, including the meeting of targets, financial issues, service reconfigurations and achieving foundation status.

Staff shortages have been a particular factor in compromising patient safety despite the enormous increase in funding and staffing across the NHS (House of Commons Health Committee, 2009). This means that other crucial factors may need consideration e.g., attitudes, knowledge and behaviour.

Care of the elderly: the Health Service Ombudsman's report (2011)

The 10 investigations into NHS care of older people have, according to the King's Fund, 'provoked an understandable, but wearingly familiar, wave of shock and media outrage' (Cornwell, 2011).

> *If the language in the report is new, the findings are not. We know that poor care occurs in health care systems everywhere. The fact that all too often it is older people who suffer, may reflect wider societal values, but from our work we know that it can happen to anyone. The fundamental problem is that the quality of health care is not reliable: the more vulnerable the patient, the greater the risk. The media always focuses on asking the question 'what has gone wrong in nursing?' The Health Ombudsman's stories are not just about nurses: they feature a wide variety of medical, nursing and support staff, in hospitals and in general practice and many are about lack of continuity and coordination between hospitals and primary care*

(Cornwell, 2011).

So many problems within the NHS appear to many to have become 'chronic'. This occurs despite awareness of the problem. Inaction is common, which can become the norm for issues that need investigation.

Patient nutritional needs

The important issue of caring for patients' nutritional status has been an ongoing scandal for years in many NHS care settings. It shows a defeatist, negligent attitude to basic needs during hospitalisation and treatment. Without involvement of family members to maintain nutritional intake, many vulnerable patients can be at risk of starvation in hospital. Patients with sensory deprivation, particularly those who are blind, poor-sighted, or deaf, have complained of not receiving help at mealtimes and some patients' inpatient experience was one of hunger.

Provision of food and drink: view of a 'dignity' ambassador

The late Sir Michael Parkinson, writing about his experience as a former National Dignity Ambassador, comments about the scandal of the denial of patient nutritional care, which sums up what has been an ongoing scandal in NHS hospitals for years.

I've been sent letters about older people being left without enough to eat and drink, food being taken away before they have had a chance to eat it, food being left at the end of the bed on a tray where that cannot reach it, food they cannot swallow or the reverse, a sloppy, unappetising blob on a plate. Now this is where the time and money arguments really fall down for me. It defies all logic to spend vast sums of money to keep people in hospital or a care home to give them expensive drugs and then to forget to ensure they get the most basic of human needs – enough to eat and drink. Absolutely barmy and cruel beyond belief.

(Parkinson, 2010)

All practitioners must examine their conscience and ask themselves: *do I give food to the hungry and drink to the thirsty and help those in need of such basic provision?*

Meeting patients' nutrition needs, an ongoing problem

This important and vital issue has been addressed by the RCN over the years with apparently little effect. All staff need to be aware of this historical scandal. Despite non-nursing staff often delivering meals to patients, nurses must consider their role as patient advocates, who will ensure their patients receive the food and drink that they need, even by delegation to competent staff. Without such expected daily oversight, patient abuse by neglect is the result.

Protected mealtimes can be ensured and are one way of deferring non-emergency clinical tasks while meals are properly supervised and patients are helped with their nutrition and hydration needs.

Patient vs task allocation

Today, nurses are generally allocated a number of patients, which means that a group of patients' individual needs are to be met by a designated nurse. This was a development away from 'task allocation', whereby all required tasks were met by any nurse who was competent to function in fulfilling the tasks. An individualised approach to care was introduced to ensure that the named nurse would meet all their allocated patients' individually assessed needs.

It is argued in discussing the NHS, that basic care is very simple and fundamentally important. If it is abandoned, with barely a whisper from so many healthcare managers and staff, then an explanation is undoubtedly called for. Something most odd must be going on (Mandlestam, 2011).

'Safe care'

The Care Quality Commission (CQC) observed in 2010 that the House of Commons Health Committee had recently called for safe care to be 'the top priority' for NHS managers (Rose, 2010). It is argued that it is extraordinary that either the CQC or the Commons Health Committee should have to stress this point to the NHS – an organisation, whose primary and indeed, only role, should be to treat and care for people, competently and safely. The observation, however, is unsurprising, because the evidence is clear that NHS policy makers and managers have been focusing on other things (Mandlestam, 2011).

The 'other things' which appear to cause a loss of true focus on the needs of patients, require scrutiny at all levels of responsibility.

NHS Funding for reform?

The UK health budget consumes close to half of all day-to-day government spending, yet health outcomes continue to languish in the bottom half of international tables. Reports from the National Audit Office and the Institute for Fiscal Studies has made clear in Autumn 2022, that productivity in the NHS is collapsing despite a big increase in funds and a ten per cent rise in the numbers of both nurses and doctors since 2019. More money has persistently failed to achieve better results.

It is argued that The UK can indeed be described as the "sick man of Europe", with more than seven million people on waiting lists for hospital treatment. The Chancellor awarded the NHS £6.6 billion of additional funding in Autumn 2022, saying that he was "asking" the NHS to tackle waste and inefficiency – but with no suggestion that the cash might be withheld if the efficiencies failed to materialise (Kirby, 2022).

It could be argued that for NHS reform, many more factors than simply funding need urgent consideration, including the important issue of attitudes.

Practitioner choice

Florence Nightingale recognised that nurses need practical skills, as well as moral qualities such as tact, respect for privacy, sensitivity and kindness. A nurse must above all be able to make the patient comfortable so that nature can do its job of healing (McDonald, 2013). It is true to assert that despite ethical difficulties within some care cultures, practitioners do have choice in adherence to the imperatives of conscience and the code of conduct.

The following notable NHS scandals are recounted as perhaps the tip of a potential iceberg of scandals. It could be argued that they have arisen where faith has appeared to give way to a tyranny of aggressive secularism. This may have resulted in health professionals becoming as disempowered as their patients. These scandals all appear to have in common the following: a disregard for patient care requirements and the length of time they continued without investigation,

- Gosport Memorial Hospital
- Mid Staffordshire NHS Trust

- Learning disability: 'Death by Indifference'
- Maternity services, baby deaths and brain damage
- Parents' rights for their children's healthcare.

Chapter 10 will focus in detail on the scandal of the flawed LCP and Chapter 11 will focus on COVID-19.

1. Gosport Memorial Hospital

The national enquiry into 450 deaths from medicinal opiate misuse was centred around Gosport Memorial Hospital from 1989 onwards.

What happened at Gosport over the years did not reflect the GMC or Nursing Council care expectations. There were a few nurses who attempted patient advocacy but were bullied, ignored and ostracised by those also with accountability for patient safety.

As with the other reported healthcare scandals, it appeared to take years for families to have their concerns and distress even acknowledged or investigated. The following is a commentary on this long-running scandal at Gosport Memorial Hospital, from the editor of the British Medical Journal (Godlee, 2018):

> The report of the inquiry into deaths at Gosport War Memorial Hospital is hard but essential reading (gosportpanel.independent. gov.uk). In cool, clear prose, it records the personal tragedies of patients, admitted for respite care and not in pain, for whom "keep patient comfortable" proved a death sentence. It describes the courage and persistence of the families and the devastating roll call of professional and institutional failings.
>
> Key players at every level have been found wanting: the hospital managers who effectively silenced the nurses on Dryad Ward; the pharmacists and consultants who failed to spot the routine overprescribing of opioids, despite the fact that this continued in plain sight for twelve years; the GMC, which failed to strike off GP Jane Barton despite finding her guilty of serious professional misconduct; the Hampshire

police force, which, despite three investigations begun between 1998 and 2002, failed to properly examine reports by families and whistleblowers.

This was a monumental collective failure, symptomatic of the prevailing culture. Gosport War Memorial Hospital was unusual, as the report makes clear: isolated geographically and professionally, an old-style community hospital in a traditional military setting. But how much else from this saga can we still recognise in today's health system? There is the uncritical deference shown to doctors, the fear of repercussions among staff raising the alarm, the unwillingness of patients and their families to question the medical and nursing teams, the lack of routine audit that could have spotted suspicious patterns, the ten-year delay in publishing the Baker report, the accumulating evidence that the General Medical Council is no longer fit for purpose.

Much has changed for the better in the past 20 years, but if Gosport tells us anything it is that the voices of patients, families and whistleblowers must be heard.

(Godlee, 2018)

The investigation is ongoing into the Gosport Memorial Hospital tragedy. The issues for the long-awaited, ongoing inquiry should include:

- understanding of 'the duty of care' by all involved at the time
- understanding of patient advocacy and overall accountability
- treating patients as individuals, as worthy of respect, rather than 'objects' to be 'managed'.

The questions that need answering are:

- Why were concerned nurses not listened to?
- Why was the empathy expected of many staff at the time so absent?
- How could there have been so many victims?

- What were the views, if any, of other multidisciplinary team members?
- What were the views and actions of tutorial staff whose students must have had discussions over the drugs and doses being routinely prescribed and given?
- What was the role of the NHS trust chief executive in this scandal?
- Why were the NMC and the GMC not more involved?
- Why were relatives treated with such disregard?
- Why were death certificates not more scrutinised?

A conspiracy of silence

What appears to have occurred was within an unbelievable conspiracy of silence. The ongoing Gosport inquiry conclusions are yet to be reported. Practices which were normalised at Gosport were synonymous with those of the LCP, where inappropriate drug prescribing was the norm in too many cases. This pathway was in use at the time of Gosport and for many years, until formal discarding in 2014, following the recommendation by an independent review (DH, 2013) (see Chapter 10).

Prescribing practices

The story of inappropriate prescribing practices at Gosport Memorial Hospital revealed the difficulty in establishing what happened and then holding anyone accountable despite considerable attempts and protests by relatives. The police had investigated several deaths at the hospital since 1998. By 2002, the Commission for Health Improvement (CHI) had reported its concerns, but the Crown Prosecution Service (CPS) had declined to proceed with any prosecution. The Department for Health had, by 2007, rejected the requests from a senior police officer and coroner for a public enquiry, over their concerns about a possible 92 deaths. This reveals the need for a Good Samaritan orientation in high authority postholders.

Relatives demanding justice decried the piecemeal investigations that had been conducted since 1998 by the police, the CPS, the local

NHS Trust, the GMC and the CHI. All of whom the concerned relatives considered had failed adequately to explain the large number of deaths (Mandlestam, 2011).

The Gosport Memorial Hospital scandal appears to be linked to the national scale of deaths due to the intrinsically flawed LCP. There are many similarities with relatives' experience of the LCP and Gosport Memorial Hospital, who were totally unaware of such ongoing betrayal of trust over years.

This hospital scandal needs resolution in terms of justice for the patients and their loved ones more than 20 years since the issues first came to light. It must result in clinical and non-clinical staff being forced to stop and think again about their inner orientation to the patients who were denied safe care, over many years.

2.   The Mid Staffordshire NHS Trust failings

The question can be asked: if Florence Nightingale's views on adequate patient care had been respected by all involved (not just nurses), would the unnecessary deaths at Mid Staffordshire NHS Trust have occurred? If her principles of monitoring results had been heeded, would not the consequences of cutting nursing staff have been found out faster and the cuts been reversed? (McDonald, 2013).

The conclusion of the Francis inquiry into the Mid Staffordshire NHS Foundation Trust was that a chronic shortage of staff, particularly nursing staff, was largely responsible for the substandard care. The inquiry, chaired by Robert Francis, KC, found that the trust was 'preoccupied' with cost-cutting and other processes. It lost sight of its responsibility to provide safe care (Francis, 2013).

Morale at the trust was low and, while many staff did their best in difficult circumstances, others showed a disturbing lack of compassion towards the patients. Nurses and others were accused of being uncaring. However, staff who spoke out felt ignored and there is strong evidence that many were deterred from doing so through fear and bullying (Francis, 2013).

Following the Francis report on the Mid Staffordshire NHS Trust, in 2012 chief nursing officers in England published a policy on compassion in response to serious criticisms of patients' care relating to the Trust. The policy document identified six values and behaviours, termed 'the six C's', required by all nurses, midwives and care staff. This is similar to 'the six C's' defined and published in 1992, by Sister Simone Roach, the Canadian nun, in her theory of caring (Bradshaw, 2016). Roach considered caring and the components of it, including compassion, to be moral virtues and an inner motivation to care.

The six Cs are: care, compassion, competence, communication, courage and commitment (NHS England, 2014).

The implementation of these values and behaviours was heralded as a new vision for nursing. Many nurses would agree that these are and always have been pre-requisites for nursing, although monitoring of their expression can be difficult. The component parts of a skill are established as knowledge, attitude and behaviour. The two latter skill components can be more difficult to evaluate than the knowledge component and so the need for courage is at the forefront of patient advocacy.

3. Learning disability: Death by Indifference

Mencap is an organisation committed to reducing stigma and discrimination for people with learning disability. Their mission is to transform society's attitudes to learning disabilities and to improve the quality of life of people with a learning disability and their families. Mencap is again calling on the government to make the NHS safe for people with learning disabilities, following the publication of their report: *Death by Indifference: 74 deaths and counting* (Mencap, 2012), which found continued institutional discrimination in the NHS. The report looked at what progress had been made since the publication of Mencap's original *Death by Indifference* report in 2007 and called on the government to ensure that:

- Annual health checks become a permanent part of the GP contract to ensure early detection of health conditions.
- All health professionals act within the law and get training around their obligations under the Equality Act and MCA so they can put this into practice when treating patients with a learning disability.

- Regulatory bodies such as the CQC, GMC or NMC conduct rigorous investigations and deliver appropriate sanctions where health professionals clearly failed in their obligations to patients with a learning disability.
- The NHS complaints process is overhauled: it is not fit for purpose; it is time consuming and defensive and it does not enable the NHS to learn important lessons quickly enough to prevent further deaths.
- Acute learning disability liaison nurses are employed by every acute service and are linked to senior leadership, who have a strategic role in supporting ward staff to make reasonable adjustments.
- A standard hospital passport is made available to all people with a learning disability
- All hospitals sign up to Mencap's *Getting it Right* charter (Mencap, 2010) and put in place the good practice that we know saves lives.

The DH published its three-year strategy for learning disability services in England titled *Valuing People Now* (2009).

Mencap's charter, *Getting it Right* (2010), asked healthcare professionals to pledge to:

- make sure that hospital passports are available and used
- make sure that all of our staff understand and apply the principles of mental capacity laws
- appoint a learning disability liaison nurse in our hospitals
- provide ongoing learning disability awareness training for all staff
- listen to, respect and involve families and carers
- provide practical support and information to families and carers
- provide information that is accessible for people with a learning disability
- display the getting it right principles for everyone to see.

Mencap's 2012 report (Death by *indifference*) confirms that, although some positive steps have been taken in the NHS, many health professionals are still failing to provide adequate care to people with a learning disability. The report highlights the deaths of 74 people with a learning disability in NHS care over the preceding 10 years, which Mencap believes could have been avoided and are a direct result of institutional discrimination.

Duty of non-discriminatory care

Equal healthcare is a legal obligation that should be embedded in the everyday running of the NHS. The publication of the *Death by indifference* report also prompted some families to contact Mencap and they continued to do so in the weeks, months and years that followed. It is these cases – a total of 74 to date – that formed the basis of the article published in the Guardian on 3 January 2012.

Mencap believes the 74 cases are only a tiny proportion of the actual number of such cases. They highlight an NHS that continues to fail people with a learning disability, doctors whose practices appear to show no regard to the Equality Act or the MCA and nurses who fail to provide even basic care to people with a learning disability.

Most of the cases made aware to Mencap have been since publishing *Death by indifference* (Mencap, 2007). Families and carers reported that they have had to carry out caring duties such as cleaning, feeding and administering medication to patients with a learning disability during their time in hospital. One parent told Mencap: 'I worry for those people who don't have families or carers who are able to stay with them'. Duty of care is a legal requirement due to all patients, but for people with a learning disability it is often overlooked.

Family concerns over lack of care

Families told Mencap that they had to give round-the-clock nursing care and that they were too concerned for their relative's well-being to leave their side. They reported that if it were not for them being there, basic tasks such as feeding, providing drinks, washing and changing would not get done in a way that would properly meet that person's basic needs. Too often, hospitals rely on family members or paid carers to take on this role without proper care plans being in place. If family carers want to take on caring responsibilities in the hospital environment, staff should support them to do so, but clear definitions of exactly what they are taking on must be drawn up. Administering medication and other medical procedures should never fall to families or carers (Mencap, 2012).

Best interest decisions

Most insidious of all is what Mencap have come to refer to as 'flawed best interest decision-making'. This happens when, despite the process being technically followed, the medical advice given in the best interests' decision meeting has been weighted in favour of a decision not to proceed with active treatment and the application of 'do not resuscitate' orders. Families, who naturally do not want to prolong the suffering of their loved one, have sometimes agreed with the decision, only later to find that there was a better prospect of recovery with treatment than they had been told. This is devastating for families who sometimes blame themselves ever after for not having fought harder for their loved one.

These shocking cases, each as serious as the six in the *Death by indifference* report of 2007, must also be seen in the wider context of the strong criticisms made about the performance of the NHS, relating to other vulnerable patients, such as older people (PHSO, 2011).

These accounts echoed Mencap's own concerns that the NHS is too often failing to provide the most basic nursing care such as nutrition, hydration and pain relief and is denying people dignity and respect, additional to poor nursing. These complaints and tragedies had occurred at the height of the practices of the flawed and now supposedly discarded LCP.

The Mencap report: Death by *indifference* (2012)

The report uncovered common errors made by healthcare professionals. These include failure to abide by disability discrimination law, ignoring crucial advice from families, failing to meet even basic care needs and not recognising pain and distress and delays in diagnosing and treating serious illness. Mencap believes that this is underpinned by an assumption by some healthcare professionals that people with a learning disability are not worth treating.

The report also shows there has been no systematic monitoring by the DH to ensure that the health needs of people with a learning disability are being met. In particular, the DH is failing to meet many of the 10 key recommendations set out in the government inquiry led by Sir Jonathan Michael, *Healthcare for All* (2008). Mencap believes that for people with a learning disability to stop dying needlessly in the NHS, it is essential that the *Healthcare for All* recommendations are fully implemented.

Abuse at Winterbourne View care home for learning disabilities and autism

Four people were arrested in 2011 after the BBC Panorama revealed a pattern of serious abuse at another care establishment, the Winterbourne View private hospital for learning disabilities and autism near Bristol. The programme set up undercover filming after it was approached by former nurse and Good Samaritan, Terry Bryan, driven to this decision following a lack of response from the CQC over his concerns.

The hospital's owners, Castlebeck, apologised and suspended thirteen employees (some were later jailed). NHS Southwest said it was 'appalled' and the CQC said there was an 'unforgivable error of judgement' in not investigating earlier abuse claims. Adequate staff qualifications to care for these vulnerable people were lacking. There seems to be a recurring theme in care scandals, of whistleblowers being ignored.

Lessons learned?

Police are investigating allegations that vulnerable patients were bullied, humiliated and verbally abused by staff at one of the UK's biggest NHS mental health hospitals in Manchester. Another 'Good Samaritan' undercover reporter brought to light the incidence of staff who were apparently filmed mocking, slapping and pinching patients at the Edenfield centre near Manchester during an undercover investigation by BBC Panorama.

Dr Cleo Van Velsen, a consultant psychiatrist, said the undercover filming showed a "toxic culture" among staff of "corruption, perversion, aggression, hostility, lack of boundaries".

Greater Manchester police (GMP) said it had launched an investigation and was reviewing the Panorama footage to identify any offenders.

It was reported that the allegations involve 40 patients and 25 staff, more than a dozen of whom have been suspended.

Greater Manchester mental health NHS foundation trust, which runs the Edenfield centre, said it was taking the allegations "very seriously" and had taken "immediate actions to protect patient safety" (Halliday, 2022).

Justice

Some practitioners appear to feel the full force of the law for their ill treatment of patients, others do not. It is also not good practice for the CQC to give warnings of their planned inspection visits.

Mark Goldring, Mencap chief executive, has said about Mencap's latest report:

> *The report confirms that five years on from our landmark Death by indifference report, many parts of the NHS still do not understand how to treat people with a learning disability. At Mencap we continue to hear heart-breaking stories of unnecessary deaths and pain. Sadly, we believe that these cases are just the tip of the iceberg. Although some significant steps have been taken within the NHS, where progress has been made, it has been patchy and inconsistent. If the government does not get to grips with this serious issue, more people will die unnecessarily. As the NHS faces many new challenges and undergoes many new changes, it is even more vital that the welfare of people with a learning disability is not forgotten.*

(Goldring, 2012)

The cavalier attitude of refusing some people with learning disability a plan for CPR is echoed in the cases highlighted by the COVID-19 pandemic. Yet again relatives are realising with shock that neither they, nor their loved ones, were consulted on these crucial life and death decisions (see Chapter 11).

4. Maternity service failings, baby deaths and brain damage

The independent review team of maternity cases at Shrewsbury and Telford hospitals, was led by midwifery expert, Donna Ockenden. They found 1862 serious incidents including hundreds of baby deaths and an unusually high number of maternal deaths. The review uncovered a pattern of grim failures that led to the deaths and harming of mothers and babies from 2000–2019. These included a lethal reluctance to conduct caesarean sections; a tendency to blame mothers for problems; a failure to handle complex cases; a lack of consultant oversight and a 'deeply worrying lack of kindness and compassion'. Urgent changes are needed in all hospitals in England to prevent avoidable baby deaths, stillbirths and neonatal brain damage, according to the report into one of the biggest scandals in the history of the NHS (Ockenden, 2021). These failures happened over many years, a factor which is shared by other UK healthcare scandals.

Ensuring maternal and child safety

The review details a series of immediate actions and 'must do' recommendations for all hospital trusts to improve maternity safety 'at pace'. These include a formal risk assessment at every antenatal contact, twice-daily consultant-led maternity ward rounds, women and family advocates on the board of every NHS trust and the appointment of dedicated lead midwives and obstetricians.

In June 2021, West Mercia police launched an investigation into the worst of the cases. A clinical review of a selection of 250 of the cases prompted Ockenden to outline the emerging findings report so that action could be taken before the full report was completed. The final review report could prove to be a landmark review in NHS history. The interim report stated that the Trust owes it to the 1862 families who are contributing to the review to bring about rapid positive and sustainable change across the maternity services at the trust (Ockenden, 2021).

As with other NHS scandals, this investigation took years. It was achieved after 20 years of maternal and baby deaths and a persisting lack of some staff compassion and kindness and the Trust's failure to have thoroughly investigated incidents of poor care by its staff. That an inquiry was finally initiated with the Trust now facing possible criminal charges is due to the determined efforts of parents bereaved by the unnecessary deaths of their children.

> *Donna Ockenden wrote to the Secretary for Health and Social Care on publication of her final report in March 2022, with the following recommendation: The Department of Health and Social Care (DHSC) and NHS England and Improvement (NHSEI) must now commission a working group – independent of the Maternity Transformation Programme – that has joint Royal College of Midwives (RCM) and Royal College of Obstetricians and Gynaecologists (RCOG) leadership, to make plans to guide the Maternity Transformation Programme around implementation of these immediate and essential actions (IEAs) and the recommendations of other reports currently being prepared.*

(Ockenden, 2022)

Lack of listening

Parents involved with failings in another NHS Trust, Nottingham Maternity services, requested the leadership of Donna Ockenden to conduct a similar review. Refusal to conduct necessary investigation and listen to patients and staff on an ongoing basis means management staff are responsible for a culture, described by one bereaved victim of the maternity scandal in Nottingham Maternity Units, over years, as 'grotesque and disgusting… where they didn't listen and have not listened' (Hawkins, 2021). This Trust's maternity service was accused of bad care and neglect from 2010 to 2020 and had seen dozens of babies dying or left with brain damage at the unit.

The chief executive of Nottingham University Hospitals Trust has said: 'We apologise from the bottom of our hearts to the families who have not received the high level of care they need and deserve, we recognise the effects have been devastating' (McDonald and Lintern, 2021). There had been a wall of defensiveness, lies and parent blaming and an inappropriate use of drugs and failure to learn from previous poor care outcomes.

5. Parents' right to question their children's healthcare

The UN, in the Universal Declaration of Human Rights, has proclaimed that childhood is entitled to special care and assistance.

The following are the four principles of the UN Convention on the Rights of the Child:

- non-discrimination
- best interests of the child/children
- the right to survival and development
- the views of the child.

The 'principle of family-based care' is also enshrined in the UN Convention on the Rights of the Child (1989). Article 7.1 states that a child has, 'as far as possible, the right to know and be cared for by his or her parents'.

The Convention also acknowledges the primary role of parents and the family in the care and protection of children, as well as the obligation of the state to help parents carry out those duties. And the Convention makes it clear that in cases such as those explored here, the decisions should not be taken out of the hands of parents without very serious reason.

Ashya King

Three years after his parents were jailed for abducting their son from an NHS hospital to seek innovative brain tumour treatment abroad, Ashya King has confounded his British doctors and has been cleared of cancer three years after his parents removed him from hospital for treatment abroad. He was due to undergo chemotherapy and radiotherapy at Southampton General Hospital in August 2014, when his parents fled with him to Spain. They feared the treatment being prescribed by his doctors would leave him badly brain damaged and believed his best chance lay in innovative proton beam therapy being pioneered in Prague.

Brett King and his wife Naghemeh were arrested in Malaga at the behest of the British authorities and jailed in Madrid for 72 hours on child cruelty charges. After surgery in Southampton to remove the tumour, Ashya underwent treatment in Prague in 2014 after the court ruled his parents, who are Jehovah's Witnesses, had the right to take their son abroad, against the advice of the boy's UK doctors.

Dr Hernan Cortes Funes, head of oncology at the HC Marbella International Hospital in Spain, who has treated Ashya for three years, told the Daily Mail: 'This isn't an exact science, but three-and-a-half years is a good time to presume he won't relapse. He is in remission and there is no sign the tumour will return, although he will need to be monitored with yearly MRIs' (Adams, 2018).

Tafida Raqeeb

The parents of a five-year-old girl with a serious brain injury expressed their relief after winning a high court battle to keep their daughter on life support and take her to Italy for treatment.

A rare victory for parents was seen in their challenging an end of life decision by doctors, when a high court judge ruled in favour of Tafida's parents, Shelina Begum and Mohammed Raqeeb, who successfully argued that their daughter's life should be preserved. Doctors at the Royal London Hospital, where the child, from Newham in East London, was on ventilation, said it was in her best interests for treatment to be withdrawn because she had no awareness or prospect of recovering. The parents believed and requested that she should be offered rehabilitation, which the hospital had refused.

The UK hospital did not appeal the judgement and Tafida is now out of intensive care in Italy, as of January 2020, three months after her British doctors said she must be allowed to die, as she was 'brain dead'.

Other parents, so upset by negative and defeatist staff attitudes to their child's care, were driven to serious disagreement with the health team. The team, in turn, made accusations of the parents' antisocial behaviour, enlisting the police to remove them from the bedside. This incident which happened recently to a couple, both medically trained, caused them deep emotional upset. Such upsetting experiences have resulted in parents resorting to legal redress. Such increasingly reported and disturbing cases are now considered to be the tip of an iceberg.

Charlie Gard

Doctors at Great Ormond Street Hospital believed they could do no more for Charlie Gard, a baby with an exceptionally rare, inherited disease known as infantile onset encephalomyopathic mitochondrial DNA depletion syndrome (MDDS). The syndrome is caused by mutations in a gene called RRM2B which was inherited from both his parents. The condition leads to severe depletion of mitochondrial DNA in his tissues. The clinicians treating him thought that he was in the final stage of the disease and that they were no longer serving his best interests by keeping him alive. But Charlie's parents, Chris Gard and Connie Yates, refused to give up. They found a professor of neurology at a mainstream medical centre in the US who was willing to give him nucleoside therapy, an experimental treatment that has never been given to a patient with the RRM2B form of MDDS. And they raised more than £1.3 million for any required financial outlay (Dyer, 2017). They continued to battle through the courts but withdrew their application for him to travel to the US for specialist treatment after experts said the damage to his muscles was irreparable.

The couple returned to court in a bid to take their son home to die, but their wish was denied with a judge approving a plan which saw their child inevitably die shortly after being moved to a hospice.

Alfie Evans

Without doubt, the greatest scandal, considering everything that happened to little Alfie Evans during his recovery at Alder Hey Hospital, is that he was intubated and ventilated for 15 months and denied a tracheostomy, because only one month from his admission in December 2016, the doctors decided that he should die without even attempting to reach a diagnosis. In fact, even if the newspapers wrote that Alfie was suffering from a mitochondrial disease, there is not a shred of medical evidence to prove it.

It is certainly disconcerting that Alfie's ventilation tubes were found full of mould, as his father demonstrated with a pile of photos (some published by the Italian paper, *Bussola*) highlighting the numerous negligence episodes at the hospital in Liverpool.

Alfie needed weaning off his ventilator

Alfie's ventilation removal would generally be part of the process known as 'weaning off' so as not to provoke his immediate death. This did not happen. Thomas (Alfie's father) was told by an Italian doctor he was in touch with that Alfie would need immediate antibiotic therapy, but he was denied treatment for a chest infection. Incredibly, despite this, he breathed unaided for hours despite being denied an oxygen mask necessary to aid his breathing. Therefore, after ventilation was removed without oxygen being available for him, Thomas Evans launched an appeal asking for someone to bring oxygen to him as orders were given to detach it. Thomas pointed out that the death protocol approved by Judge Hayden spoke neither of oxygen deprivation nor of suspending nutrition. On the same grounds, Thomas forced them to feed his young son deprived of nutrition for a good 36 hours, a considerable time for such a small child, whose heart had already sustained a huge strain after his ventilation was removed without weaning.

Moreover, when the nutrition was at last supplied, it was kept at minimal levels. Still Alfie continued to live for four days, defended by his parents from the doctors' threats, opening his eyes from time to time and reacting. Then, in exchange for press silence, the hospital promised more oxygen and more life support. Two hours before dying, the oxygen saturation was about 98% and Alfie's heart rate approximately 160 beats per minute (bpm) so he was stable to the point that Thomas was convinced he would be allowed to take his son home soon (as the hospital administration had told him). Before Alfie died, while his father had left the room for a moment, a nurse entered and explained to those present that she was going to give Alfie four (unspecified) drugs to treat him. No more than 30 minutes later, his oxygen saturation level dropped to 15%. Two hours later, Alfie was dead.

It is difficult to say how long Alfie would have lived if he had been supplied with ordinary means of sustaining life or whether additional tests would have resulted in a diagnosis and led to a cure, rather than the ready prognosis becoming a self-fulfilling prophecy of death. It is also difficult to say that removal of ventilation was the cause of death. An Italian journalist commented, 'following the case of Alfie Evans, the brutality of a eugenics system can be disguised as democracy' (Frigerio, 2018).

The clinician Treloar writes:
The cases of Alfie Evans, Charlie Gard, Ashya King,
Tafida Raqeeb (and others), have all hit the headlines and
reverberated around the world. Many have been shocked to see
doctors applying to the courts, in order to curtail treatment
against the clearly expressed wishes of the child's parents. Fierce
public debates have raged about the appropriateness of
withdrawing treatment but even more strongly about also the
denial of parents' wishes, when plans they have made for their
child do not appear unreasonable. While public debate on the
appropriateness of withdrawing treatment from the child has been
fierce, the debate has been yet more fierce on the denial of the
parents' wishes to have the treatment continued even though their
wishes do not appear unreasonable.

(Treloar, 2018)

Archie Battersbee

The very first night, after admission to hospital, unconscious, following a tragic accident at home, the doctors told the family that Archie was not going to survive another 24 hours. Two days since his admission to hospital, the doctors said he was 'brain-dead' and invited the family to discuss organ donation. The doctors were pessimistic, but Archie's parents refused to give up on him – even after the hospital took them to court. Yet, over three months later, Archie was still alive, at which point his ventilation was withdrawn which resulted in his death.

The unsuccessful legal battle for his life has highlighted serious flaws in the UK's 'end of life' practices and has given some of the top legal minds in the country much to think and argue about. How many more times will the nation be witness to such tragic dramas as these cases represent? The precedent that Archie's case set can go an incredibly long way to fixing a system which has no room for error.

A Christian lawyer has argued that the theory of 'brain stem death' is now clearly disputable in UK courts.

A challenge to that theory is no longer a legal heresy. It is now a matter of time before that whole concept is questioned in another case by a family who disagrees with it and it is debated at the Court of Appeal level and perhaps at a higher level. The Courts and/or Parliament will at last have to grapple with the scientific controversy and grapple with a proper legal definition of death.

What Archie's case has shown is that systematic reform is needed to protect the vulnerable and their families in end of life matters. The lives of Archie, Alfie, Charlie, and other children have value. Their legacies need to be honoured.

Legislation must be passed reforming the system

(Williams, 2022)

Medical, nursing, and parental conflict

Trust between parents and medical staff can only be diminished by such recounted cases. Nurses are expected to carry out the orders of doctors or make a conscientious stand against such orders, a very painful position in which to hope to care for patients in line with the highest possible care standards.

The issues that have arisen subsequently to these recent high-profile cases include both mediation and parental access to legal advice. The Medical Mediation Foundation exists and will need to be considered in future cases.

What people say about medical conflict

Senior family law solicitor: 'I think I would offer mediation in every case where there is a potential for major decisions about care and treatment to be made'

A mother: 'The last place you want to get annoyed is a hospital where there are so many kids in pain. I like a doctor who explains everything, gives you options, speaks to you and understands you need to know everything'.

Physician:

> … *cases of dispute over withdrawal of life sustaining treatment from children, obviously require safe and ethical management for both the patient, his or her family and the hospital. The role of medical mediation and parental access to legal advice, is a pressing issue following recent conflicts between parents and hospital staff. Alfie Evans' parents clearly suffered greatly, because of the decision to stop treatment and to prohibit the opportunity of a transfer to Rome. Surely that reality should, at least a little, affect judges' decisions in cases such as these.*

(Treloar, 2018)

The BMA will need to continue to explore the role of mediation and the availability of legal advice to parents in these and other cases. (For further information see the website: http://www. medicalmediation.org.uk/)

Conclusion

These narratives reveal that the role of the nurse advocate must be supported by all available means. These stories can enable nurses to be better prepared, in future and ultimately on reflection, may be viewed in retrospect, as opportunities for learning.

A legal view on NHS care scandals

An appeal court judge (at the time), Lord Justice Munby, had noted, in 2010, in relation to dignity, the following about the various NHS scandals:

> *One reads too often, for comfort, accounts of*
> *conditions in various institutional settings – hospitals*
> *and care homes – which are a disgrace to any country*
> *with pretensions to civilisation and which ought*
> *to shock the conscience of any decent-minded person.*

(Lord Justice Munby, 2010)

Enabling staff to feel and be consistently compassionate towards patients in their care requires action by managers, educators and staff support to maintain a commitment to compassion and empathy.

Reflection in nursing is a tried and tested means of critically examining actions, constraints on action and the required educational and other available support for future similar situations. Ethical codes, communication skills, confidence, ethical principles, and conscience can be a firm foundation for nurses acting in line with the expected role of patient advocate, rather than a helpless, individual practitioner.

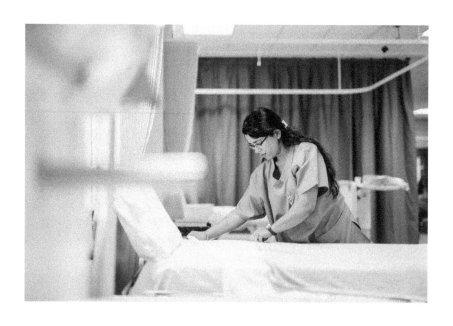

Chapter 10
NHS healthcare scandals – B: The Liverpool Care Pathway

You have not strengthened the weak, healed the sick,
bound up the injured, instead, you have ruled them
with violence and cruelty.

(Ezekiel 34:4)

Introduction

The Liverpool Care Pathway (LCP) for the dying patient was an integrated care pathway originating in the 1990s and recommended by successive governments in England and Wales to improve end of life care. It was discontinued in 2014 following mounting criticism and an independent national review.

The LCP has been described as an iconic example of what happens when 'gold standard' evidence from randomised controlled trials is not gathered before adoption of a complex intervention. Understanding the problems encountered in the roll out of the LCP has crucial importance for future policy making in end of life care (Seymour and Clark, 2018).

History

The LCP is known to have originated in the palliative care setting with apparently good intentions. However, it was flawed from the outset where a non-individualised treatment approach was common practice and use of strong sedation, opioids and dehydration would be lethal. None of these practices appeared to have been recognised by many trusting families as unethical treatment and care at the time and patient and family consent was often sadly lacking. There are reports of some families demanding patients were taken off the pathway when it was realised that benefit was not apparent for their loved one. The decision for the pathway was often reportedly explained as a planned 'comfort' process.

The lead responsibility for placing patients on the pathway was commonly devolved to nurses without due recognition of accountability for actions or omissions.

Care pathways may be an attempt to 'level up' so that individual patients all receive the best standard of care available, but the counterargument is that they are contrary to the concept of person-centred care, do not allow sufficiently for non-standard situations such as the presence of complex comorbidities and can become a tick-box exercise with too much pathway and too little care. This was noted by Rabbi Julia Neuberger who chaired the independent review of the LCP in 2013, titled *More Care, Less Pathway* (DH, 2013).

Press exposure

The LCP was in operation since the 1990s and its flaws were exposed as late as 2012 at a meeting of the Medical Ethics Alliance. A journalist at the meeting, reported in the national press, about practices which were harming patients. Relatives, on reading this in the press, were devastated to discover what had happened to their loved ones, placed on the pathway, without their knowledge, understanding, or consent.

There are many issues associated with the pathway: self-fulfilling prophecy, lack of an evidence base, defeatist attitudes, professional power, lack of informed consent, unethical practice and eugenics.

Incurable cannot mean that care has come to an end.

(Congregation for the Doctrine of the Faith, 2020b)

Initial intention of the LCP

The pathway's development in the late 1990s by the Marie Curie Palliative Care Institute, Liverpool, was originally to care for people with cancer, and then later, the principles of hospice care were transferred to non-specialist palliative care services in hospitals continuing LCP practice.

This proved, overall, to be a ruinous process for vulnerable patients who often were not dying but were nonetheless, placed on the pathway. Some have argued that even within palliative care, the pathway is problematic, as its blanket approaches to care can mean both unnecessary sedation and opioids (often used regardless of pain incidence) and without means of either oral intake or CANH.

Inappropriate LCP use in general care settings

In 2000, a National Cancer Plan was published by the government as part of its NHS modernisation programme, in which it was stated that one aim was to 'improve the care of the dying to the level of the best'. Implicit here was that such care, as delivered across hospitals and nursing homes, would be elevated to standards more typically found in the specialist settings of hospices and palliative care units (DH, 2000b).

Having originated in palliative care settings with apparently the best of intentions, the LCP was then used in all care areas as part of the UK government's 'end of life' treatment programme, which includes the Gold Standard Framework (GSF).

Grief of relatives following whistleblower revelations

Many relatives are still haunted by the fact that they were so often sadly oblivious to what was happening to their relative, covertly or in plain sight. Without consent to the pathway plan, they learned later that their unsuspecting loved ones had died as a fait accompli once placed on 'the pathway' – a term often withheld from them.

Truth telling

The serious flaws in the pathway had been highlighted at a conference in 2012, organised by the Medical Ethics Alliance (MEA) and attended by the press. There was analysis of the dangers of the pathway. After which, the discussion was written up in the national press.

Relatives who read about the meeting, whose loved ones had been arbitrarily placed on the pathway without consultation, explanation, consent, or justification, at last understood what had happened to their deceased family members.

Many incredulous relatives recount having to beg the health team to hydrate their family members who they knew were not dying on admission to hospital but would succumb to death if not given proper care. Some were successful in such desperate entreaty, others not so.

Some accused of such 'interference' were even threatened with the police for obstructing the 'work' of the care team. Many now suffer from complicated grief by the realisation that their relatives had died suddenly by use of the pathway (LCP) and the realisation of their misplaced trust in those charged with care of their loved ones.

A culture of death?

The practices employed by this pathway since the 1990s, are now considered by many to be a blot on the healthcare landscape for many years. Its dangers were surprisingly unacknowledged until 2013 when it was recommended for discarding by the government commissioned, independent LCP review, *More Care, Less Pathway* (DH 2013). This review was the result of a whistleblower neurology specialist clinician and the public becoming better informed. Subsequently, the grieving relatives, who for so long had been kept in ignorance about the intrinsically flawed nature of the pathway and its implementation, voiced their concerns. Vulnerable old people and the disabled, began to be fearful of admission to hospital.

The pathway had been used for years both for those patients who were in the dying phase and those who were not. The basic premise of the pathway was, for so many patients, often unnecessary sedation, opioid drugs, without hydration.

Professional disengagement

The LCP review panel members heard from numerous relatives that once the LCP decision was made, the following happened:

- Doctors and nurses stopped engaging with the person's clinical needs.
- These needs were no longer considered relevant, as care was deemed 'futile'.
- Some families were left to carry out as much as they could themselves, giving such care as suction for secretions, washing and mouth care (DH, 2013).
- The LCP was judged as not evidence-based by the independent review (DH, 2013), which exposed practices, in many cases, to be lethal for many vulnerable people.

Decision makers

Such common practice saw patients being placed on the LCP without proper, ethical decision-making by the head of the care team. Nurses were making decisions about such practice, which involved unnecessary sedation and dehydration for many non-dying patients. Such practices appeared to infiltrate many care areas. It took years to be investigated and exposed. Despite the number of cases involved, this should not preclude the need for serious investigation.

Care or killing?

The identification of one third of deaths in hospital, with deaths occurring within days, involving the LCP cannot exclude a direct euthanasia intention, especially when fluids are deliberately and permanently withdrawn as was more often the case according to what reviews of the LCP were conducted. One audit revealed that for patients on the LCP, assisted fluids were continued in only 16% of cases and were virtually never started (MCPIL, 2011). An obvious conclusion is that if the LCP system had become an embedded and uncritiqued, familiar part of healthcare culture, then death by dehydration, would have increased, rather than by true patient decline.

Such practice, it is known, can still occur and still with little consultation with both the patient and family as occurred for so many years with this now, supposedly 'discarded' pathway. Doctors and nurses must be prepared to become educated in the art and science of medicine and nursing. We cannot be reliant on a soulless (lethal) pathway, which disregards individual need.

Department of Health monitoring responsibility

It was apparent from the inception of the LCP, that it was accepted uncritically by NHS trust health professionals and that its roll out had been actively pursued to the detriment of patients. Despite my representation to the Department of Health (DH) at the time about grave misgivings related to the LCP, they were not accepted. This allowed the pathway to continue in use for many years. It resulted in many terrible and unnecessary patient deaths until eventually condemned by the independent review of the pathway (DH, 2013), in large part instigated by the public and true care-oriented health professionals.

Following the recommended discarding of the LCP, by the Neuberger review (DH, 2013), further attempts at communicating the dangers of its known continuing practices, to a successive health minister were again blocked.

The LCP – quality care?

Further to approaching the Department of Health, a response received from the Minister's spokesman, appeared to recognise that the LCP was not of itself a guarantor of the best quality care nor a replacement for clinical judgement and should not be treated as a simple tick-box exercise. It became recognised that staff should receive appropriate training and support to ensure proper use of the LCP. However, there were ongoing problems with it and it cannot be denied that many people who were placed on the LCP received poor care.

Problems

- The LCP was clearly a treatment rather than a care pathway.
- The word 'treatment' was conspicuously absent from LCP descriptors.
- Consent to the pathway was significantly under-discussed or denied.
- The patient/family members/patient advocate were often unaware of any consent sought for the powerful cocktail of drugs involved and general lack of fluid provision or its continuation
- There was a duty of optimum care denied to patients.

Individualised care

Experience of working within palliative care and general nursing for years taught me that non-individualised, 'blanket' approaches to treatment and care are neither appropriate nor ethical. Any suggestion of inappropriate prescribing would be questioned as part of the duty of care to the patients and to sometimes, inexperienced medical staff.

- Pathways, such as the LCP, can so easily deskill both doctors and nurses.
- Every patient is different, with variable symptoms and needs within the holistic philosophy of care.
- Every experienced practitioner must understand the need to improve, maintain and teach theory and practice skill requirements within any specialty.
- Healthcare professionals must understand the difficulty of making a prognosis and the potential dangers of labelling patients.
- Practitioners must never again feel they are unable to function without such an obviously flawed 'pathway'.

Prognosis

Treatment and care must be needs-driven, rather than prognosis-driven. The difficulty in predicting death within the next few weeks, days or even hours, should be well accepted by health professionals. Prognosis is known by most wise doctors to be a difficult art.

'Poor prognosis' can be a useful term to employ when the aim of practitioners is not to cherish life that is still to be lived, regardless of age.

Nurses and doctors need to be aware and accept that the art of issuing a prognosis is notoriously difficult and, in my experience, patients so often can confound such medical declarations. The LCP was regarded as providing evidence-based guidelines for the management of the terminally ill, based upon a prognosis of imminent death. There is no such evidence base in the medical literature.

The inherent dangers of the LCP spell out the overdue need for ethical and rational, evidence-based discussion among health professionals about any care pathway's relevance to optimum and compassionate treatment and care.

Pathway patient selection

The LCP independent review team found dissatisfaction with how patients were placed on the pathway. The LCP did not attempt to use any prognostic index to determine who was placed on the pathway. The fact is that entry onto the LCP was purportedly decided by the multidisciplinary team, with the prediction that the patient was in the last few hours or days of life. This became, in many cases, a self-fulfilling prophecy.

Moreover, according to an audit of the pathway, its commencement for patients was not always endorsed by the senior healthcare professional in 28% of cases (MCPIL, 2011). Therefore, entry onto the LCP could be interpreted as a management decision that the patient's life should end within days once placed on the LCP.

A pathway of no return

Once placed on the LCP, very few patients were taken off the pathway and when some were taken off it, it was usually at the request of relatives who saw their loved one go home without need for the LCP. In the 2007 audit conducted by the Marie Curie

Palliative Care Institute, 2,672 patients were included and 2,664 patients died within a median time of 33 hours. This means that only 0.29% came off the pathway or that 99.7% of enrolled patients died on the LCP (MCPIL, 2011).

Admitted NHS guilt over prognosis and dehydration

A London NHS trust has publicly admitted to failings in both a lack of adequate provision of hydration and in making a diagnosis of 'dying' of a war veteran. The trust admitted that without these errors, the patient, Mr Joseph Boberek, who was a patient at the Hammersmith Hospital, West London, would not have died.

In what is believed to be the first time, hospital chiefs have publicly accepted that the LCP had 'killed' a patient, the Imperial College Healthcare Trust told his daughter that 'if the failings had not happened, on the balance of probabilities your father would have survived and returned to his nursing home' (Petre, 2016).

After five days in hospital, Mr Boberek was becoming drowsy and confused, but his daughter was reassured by doctors who said they would give him a further two litres of fluid – though she later found he had been given less than a quarter of that. A week after his admission he was vomiting and the following day – 6 June 2013 – Mr Boberek's daughter told the specialist registrar, who was the most senior day-to-day doctor on the ward, of her concerns.

Consent to the pathway?

The hospital trust had noted in their communication to Mr Boberek's daughter, Jayne, that the doctor 'explained to you that your father was deteriorating and it was agreed that the aim of the treatment was to keep him comfortable'. Jayne Boberek said that she did not commit her father to the LCP. Nevertheless, she found that the registrar had authorised the protocol and he told her it was the 'best thing' for her father and had been agreed by the consultant in charge (Petre, 2016).

The damning report by the PHSO in 2016 found a litany of failings at the hospital. Doctors claimed Mr Boberek was suffering from terminal heart and kidney failure when this was not the case. Jayne Boberek was later told by the PHSO there was no evidence that her father had a new infection. The report also found untrue, the trust's explanation that Mr Boberek was immediately dying on 6 June 2013. The report added: 'His hydration had been inadequate and there is no evidence he was encouraged to drink fluids. There is no evidence he needed any more antibiotics or that the clinical situation had changed on 6 June 2013' (Petre, 2016).

Although he was frail, he would almost certainly have lived if he had been properly treated. He was not suffering from dementia, as stated in his medical notes (PHSO, 2016).

Chief executive apology

In a letter to Ms Boberek in 2016, trust chief executive Dr Tracey Batten admitted the Trust should have provided more hydration and oral fluids. She said the Trust was sorry it had made 'a number of incorrect diagnoses' and 'incorrectly told you that your father was dying and placed him on the LCP'. She added, 'Please accept my unreserved apology that this happened and for the emotional impact that this has caused you. Our complaint responses were not supported by evidence and, if the failings had not happened, on the balance of probabilities your father would have survived and returned to his nursing home'.

Ms Boberek, who has refused an offer of compensation, said: 'Until recently I had a lot of rage in me, constant rage. I feel that has gone now that I have got some of the answers. But I do feel anger. I feel most of all I don't want this to happen to others' (Petre, 2016).

The PHSO's report about the failures of this patient's treatment was achieved by the campaign for an investigation by Mr Boberek's daughter. Several families across the country have complained to the police that their loved ones were unnecessarily put on end of life regimes and died at NHS hospitals. Those cases are yet to be resolved.

Referring to the case, a clinician who was instrumental in the LCP review commented, 'It is important that the findings of this case are the impetus for ending the intentional dehydration of sick, elderly patients in the NHS' (Pullicino, 2016).

Learning from deceitful, unethical practice

The Boberek case highlights the need for questioning of colleagues about use of 'care pathways', unethical practice, honest and ethical communication with patients and their relatives. Failings in these areas are clearly revealed in this case (and others), which caused the death of a patient and immense suffering to a relative.

More Care, Less Pathway – Neuberger LCP review (DH, 2013)

Such failures were among the main concerns of the Neuberger independent review of the LCP in 2013 which recommended its phasing out.

There is no precise way of diagnosing if someone is dying and patients should be supported with hydration and nutrition unless there is a strong reason not to

(DH, 2013)

The LCP review found many examples of patient drug management which was not appropriate or exemplary. Opioids and other drugs used in terminal care are well known to cause overwhelming thirst and dryness. All drugs, if needed at all, must be used appropriately and not in a 'blanket', thus unethical way.

The following is an extract from the Foreword of the independent review of the Liverpool Care Pathway, *More Care, Less Pathway* (DH, 2013).

It was clear to the review team, from written evidence received and what was heard at relatives' and carers' events, that there had been repeated instances of patients dying on the LCP, being treated with less than the respect that they deserved. It seems likely that similar poor practice may have taken place in the case of patients with no close relatives, carers, or advocates to complain, or where families have not felt able or qualified to question what has taken place. The committee were led to suspect that this became a familiar pattern, particularly, but not exclusively, in acute hospitals. Reports of poor treatment in acute hospitals at night and weekends – uncaring, rushed and ignorant – abound.

The LCP review recommended change, despite the obvious difficulties in staff numbers and oversight: 'It was appreciated by the committee that hospitals are often short staffed and that senior staff may often not be present at night, over weekends and on Bank Holidays. This is perceived by many as one major cause of poor levels of care and communication'.

In order that everyone dying in the acute sector can do so with dignity, the committee recommended that the present situation had to change. It is for this reason that the review committee made seven pages of strong recommendations for change (DH, 2013). See Table of Recommendations (pp. 53 – 59 of the Report): https://assets.publishing.service.gov.uk/government/uploads/system/uploads/attachment_data/file/212450/Liverpool_Care_Pathway.pdf

Continuous deep sedation

A notorious practice of the LCP was the use of terminal sedation. This involved, as has been commonly reported by relatives, the sedating of patients who were not terminally agitated, delusional, or psychotic and had no clinical need to be sedated. Families reported that patients, immediately before being placed on the LCP, often were eating, drinking, talking and even walking, before being sedated and suddenly becoming comatose (without staff communication to the patient or the family).

Mortality – inevitable death without sustaining life

The strongest patient who is sedated and dehydrated will die. Where the practices of this discredited pathway persist (and this is still reported today), the inappropriate combination of opioids, sedation and dehydration will kill the patient. It is difficult not to regard this practice as part of a eugenic culture which meets management targets and which is reliant on the fear of staff not to voice concern or refuse to undertake such practices.

The review committee of the LCP strongly felt that 'if acute hospitals are to deal with dying patients – and they will – whether or not they are using the LCP, they need to treat patients, their relatives and carers with more respect. Hospitals and other institutions need to make more time available to them at any hour of the day or any day of the week' (DH, 2013).

Deep sedation

In the Netherlands, since legalisation of euthanasia in 2002, the numbers dying after continuous deep sedation (CDS) had risen from 5.6% in 2001 to 12.3% in 2010 (Onwuteaka-Philipsen et al., 2012).

In Belgium, nurses involved in administering CDS thought there was an implicit or explicit intention to hasten death in 77% of cases and a possible or certain life-shortening effect in 96% (Inghelbrecht et al., 2011).

A UK study by Bart's and the London School of Medicine and Dentistry found continuous deep sedation was used more frequently in Britain – in 16.5% of cases. The study's author, Professor Clive Seale, suggested that could be because euthanasia was (and is) not a legal option here in the UK (Seale, 2009).

Sedation prevention

A retired NHS geriatrician suggests that the ethical and legal risks of sedation would be greatly reduced if palliative carers took a more active approach to hydration. The legal and ethical problems of terminal sedation could be overcome quite simply by providing hydration for a matter of days until life ends naturally (Craig, 2002). Dr Craig shows how advocates of euthanasia in the UK and elsewhere are exploiting the practice of 'terminal sedation'.

Palliative care specialists have argued that with careful assessment of reversible factors and alternative management for problems like delirium, some of the need for sedation may be avoided (Thorns and Sykes, 2000).

The LCP – a 'care quality innovation' (CQUIN)

Adoption of the LCP was considered as an indirect indicator of the quality of care received by dying patients (but not all patients were truly dying). Therefore, NHS Trusts were commissioned to performance manage staff to assure that the pathway was implemented and at least in some regions, hospital trusts forfeited income under the CQUIN process if they did not implement the LCP. Could this have contributed to so many patients being prematurely placed on the pathway? Is this why post holders were employed to facilitate (enforce) its implementation?

Spiritual care

Intentionally creating a culture of spiritual care supports the provision of holistic nursing. Equal emphasis on caring for the body, mind and spirit of patients fosters the development of caring relationships and interconnectedness and promotes spiritual health and well-being. This is part of holistic care as advocated by the NMC (2010):

> In partnership with the person, the carers and their families, all nurses are expected to make holistic, person-centred and systematic assessments of physical, emotional, psychological, social, cultural and spiritual needs, including risk and develop a comprehensive, personalised plan of nursing care.

Opportunities for completion of 'unfinished business', are treasured by most patients whether or not they may be dying, this may include attending to spiritual needs. The NMC expects, as stated in the nurses' code of conduct, that nurses will: 'make sure that those receiving care, are treated with respect, that their rights are upheld and that any discriminatory attitudes and behaviours towards those receiving care are challenged' (NMC, 2018).

The obvious conclusion is that inappropriate and speedy sedation is unethical and denies the patient the right to spiritual care as an integral part of holistic nursing.

Consent

The nurses' code of conduct also states that the nurse 'must make sure that you get properly informed consent and document it before carrying out any action' (NMC, 2018). The following is another pertinent extract from the independent review of the LCP, concerning lack of consent:

Where care is already poor, the LCP could sometimes be used as a tick box exercise and good care of the dying patient and their relatives or carers may be absent. Whether true or not, many families suspected that deaths had been hastened by the premature, or over-prescription of strong pain killing drugs or sedatives and reported that these had sometimes been administered without discussion or consultation. There was a feeling that the drugs were being used as a "chemical cosh" which diminished the patient's desire or ability to accept food or drink.

(DH, 2013)

Care accountability

With sedation drug regimens and no hydration, patients have no chance of return from the point of oblivion due to these drugs and the associated deliberate dehydration. Such practice perpetuates unethical, non-individualised, non-holistic care. Patients warrant effective assessment throughout every stage of their illness. Blanket prescriptions for symptoms which may not be intractable or even exist, is unethical medicine. Unquestioned, unchallenged administration of such drugs and dehydration is unethical nursing. Such practice would be considered indefensible by professional bodies and a court of law.

Hydration

There were several revisions of the LCP and by version 12, still not enough attention was being paid to hydration needs.

Clinically-assisted hydration, when required, absorbable and practicable, will not harm patients and should be included as part of fundamental and humane care of patients who may or may not be at the end of life. Competent practitioners can monitor the potential risk of fluid overload. Careful attention to hydration, in skilled hands, means sedation need not and should not, shorten life (Craig, 2002).

The LCP review panel recommendations for staff education on hydration

- All staff in contact with patients should be trained in the appropriate use of hydration and nutrition at the end of life and how to discuss this with patients, their relatives and carers.
- There should be a duty on all staff to ensure that patients who are able to eat and drink should be supported to do so unless they choose not to.
- Failure to support oral hydration and nutrition when still possible and desired should be regarded as professional misconduct.
- Specialist services, professional associations and the Royal Colleges, should run and evaluate programmes of education and training and audit how to discuss and decide with patients and relatives or carers how to manage hydration at the end of life.

An addition to the above recommendations: where oral nutritional and fluid needs are becoming difficult for the patient, it is the duty of the care team to organise the most appropriate route (with required monitoring) to clinically assist optimum intake for the patient to prevent the risk of starvation and dehydration.

One of the recommendations of the LCP review

Given the very strong links between the vulnerability of older people and the quality of care for the dying, the Vulnerable Older People's Plan should include a strand on care for the dying and that NHS England's contribution to it should be specified also as a priority in the NHS Mandate (Paragraph 311, p. 59).

(DH, 2013)

A general nurse's experience of the LCP

On a return to practice course at University, I had a placement on a busy acute elderly care ward. The nursing staff with their dedicated assistants were very hard-pressed workwise. *The target for discharge was thirteen days.* Consequently, on admission, discharge was discussed.

On one shift, I was instructed to monitor side-ward patients, one of whom had a "Nil by mouth" sign above her bed. I overheard the Consultant instructing the House Doctor to inform the relatives that this lady was not responding to treatment, had developed pneumonia and so treatment was being withdrawn. Neither the relatives nor the patients were consulted nor were they told that "treatment" included food and drink.

The dear old lady was rational and able to talk. As she had a naso-gastric (NG) tube, I gave fluids via this route and noticed an improvement in her vital signs. On confessing to the senior staff nurse, of my disregard for the instruction not to give fluids, she admitted that she had also done the same. I fed the patient some ice cream and jelly, which she devoured eagerly.

The House Doctor appeared with the medication chart and told me he was writing her up for diamorphine. I asked why, because she was in no pain and I informed him that her condition was improving (no doubt the fluids had relieved her symptoms somewhat and reduced her temperature but did not mention the fluids nor the food). He walked away without writing the prescription. Next day, the lady was returned to the main ward and two days later was discharged to a nursing home. If the fluids had not been given and the diamorphine had been given, she would have died within the time of her supposed discharge date.

Another lady who was side-warded at the same time, but not in my care, died on the day the other patient went to the nursing home, both just inside the 13-day deadline. I concluded that the only reason she, and others like her, were side-warded was because they could not be discharged quickly enough, so they were being treated in such a way as to allow the discharge date to be met by any means, even death.

A paediatric nurse's experience of the LCP

A paediatric nurse, exasperated and dismayed by seeing similar cases, had written to the Minister of Health, denouncing the ways in which children and babies die:

Dying of thirst is terrible and it is inconceivable that children should die like that. Their parents stand at a crossroads and feel almost forced to choose this path because the doctors say their children have only a few days to live. But it is very difficult to predict death and I have also seen a few children come back to life after the LCP had been started and then stopped'.

I have also seen children die terribly of thirst because hydration is suspended until they die. I saw a 14-year-old boy with cancer die with his tongue stuck to his palate when the doctors refused to hydrate him. His death was experienced with anguish by him and us nurses. This is euthanasia being introduced through the front door.

The National Health Service responded to this nurse's concerns without addressing the matter: 'Care for the end of life must meet the highest professional criteria and we must know how to stand next to the child's parents during the decision-making process'.

Doing no harm?

The same paediatric nurse has summarised her experience of trying to reconcile the LCP with ethical nursing practice and the concept of doing no harm and narrated to me the following:

> I think this is best summed up as a feeling of complete "moral distress", due to not being able to give children fluids and watching children suffer effects of dehydration and potentially dying from dehydration before the natural disease process, feeling powerless to help with this, despite raising concerns. Overwhelming concern that your patient is being over sedated and dying too soon as a result and with no way back for patients should things turn around (as can sometimes happen). Alongside oversedation, further distress results for nurses with a system where there are no upper limits on morphine doses.

> The nurse suffers the effect of giving extremely high doses of morphine/sedatives not knowing whether the dose they give will potentially end the life of the patient. As a nurse I wanted to care for the dying child, giving them a drink when they needed it, relieving their suffering with pain relief without the terrible burden of whether we are crossing the fine line between where palliative care ends and euthanasia begins. I also had to endure being treated very badly for raising concerns about the LCP in the workplace.

Such moving narratives cannot be dismissed as mere anecdotes. Many compassionate practitioners must have felt similar distress due to their experiences of the LCP.

The Care Quality Commission

A former neurology specialist clinician has suggested that a way to stop intentional dehydration, for any reason, would be to require NHS Trusts to report to the CQC any instance of a patient not having fluids for more than 24 hours and if so, for significant penalties to be instituted. Moreover, a diagnosis of 'dying' should never be the basis for limiting care which too easily can become a self-fulfilling prophecy for the patient who died but could be saved with more hydration and more care (Pullicino, 2016).

Department of Health awareness of the LCP flaws

The DH appeared to have implicit faith in the worthiness of the LCP until it was discredited and discarded. It would be interesting to know why ministers for health do not want to engage with concerned clinical staff who attempted to share their rightful concerns about the dangers to patients at the height of the pathway use and even following the recommended discarding of the LCP practice. All politicians must take seriously, as parliamentarians, their overriding mandate which is to protect the public.

Fake compassion

It needs to be understood also that declared compassion by some practitioners can be fake. Some practitioners must have believed that patients placed on the LCP, who were not dying, were better off dead. This is reminiscent of Dr Shipman's pathological mindset. Has nothing been learned from the tragic loss of life due to his covert and murderous activity?

There can be a lack of awareness of the presence of those in healthcare who are eugenically driven. Such practitioners may be allowed 'free rein' by a door opened to them, such as the LCP or practices (by another name) by which numerous patients and families were and may continue to be failed within the NHS.

Quality of practitioner and practice

A history of medical crime in the caring professions should be taught within medical and nursing education programmes. These should also include the need for vigilance and how to report concerns and to intervene when suspicions are raised.

It has been argued, refreshingly, that the concerns about the questionable evidence base of the LCP should have a more objective focus in discussions. The performance of the pathway is less an issue than the performance of the pathway user (MacKintosh, 2015). Evidence from a study in Italy (Constantini et al, 2014) highlights this point. However, any practice development should never be accepted as an easy, 'blanket' and unchallenging tool for some practitioners to fail their patients. Some relatives may have viewed the LCP as of benefit to their loved ones. It appears, however, that the experience of most people was negative.

Study criteria

When it is suggested that LCP practice compared with non- LCP care appears to find no difference for patients, it is necessary to list the necessary comparison criteria. Are these: length of life, reported comfort of patients themselves and relatives' satisfaction with care, type of sedation and other drugs employed, possible side effects and whether hydration was provided. Possibly lengthening life due to hydration should not be an overriding concern in care of any patient. Moreover, experience of side effects of medicines given to dying patients or to those not dying but sedated, cannot always be expressed. Nor can family members ascertain this information. However, effectiveness of pain relief can be expressed by patients who are not sedated to be able to report this.

Conclusion

This chapter has explored a culture which can exist where deception of patients and their loved ones can be rife and the words 'patient care' are shown to be shallow, hollow and meaningless. Defining both the concepts of compassion and dignity may be difficult, but it is clear when they are absent from care.

The perceived loss of the ability to 'care' in nursing is controversially suggested that it is perhaps due to the somewhat evangelical search for 'professional' status. This has meant that nursing has slipped into the same trap that befell other professions and has created a professional mystique all of its own, with its own complex language and behaviour (Fletcher, 2000).

Current practice, ongoing neglect and practitioner accountability

Nurses' and doctors' professional registering bodies, the NMC and the GMC, invite feedback from their members and from the public who have concerns or complaints about perceived neglectful practice, attitude, or lack of perceived evidence on clinical decisions.

LCP pathway practices are still being reported, involving blanket prescription of opiates, sedation and dehydration. Where patients are unable to swallow safely, the need for ensuring adequate hydration must be investigated and employed as part of the duty of care. This can require the expertise of the speech therapist to ascertain a patient's possible unsafe swallowing ability.

The Independent review of the LCP cautioned that,

... if fluids are stopped without review over many days, death from dehydration will be inevitable, the lack of hydration having accelerated the dying process. Inadequate hydration is a real vulnerability for old and frail people and may resemble dying.

(DH, 2013)

Patient abuse

Neglect in any area of patient care such as inattention to nutritional and hydration needs is equated in safeguarding as a form of abuse. Regular review of the code of professional conduct can maintain the focus on the duty of care. The nurses' registration body reminds nurses that they will be at risk of disciplinary action if they do not follow their professional code of conduct. The code insists on holistic care (which inevitably includes required nutrition and fluids) and the need for advocacy and evidence-based nursing.

Prescription checks

Questioning is an expectation of all involved in care and in particular, the medication process. This can include the prescriber (who may be the pharmacist as an independent prescriber for certain drugs today), the nurse in some circumstances, the dispenser and lastly, the practitioner who administers the drug. This questioning and checking system have always been part of accepted, safe and accountable practice.

Questioning of drug prescribing and administration appeared limited at the outset and throughout the time of the overt and covert LCP practice. This prerequisite of safe practice cannot be abandoned due to expediency.

Protection for patients and nurses

The right to conscientious objection and the nurses' code of conduct are means of assisting the nurse with the profession's expected role of patient advocate. The uncritical acceptance of the LCP by NHS Trusts and the associated financial incentives, appear to have provided a degree of credibility and apparent protection for practitioners in its implementation. The created nursing role of LCP facilitator needed questioning. The subliminal message through the strict implementation, the silence and acceptance that this was a good 'care' development was compounded by its designation as a care quality innovation for Trust remuneration.

Practitioners, despite their possibly troubled conscience and misgivings, may have been forced into what they believed to be unethical practice. However, the professional code of conduct can and must be used by practitioners, acting to protect both patients and their conscience. Making the right choice for vulnerable patients, must be remembered, is always an option which should be considered as a human right.

The future

LCP practice has not gone away. Many pro-LCP practitioners refuse to accept that the pathway is inherently flawed. It has revealed an implicit undercurrent of issues such as health economics, ageism and consideration of 'worthwhile lives' rather than the care benefits to be conferred on each individual patient.

Many relatives remain heartbroken and traumatised by the realisation that their loved ones did not receive true care at the height of the LCP project. Post-traumatic stress disorder is reported by affected relatives, who, too late, were made aware of the failed care for their loved one. The same pathway practices are still being reported although sometimes disguised by another name.

Support for the Good Samaritan

It is argued that what happens in both patient/client care and nurse-doctor relationships depends very much on what nurses do with their opportunities (Ashworth, 2000). However, practitioners who are not in agreement with a lack of true care apparent in any care setting, may feel vulnerable and unsupported when questioning incidence of poor practice and negligence as discussed in Chapter 7.

Corporate responsibility

Bad healthcare culture must be fought against by practitioners, managers and the public to prevent numerous patients and their families being repeatedly failed by those they trusted. Positions of power, disengagement and inaction, must not be adopted in future. Those who tried to alert management and parliamentarians to their concerns must not be failed again due to a lack of listening and owed support.

Deskilling of practitioners?

*The LCP did not in fact, attempt to use any
published prognostication index to determine
eligibility for the pathway.*

*For this reason, being "within the last hours
of days of life" is a prediction it is
not a prognostication.*

(Pullicino, 2012)

Practitioners must not believe that they are unable to operate in care settings without a care pathway to follow, particularly where the content is not evidence-based. Health professionals can so easily become deskilled when reliant on such a pathway. All must share with less experienced staff, their theory and practice knowledge for the patient's benefit, irrespective of the care setting.

Outcomes

Ethically-minded health professionals would all agree that care of patients towards the end of life should always be needs-based rather than protocol-driven, to ensure optimum care (Kearney, 2013).

Whether murder charges will result from investigation of the unethical practices of the LCP, or its similar replacement care practices, remains to be seen. Families' questions have remained unanswered. Many have had an unbearable and unacceptably lengthy battle to achieve even an investigation in cases of the unexplained, sudden death of their loved ones.

There is a need to develop good practice in palliative medicine, and disease specific treatment for people with non-cancer conditions.

It is noteworthy that the LCP was endorsed by 'Compassion in Dying', an organisation, which has strong affiliation to Dignity in Dying' whose current name replaces several prior, discarded titles, one of which was the Voluntary Euthanasia Society.

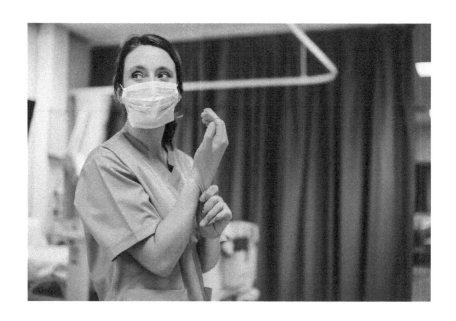

Chapter 11

NHS healthcare scandals – C:
The COVID-19 pandemic

*Many of us have become aware of how much
we need other people.*

(Juthani, 2021)

Introduction

The failings for elderly people during the COVID-19 pandemic included little evidence of appropriate efforts to treat or to resuscitate them at the outset of illness. Such a culture is in marked contrast to all the professions' expectation of questioning issues in practice and to act as the patient's advocate in line with the professional codes of conduct. Orders for 'do not attempt cardiopulmonary resuscitation' (DNACPR) were often arbitrarily given without consultation or communication with either the patients or their families.

The coronavirus pandemic has resulted in initial public displays of gratitude for the NHS staff. The NHS, however, cannot become sacrosanct to the point that its failings continue to be ignored, despite the wonderful work of so many of the NHS staff on a daily basis and particularly during the coronavirus pandemic.

Care homes and the vulnerable elderly

The UK, which has a population of 67 million, has the second highest recorded coronavirus death toll in the world after the US. The pandemic has highlighted the pre-existing problems within the system. These were again reflected in the mismanagement of the vulnerable elderly.

A fundamental mindset problem

Elderly people have been described as 'hospitals' core business' by Dr Finbarr Martin who cited past research conducted by the DH (in collaboration with Comic Relief (DH, 2008). This research found that most of the people looking after frail, older people in hospitals believed that they shouldn't be there. The mindset of the service is that this isn't something for which I legitimately ought to have the knowledge or skills. This desire to either transfer responsibility for the patient to someone else, or have the patient discharged as soon as possible, represents a fundamental mindset problem (Martin, 2012).

The issue has been increasingly appearing in the media, with many dire warnings of the size of the challenge the NHS is facing. But Dr Martin, nearly 10 years ago, stated that it could be tackled and that organisations such as the British Geriatrics Society can offer help and support to meet this need (Martin, 2012).

Original vision for care of elderly people

The vision which first inspired the work of the hospital and the vocation of the medical and nursing professions, was the belief that the lives of those most frail and dependent were to be revered and respected, being loved and needed and certainly not to be considered as burdens. The transfers of untested COVID-positive patients to care homes to free up the hospitals for an anticipated influx of COVID-19 admissions, appeared negligent. The inevitable result was the many unnecessary deaths.

Evidence of risk.

It was emerging at the early stage of the pandemic that asymptomatic patients could be incubating the virus. NHS care home managers had no choice in the transfers of hospital patients infected with COVID-19 to their care homes until some managers, as Good Samaritans, realised what was unfolding and tried to prevent an ongoing systematic infection of their residents.

Further transfers of patients from hospital to care homes continued in order to 'save' the NHS from being overwhelmed by patients with COVID-19 needing hospital care. One conclusion about the way elderly patients were put at risk in their care homes could be that they are considered expendable in this secular age, rather than people to be cherished.

Elderly people and care discrimination

The National institute for Health and Care Excellence (NICE), issued a set of guidelines for the NHS. The document *COVID-19 rapid guideline: critical care in adults* (NICE, 2020), presented a flowchart, updated on 27 March 2020, helping doctors to decide whether adults admitted to hospitals with coronavirus symptoms qualified for critical care, which usually takes place in intensive care units. A path on the flowchart concluded with *'end of life care'* if a patient's condition worsened after they were determined as being 'frailer' but not suitable for critical care.

A lack of humanity

A former neurology specialist clinician who exposed the truth of the LCP, argues that this flowchart encouraged doctors to treat sick, elderly people who fell into this category, as if they were dying, rather than as if attempts should be made to treat them:
A major problem with those guidelines was that they said that those people who were not appropriate for ventilators, if they were over 65 and if they deteriorated, there was a line going to "end of life care," which was really wrong. When this whole COVID-19 crisis started, people realised that there were not enough ventilators compared with other countries. We did not have a lot of NHS beds either because the number has been run down over the last number of years. So, I think there was panic.
They decided to clear the hospitals to make a lot of space ready. The hospitals were cleared of the elderly and many of them were sent to nursing homes. Some of those moved to care homes could have had the coronavirus, which has an incubation period of up to 14 days during which carriers have no symptoms of the disease.
In the nursing homes there was no testing available, no personal protective equipment. The situation then became that if somebody got sick in the nursing home, there was nowhere for them to go.
And I think this is what has happened. The Nightingale and other hospitals did not reach capacity even at the height of the

pandemic, so the free beds should have been opened to the elderly. It's a terrible situation and there's a total lack of humanity for the elderly – and the disabled are included, too, in many cases in this thing.

(Pullicino, 2020)

Government action on COVID-19 testing

In a policy paper, updated 16 April 2020, the government acknowledged care providers' concerns about the difficulty of isolating COVID-19-positive care home residents and confirmed a policy of testing all prior to admission to care homes which was further updated, 3 May 2022 (Department for Health and Social Care, 2022).

Calls for care homes inquiry

Catholics are calling for a public investigation into why so many elderly people have died in UK nursing homes during the coronavirus crisis. Lord Alton, a crossbench peer who has no party affiliation, said during a virtual House of Lords debate on 23 April 2020, that an inquiry into nursing homes was 'inevitable'. He called for the creation of,
… a national care service' to work alongside the NHS. He argues that the deaths in our care homes have made abundantly clear that, alongside our National Health Service, we need a National Care Service. If a national care service emerged from the wreckage of COVID-19, it would represent a gain, among so much loss, comparable to the gain of the National Health Service post-1945.

(Alton, 2020)

Clinicians' views on the care for the elderly and COVID-19 practice

It has been argued that the treatment of the elderly has deteriorated within the healthcare system:

We're building on a mindset within the NHS that has gone on for more than 10 years. It has been built on the Liverpool Care Pathway and more recently you have had these end of life pathways which are still going on, still unchanged basically, from the Liverpool Care Pathway. So, the elderly, I'm afraid, have been devalued in the NHS. This was partly due to a lack of beds and partly to a lack of staff.

I don't think individuals are to blame. The individuals work extremely hard. But the 65s and over, represent almost a fifth of the population. You cannot short-change them. These are the people that need medical care. They need it most. You cannot just say to the elderly, no more healthcare and that is it… These end of life care practices that are going on in the NHS have to be looked into. We have to look into what is happening, how the elderly people are being treated and there has to be a change. Because I do think it is partly a question of how people view the elderly sick as a burden rather than as a challenge and that we have to support them and look after them in the correct way if we're a humane society.

(Pullicino, 2020)

Lethal guidance?

Dr Adrian Treloar, a consultant in geriatric psychiatry, told the Catholic News Agency that he shared some of Professor Pullicino's concerns.

Referring to NICE guidance on COVID-19, updated 8 April 2020 (NICE, 2020), he said:

The guidance on "caring for someone who is dying at home from COVID-19 infection" is in fact, very carefully written and very compassionate and only to be used, when absolutely certain that the person is dying and does not want to go to hospital. It is basic palliative care. But if it is used inappropriately for someone who has COVID-19 (and respiratory depression) it may be rapidly lethal. Care homes saw considerable efforts to prepare for the pandemic by promoting end of life care planning, alongside a NICE guideline which denies critical care for people with mild to moderate dementia

> *and which promotes end of life care as the alternative.*
> *The promotion of end of life care and the high death toll in care*
> *homes sits worryingly alongside a system that simultaneously*
> *omitted to do even the minimum it should have done*
> *to protect the vulnerable from the virus.*

> (Treloar, 2020a)

Cardiopulmonary resuscitation (CPR)

Resuscitation is a sensitive question at the best of times. Not all patients who undergo CPR in hospital survive, with survival rates dropping to between 5–10% outside of a hospital setting. But consent is a precious right for all patients and to obtain it is a skill required of nurses and doctors with each patient admission where appropriate and possible. CPR can cause punctured lungs, fractured ribs and severe bruising but failing to fully appraise a patient or their loved ones of their options is a breach of their human rights. Not all CPR attempts fail, even in the elderly who can be very fit.

Do not attempt resuscitation orders

Do not attempt cardiopulmonary resuscitation (DNACPR) orders only refer to CPR, they do not cover any other type of treatment that someone may need for their condition or care that helps people feel comfortable and pain-free.

The following is an extract from Resuscitation UK (RCUK) on DNACPR:

> DNACPR only specifies whether a person will receive CPR or not. Patients will still receive appropriate treatment for their health issues and all personal care needs will be attended to.
>
> (RCUK, 2022)

DNACPR orders can compromise treatment and care

It is reported that once a DNACPR notice is in place, ordinary care can be compromised. In 2020, the CQC found examples of routine care not being provided in homes, such as an ambulance or doctor not being called, due to the existence of a 'DNR' order (CQC, 2020).

Fair resource allocation

Coronavirus demands on the NHS resources were outstripping supply and those responsible for care and well-being are facing challenging decisions. The question arises about the type of provision which will be available if treatment and life support is needed in these circumstances. While the allocation of resources must be done as fairly as possible, the criteria of fairness must be clear and shared by all. These principles apply both morally and in law, which governs our expectations and rights on health and social care.

'Blanket policies' on cardiopulmonary resuscitation

'Blanket' DNACPR notices are reportedly being issued in UK hospitals and nursing and care homes. The practice has become more widespread during the COVID-19 pandemic. The Parliamentary Joint Committee on Human Rights (JCHR) pointed out the increased use of the practice in a September 2020 report, which particularly criticised the issuing of DNACPR notices for persons with learning disabilities or other similar impairment, solely, or primarily, on that basis (JCHR, 2020).

> *It is discriminatory to apply DNACPR notices in a blanket manner to groups, on the basis of a particular type of impairment, such as a learning disability, or on the grounds of age alone.*

(Cole and Duddington, 2021a)

The Care Quality Commission findings on DNACPR notices

The CQC interim review (2020) found that unacceptable and inappropriate DNACPR orders were made at the start of the COVID-19 pandemic. The findings come after the CQC raised concerns that older and vulnerable people may have had DNACPR decisions made without their consent or may have made them without enough details for an informed decision (Hackett, 2020).

The number of complaints that the CQC received about the DNACPR orders jumped to 40 between March and September 2020, during the first year of the pandemic, compared to just nine similar complaints in the previous six months.

One example of the pressure and confusion during the early days of the pandemic noted by the CQC was that that guidance, intended to help clinicians assess frailty as part of a wider, holistic assessment around the appropriateness of critical care, may have been interpreted as the sole basis for clinical decisions in some instances.

Lack of family discussion or consent to DNACPR

Despite reminding care providers of their obligations, the CQC said it received evidence from staff and patients' families that DNACPR orders had been applied without consultation. One carer told the CQC an on-call doctor had informed care home staff that if a resident were to catch COVID-19, a DNACPR order would automatically be put in place (CQC, 2020).

Another witness said some care homes and learning disability services had been told by GPs to place blanket DNACPR orders on everyone in their care.

Some families of patients said they were not made aware that a DNACPR order was in place until their relative was quite unwell. Others said they had been told their loved one had agreed to a DNACPR, but they had concerns over their understanding due to factors such as deafness or language barriers.

The British Medical Association 2020 COVID-19 guidance for members

The BMA guidance of 2020 recommended action for its members during the COVID-19 pandemic. The guidance recommended that during the peaks of the pandemic, it is possible that doctors may be required to assess a person's eligibility for treatment on a 'capacity to benefit quickly' basis. As such, doctors may be called on to deny some of the most unwell patients access to life-sustaining treatment such as CPR, intensive care, or artificial ventilation.

The guidance of the CQC states that decisions on DNACPR orders must never be dictated by blanket policies, must be free from discrimination and not made on a clinician's 'subjective view of a person's quality of life'.

BMA guidance for GP access

BMA guidance for GPs was issued in 2020 for the safety of patients and staff. The following recommendations came into force despite many concerns of GPs over supervision and technology:

- Practices must now move to a triage first model for consultations. NHS England have developed a range of resources to help practices implement this approach. Practices in other nations are also moving towards this model.
- Practices are asked to use telephone, video and online consultations to support triage and remote management of patients.
- In particular, you are encouraged to promote online consultations to patients and introduce this service where they do not already have it.
- Video consultations should be used where possible; however, telephone access will be used where there are barriers to digital access' (BMA, 2020).

Nursing staff appear to be more accessible and visible as Good Samaritans for patients, seeing them face to face and home visiting. The BMA guidance is a good example of where it may be overwhelmingly difficult for clinicians to be seen to be going against professional 'guidance' in order to act as the Good Samaritan.

Lack of patient access to investigation and treatment

Elderly patients report being told by receptionist staff that the GPs are too busy to see them and even online or phone consultations are not possible until weeks ahead. Notwithstanding the easing of lockdown for many weeks and the fact that many hospitals had prepared for returning patients by compartmentalising areas for enhanced safety, patients report being told that they must wait for many months for a phone appointment. 'That is moving beyond mere neglect, into the realms of manslaughter' (Pearson, 2020).

The *Daily Telegraph* 'Help Us to Help You' campaigned for patients to access personalised and face-to-face medical interaction, which resulted in 'total telephone triage' being abolished. This was the NHS system where those wishing to see a GP were told to have an online or phone discussion first.

Lack of GPs?

Many GPs account for this situation by explaining the lack of GPs to cope with the number of patients. It is interesting, however, to note that many GPs now work part time which may be attributed to stress of the role.

Many patients report that accessing face-to-face GP appointments has been a battle, including attempts to secure even online consultations. Forecasts that online GP consultations are the way forward as part of the remit of a GP are a concern to many, particularly for those patients without computer access or technical ability. For some, with confidence in such technology, such a system can be convenient. Accounts vary of the situation. GPs insist that they continue to provide opportunity for face-to-face appointments together with initial assessment appointments either by phone or online interaction. NHS dentistry is a rarity. Is the future for NHS medicine to be provided by the private sector except for emergency treatment if diagnosis can still occur in primary care?

Treatment disparity

Tension between the appropriate treatment and scarcity of resources has, in most people's experience, never been so visible. A decision against offering a certain life-prolonging treatment to an individual must never be a judgement based on the worthwhileness of that person's life, including their age or other social characteristics, but a pragmatic decision about the likelihood of benefit from the intervention, given their medical condition. The NHS Constitution itself is clear that we should deliver care and support in a way that achieves dignity and compassion for each and every person we serve (DH, 2021).

Protecting the NHS

The desire to protect the NHS has distorted its mission, as during the pandemic, many patients have stayed away for fear of being a burden (but also due to fear of catching COVID-19). It has been suggested that the NHS has been relegated to a service only for COVID-19 cases. Many thousands of required hospital treatments have been deferred or cancelled. A book recently published by a former Director of Public Health, Dr John Ashton, is aptly titled *Blinded by Corona* (Ashton, 2020).

Protecting the NHS has, in fact, almost destroyed it due to the thousands of patients who are now in need of care for conditions which have become inoperable, beyond cure and in some cases, terminal. Moreover, millions of people have become part of a huge backlog to be treated in the months and years to come.

COVID-19 effects on patients in general

The core work of the NHS has been almost extinguished in some areas and specialties. In early 2020, Prostate Cancer UK announced that prostate cancer had become the most commonly diagnosed cancer in the UK, thanks largely to a greater awareness of the disease in recent years (UK cancer incidence data, 2020). In the specialty of urology alone, urgent referrals for urological cancers in 2020 had dropped by half in England (49.5%) compared to the same period in 2019.

Disease risk awareness

The COVID-19 pandemic made it harder for men to visit their doctor, according to the latest statistics shared by Prostate Cancer UK from NHS England (Urology News, 2020). This leading men's health charity, is encouraging all men at increased risk of prostate cancer to contact their GP to discuss the advantages and disadvantages of a prostate-specific antigen (PSA) blood test, which can give them an indication of any problems with their prostate. Men at risk include those over 50, particularly Black men and those with a family history of the disease. As most men generally do not experience any symptoms until the disease has spread and become incurable, it is critical that men with these risk factors act (Culhane, 2020).

Do patients really prefer digital GP consultations?

The COVID-19 pandemic crisis has identified and exacerbated the pre-existing flaws of the NHS system. It is suggested by the psychiatrist Dr Max Pemberton that there was something rather disingenuous about the former Health Secretary, Matt Hancock's claim that Skype communication is what patients want for their medical consultations.

I suspect he is trying to justify the increasing push for doctors to work remotely, with the majority of consultations taking place via the internet, becoming a permanent fixture. This is actually a much bigger issue to do with a lack of flexibility when it comes to patients' needs and preferences, with coronavirus a convenient fig leaf for administrators and managers to achieve their own goals, be it savings in cost or time. There are times when we all need a degree of physical intimacy to reassure us and show support – a touch that says more than words ever could: "I'm here, I'm with you. You are not alone." He concludes that: "It saddens me that so many of my colleagues are becoming so risk averse because of this wretched virus. We are in danger of forgetting the most powerful thing medicine has to offer – care and compassion. COVID-19 and its risk averse culture, risks turning doctors and other healthcare workers into box-ticking, emotionless avatars.

(Pemberton, 2020)

Study of nursing views of their pandemic experiences

During the COVID-19 pandemic, considerations of populations disproportionately exposed to risk is crucial. Often termed 'vulnerable populations', this group not only includes older individuals, those with disabilities, ill health and comorbidities but also those from any socioeconomic group who might have difficulty coping mentally, physically, or financially with the pandemic (Lancet, 2020).

Advanced nurse practitioners

A small quantitative and qualitative study (124 respondents) was conducted to understand the experiences of advanced nurse practitioners across both the primary and secondary care settings. Topics chosen were based on contemporary, anecdotal reports from healthcare professionals in the UK about the issues that COVID-19 had caused in the NHS.

Findings revealed that they had experienced during the first three month of the pandemic, short staffing (51%) and inadequate infection prevention resources, personal protective equipment (PPE) (68%). Shortages of PPE during a pandemic are known to be a risk factor for increased staff turnover and retention issues.

Concerns about the long-term impact of reduced services on patient care have contributed to the distress felt by the nurses. Almost half of the nurses surveyed (47%) were considering a change in job. The impact of these challenges on the mental health of the nurses has significant implications for staff retention across the UK.

Despite difficulties, there were reports of positive changes to working practice that had enhanced care. Examples of innovations they considered that had worked well for them as practitioners, were remote consultations which they suggested should be explored in future research from the patient's perspective. Where there are shared benefits, these can be carried forward into future nursing practice (Wood et al., 2020).

A nurse whistleblower on COVID-19 Care in America

Good Samaritan American Nurse, Erin Maria Olzewski. made headlines in 2020 when she revealed how patients who repeatedly tested negative for COVID-19 were being described as 'COVID-19 confirmed' in their charts, which triggered a higher compensation from US government pay-outs. She contrasted the treatments that they had provided in Florida to what was happening in New York. Olzewski said "Florida Governor, DeSantis didn't ban medication that saves lives. And that's a big deal. In Florida we treated our patients with hydroxychloroquine and zinc, sent them home and they were fine. In New York, they were banning alternative treatments like hydroxychloroquine. The only thing they could do was to put people on ventilators.

And that's one of the things that you see across the US, and many of the blue states, is the governor got in between the doctor patient relationship. And that should never happen. That is where we saw the most deaths, in those states where they banned treatment protocols" (Knight, 2020b).

Hospital financial incentives

At the time, the US Department of Health and Human Services (HHS) provided what some called 'perverse incentives' instituted by government COVID-19 relief funding. This awarded significantly more compensation to hospitals should patients be classified as COVID-19 positive ($13,000) or if they are put on a ventilator ($39,000).

Olzewski indicated these incentives dramatically impacted what was happening at Elmhurst Hospital, New York. "You know, $13,000 to admit [COVID-19 classified] patients and they were just admitting everybody". She further alleged that with the $39,000 incentive, the hospital would then put admitted patients on a ventilator that they knew would kill them. Additionally, "in some cases, there was an incentive of $10,000 [for] every death, with families kicked out and not being able to monitor, it was the perfect storm and people took advantage of it" (Life Site News, 2021).

Such a narrative brings into question what occurs by commission or omission in UK care settings, mindful that the practices of the LCP have not disappeared. This is a particular concern when relative visiting was non-existent, except in exceptional circumstances during the height of the COVID-19 pandemic in the UK.

Elderly people's isolation

The vision which first inspired the work of the hospital, and the vocation of the medical and caring professions, was the belief that the lives of those most frail and dependent were to be revered and respected. They were to feel loved and needed and certainly were not to be considered as burdens which impacts on their own feelings of self-worth.

COVID-19 increased the number of deaths for people with learning disabilities by a greater margin than for the general population across the adult age spectrum. The vast majority of alleged COVID-19 deaths are people over the age of 85. And three in every five alleged COVID-19 deaths occurred in those who suffered learning difficulties and disabilities. Age specific COVID-19 death rates per 100,000 population were higher for people with learning disabilities in all adult age groups but by a greater margin in younger age groups (Public Health England, 2020).

COVID-19 'end of life' care

DNACPR orders were used as permission to begin end of life care which involved the denial of medical treatment, questionable amounts of midazolam and deprivation of food and water. The discarding of such LCP practice had been recommended seven years prior to the pandemic.

Sedation

End of life care guidelines for COVID-19 involved the injection of high doses of midazolam. The UK purchased a two-year supply of midazolam in March 2020 and then went back to France for more. Inappropriate doses of midazolam causes the same symptoms as in the serious complications due to COVID-19.

The Coronavirus Act (2020) on certifying death

This new Act meant that any doctor could certify a death, even if they were not the attending doctor. The Act stated that COVID-19 could be listed as a 'direct' or 'underlying' cause of death for the purposes of the medical certificate of cause of death.

The new law also stated that COVID-19 deaths do not need to be reported to the coroner, despite COVID-19 being listed as a notifiable disease. Did the doctors need proof under the new law that COVID-19 was the official cause of death?

The Act also allowed the cause of death to be verified remotely. The guidance explains that the person physically attending the body of the deceased need not be a medical professional but that they should 'usually and normally' be independent of family members. This is precisely what happened in care homes, as GPs refused to visit. Medical practitioners were required to certify causes of death 'to the best of their knowledge and belief', without diagnostic proof, if appropriate and to avoid delay (Coronavirus Act, 2020).

Patient protection must include compassion

It has been argued that the miseries for the elderly in their care homes, to ensure their safety from COVID-19, including being unable to see even one of their family members for visits, should be weighed against the need for love and compassion. It has been realised how hard it is for the elderly in care to be without visitors, so a pilot study of one named relative being allowed to visit with regular testing was initiated.

One journalist remarked:

… every last, precautionary measure of infection prevention should not trump the deaths in loneliness of tens of thousands. When the elderly people are no longer with us, due to their deaths by COVID-19, we shall look back on how we treated the institutionalised elderly in this year of COVID-19 and be ashamed.

(Parris, 2020)

This criticism cannot overlook, however, those dedicated staff, the Good Samaritans, who tried their very best to care for the vulnerable elderly in care homes, which involved being apart for considerable periods from their own families, to protect their residents from the risk of COVID-19.

Calls for an independent COVID-19 inquiry

The vice president of the Association of Directors of Public Health, UK, Jim McManus, has documented his concerns to government about disparity in treatment access. Lord Alton and Professor Patrick Pullicino, a former specialist in neurology have called for an independent inquiry about the whole approach to this scandal of non-parity of access to critical care related to the COVID-19 crisis.

The common good

The Catholic tradition views the worship of God as rooted in fundamental justice. Justice is classically defined as giving to another his or her due. God and God alone, is due our worship. Thus, we act justly, both individually and corporately, when we worship God. When our worship is other-directed, we commit an act of injustice toward God. Thus, the good that orders our lives is not the freedom to be able to worship God, but the actual worship of God. Thus, common good is the sum of the conditions that make that not only possible but facilitate it – to reach it 'more fully and easily'. In summary, the common good is a particular, substantive set of conditions that facilitate the worship of God (Craycraft, 2022). The aggressive secularists may argue with this belief which involves concepts of justice, equality and charity.

Care disparity for the elderly

Three Catholic bishops with responsibility for health and social care have written about care disparity for elderly people. Those with underlying health conditions should discuss the sort of treatment they may want with their families so that effective communication is possible in a crisis. Each of us may be presented with clinical scenarios which are both unwelcome and distressing, yet doctors are faced with making the least-worst decisions. This approach helps us to focus on the common good. Similarly, Catholics will focus on the benefit of a particular treatment for the person, taking into consideration all medical factors. This, again, helps us to focus on the common good of all and best meets the principles of justice and equality (Moth et al., 2020).

Until the current pandemic, resources have always been allocated according to medical need and benefit to the patient. Today this approach must be complemented by maximising scarce resources for the common good and so prognosis and the likelihood of benefit, become the overriding criteria.

Appointment of Rt Hon Baroness Heather Hallett to lead UK-wide COVID-19 inquiry

Following the announcement by the UK government of the appointment of Rt Hon Baroness Heather Hallett to lead a UK-wide COVID-19 inquiry, the First Minister of Wales, Mark Drakeford said:

> *I have long argued the importance of this being a Judge-led inquiry and Baroness Hallett has extensive experience of dealing with high profile, sensitive and complex inquiries, including within a devolved context. This understanding of devolution is important if the inquiry is to fully scrutinise the decisions and actions*

*taken by the Welsh Government and other Welsh
public services in response to the pandemic.
I am also pleased that the UK government has
confirmed that Welsh Ministers will be involved in
setting and agreeing the terms of reference for the inquiry.
The pandemic has been – and continues to be – one of
the most difficult periods this country has ever faced.
The appointment of Baroness Hallett will ensure the
inquiry is handled sensitively and families who have lost
loved ones are able to receive answers to the questions
they have been asking.*

(Drakeford, 2020)

COVID-19 vaccines

Health professionals and lay people are reporting coercive pressure to receive the vaccines. They should understand that it is illegal under various international treaties to coerce somebody to receive a medical treatment that is experimental. This standard derives from the trials following the defeat of Nazi Germany, where Dr Josef Mengele and other doctors performed experiments on living humans (who, of course, were not volunteers), sometimes killing them.

COVID-19 vaccine side effects

Many people are also reporting that no real communication was given about the vaccine's possible side effects, which needed an alert as soon as serious effects were emerging, before public trust began to falter about both the first, second and subsequent vaccines. No one should be put in a position and our law prohibits coercion or mandating, to take something that is an experimental treatment, where the outcome is not reasonably certain. This is true of the new COVID-19 vaccines (Yeadon, 2021).

Patients, friends and acquaintances have reported serious side effects from both the main vaccines (Astra Zeneca and Pfizer). No one should be forced to take a vaccine (described as 'safe') which did not go through the usual safety protocols. There is debate as to whether the COVID –19 vaccines are 'vaccines' in the normally accepted sense of the term but experimental drugs for emergency use. Therefore, they are not fully approved by the Food and Drug Administration (FDA) or the European Medicines Agency (EMA).

GPs had reported the need for them to go and deliver the second vaccine due to their elderly patients being unable to walk since receiving the first injection. This needs to be taken seriously by all practitioners who wish to act as the patient advocate since it is now known that there is no guarantee that the vaccines can prevent contraction of COVID-19 or transmission. Lessening of severe infection and hospitalisations is thought possible by their use. While it is believed that natural immunity derived from COVID-19 infection is superior.

'Big Pharma'

There is nothing new about criticising methods with which big pharmaceutical companies operate and market their products. During the 'golden age' of drug discoveries, drug companies were highly ethically, scientifically and scrupulously driven. This golden age preceded the massive fines imposed on virtually every big drug company (Pfizer, Eli Lilley, Abbott, Merck and Astra Zeneca), which have incurred fines in excess of £10 billion following judgements over the past three decades. This would suggest, to paraphrase Shakespeare, that there must be 'something rotten in the state of the pharmaceutical industry' (Le Fanu, 2012).

> *A disturbing case involved Glaxo Smith Kline (GSK), … which pleaded guilty to promoting its drug, Paxil, as a "highly effective" treatment for adolescent depression when the relevant clinical trials demonstrated it to be no better than a placebo. In addition, the company failed to disclose that those taking it reported, paradoxically, being more prone to suicidal thoughts – subsequently implicated by several groups of bereaved parents at a public hearing, as the cause of their child's death.*

(Le Fanu, 2012)

The impact of the COVID-19 vaccine programme in years to come in terms of serious side effects will be revealed. All health professionals as Good Samaritans must be prepared to question any drug that is being ordered, in terms of side effects and must communicate clearly, such information to patients.

First do no harm

Doctors who are speaking out on behalf of their patients who, in their professional opinion, have been harmed by the COVID-19 vaccine, are reported to have been side-lined, suspended, or sacked and treatment discussions have been discouraged.

Informed consent and ethical decision-making

True choice can only be made with informed consent. The decision to receive the vaccine has been described as more than a civil liberties matter. It is existential for the nation and possibly the world to take that attitude (Yeadon, 2021).

People's decisions on ethical grounds must be respected. Aborted foetal cells are part of the constituents of these vaccines (or in the early test development process) which is proving controversial and causing ethical conflict among the public and those expected to deliver the vaccines. Pressure from the public about the constituents of these vaccines may force the manufacturers to think again about these and other medication where such unnecessary constituents cause conscientious objection in receiving and administering them.

The COVID 19 narrative

It is argued by the co-Director of the Organisation for Propaganda Studies, that a preliminary examination of events over the last two and a half years indicates that information suppression has operated in at least three different ways: direct censorship through removal of content and de-platforming, sponsoring of hostile coverage designed to smear and intimidate anyone raising critical questions regarding the COVID-19 narrative, and coercive approaches involving threats to livelihood and employment.

Those questioning COVID-19 policies have sometimes been described as far right or fascist whilst pejorative use of the term "conspiracy theorist" is frequently employed to describe those questioning official narratives.

Furthermore, censorship and suppression of academic debate has been reported with respect to academic journals whereby articles and research running against the so-called scientific consensus appear to have been unfairly removed or blocked. For example Dr Peter McCullough reports unjustified censorship of a peer reviewed and published article relating to COVID-19 whilst, more broadly, undue suppression of legitimate research findings was reported by Dr Tess Lawrie with respect to Ivermectin trials. All of these are worrying indications that academic processes themselves have become subject to nefarious censorship and control.

Whilst detailed and systematic research should be conducted in order to identify the scale and range of the censorship that has been occurring, it is reasonably clear now that, relative to pre-2020, the levels are unprecedented and represent a normalization, or routinization, of censorship.

Coercion acts as a final block for anyone entertaining the possibility of risking talking about censored issues and riding out the smears that will result.

The potential unpleasant consequences of discussing such issues, e.g., possible loss of job and income can appear simply too much to bear. Overall, the role of authorities in enabling censorship and coercion results in, broadly speaking, an institutionalised culture in which suppression of opinions and debate becomes the norm (Robinson, 2022).

Remote cooperation

The Congregation for the Doctrine of the Faith cautions that both pharmaceutical companies and governmental health agencies are encouraged to produce, approve, distribute and offer ethically acceptable vaccines that do not create problems of conscience for either healthcare providers or the people to be vaccinated due to the use of aborted foetal cell lines (Congregation for the Doctrine of the Faith, 2020a).

The doctrine of papal infallibility does not relate to this subject. It relates to defined dogma which is not relevant to the declaration by Pope Francis on the use of these particular vaccines. He has said that receiving these vaccines can be considered as 'remote' cooperation only, yet he emphasised that conscience is to be considered and respected on whether to take the vaccines.

Conscience

St John Henry (Cardinal Newman) developed an understanding of conscience as our antenna for objective truth, as the voice of God echoing in the heart of every human being. This human capacity, Newman stressed, is fragile and open to distortion by personal and cultural forces. The Church's God-given authority to speak the truth in season and out of season is thus needed to awaken conscience as much as God's grace is needed to follow it (Twomey, 2019).

For Newman, conscience is the human capacity to recognise the objective truth about good and evil. Newman wrote at the end of his exposé on conscience: 'Certainly, if I am obliged to bring religion into after-dinner toasts (which indeed does not seem quite the thing), I shall drink – to the Pope, if you please, – still, to Conscience first and to the Pope afterwards' (Twomey, 2019).

Treatment for COVID-19

When people were diagnosed with the virus, it was rare to treat it, when in the early days there were treatments but which were generally not given when symptoms were first apparent until it was too late. Most people were told to stay at home with no treatment offered.

Investment in COVID-19 treatments (of which there are several) should have been considered equally as important as the vaccine rollout, which has been described as 'premature and reckless' by scientists and clinicians in an open letter addressed to the EMA in February 2021.

The letter set out in worrying detail what they say are the dangers of continuing with the inoculation programme but has not received the attention it deserves. They warn of possible autoimmune reactions, blood clotting, abnormalities, stroke and internal bleeding and highlight side effects in previously healthy, younger people. They state that the administration of the vaccines constituted and still does constitute, 'human experimentation', which was and still is in violation of the Nuremberg Code.

The signatories of the letter demanded conclusive evidence that an actual emergency existed at the time of the EMA granting conditional, marketing authorisation to the manufacturers of all three available vaccines to justify their approval for use in humans, purportedly because of such an emergency. They conclude that if these concerns are not addressed by the exercise of due diligence by the EMA, they demand that approval for the use of the gene-based vaccines be withdrawn (TCW defending freedom, 2021).

Care workers threatened with job losses if refusing the vaccine

Those unwilling to accept a vaccine (often described as 'experimental') that has not been examined by the usual procedures should not be under threat of losing their jobs.

New UK government legislation meant that from November 2021, anyone working in a CQC-registered care home in England for residents requiring nursing or personal care, must have two doses of a COVID-19 vaccine unless they have a medical exemption. It applied to all workers. These included those employed directly by the care home or care home provider (on a full-time or part-time basis), those employed by an agency and deployed by the care home and volunteers deployed in the care home.

Those coming into care homes to do other work, for example healthcare workers, tradespeople, hairdressers, beauticians and CQC inspectors, also had to follow the new regulation unless they had a medical exemption.

The responses to the consultation on compulsory (yet still experimental) COVID-19 vaccination made a case for extending this policy beyond care homes to other settings where people vulnerable to COVID-19 receive care, such as domiciliary care and wider healthcare settings. Such plans were then reconsidered for all Care and NHS staff, due to predicted huge staff shortages as a result of those unwilling to take the vaccine, generally due to emerging side effects and lack of the long-term data and also the ethical issues.

Vaccine passports

Further moves are being planned for driving up vaccination rates by the creation of a vaccine passport confirming two vaccines for being allowed admission to crowded venues. Many results are anticipated from such a draconian move, most concerning is definitely staff attrition from the care sector and fears about further erosion of UK civil liberty. People who cannot engage with forced vaccination due to ethical or safety concerns will experience the full force of the implications for their lives.

This is the driven plan, despite the well-known fact that vaccines do not prevent transmission or contracting of the virus, even though the vaccine 'benefits' may last for only a few months while it is considered to be effective.

Conclusion

We are all made equal. As Christians, our starting point is that we are all made equally in the image of God. Human value is not a measure of our mental or physical capacity, societal function, our age, our health, or of any other qualitative assessment. God made each of us and in so doing gave us all equal dignity and value. This is never lost during sickness or dying.

Those who act on their conscience don't simply follow the majority opinion – they suffer for it, as did Sophie and Hans Scholl (of the While Rose resistance movement opposed to Nazism). Acting in conscience, under the influence of Newman, they paid for it with their lives. Conscience calls for courage and faith (Twomey, 2019).

The figures on the fatal, injurious and long-lasting side effects of the vaccines, in years to come will reveal whether world-wide vaccination and its accompanying marketing and media promotion rather than use of known available treatments for this viral infection and threats to liberty, world-wide, were necessary.

Through exploration of the diverse healthcare scandals, recounted in Chapters 9–11, we see attempts to repeatedly 'shut down' complainants in their efforts to disclose care that was suboptimum at best and harmful or lethal at worst. Negative effects of an unsafe health culture need top-down root cause analysis for resolution, restitution and prevention of future harm.

Good Samaritan practitioners at all levels of care, have their conscience and codes of conduct to rely on to help them. Perseverance and courage are required for patient advocacy for safe, compassionate and patient-focused practice.

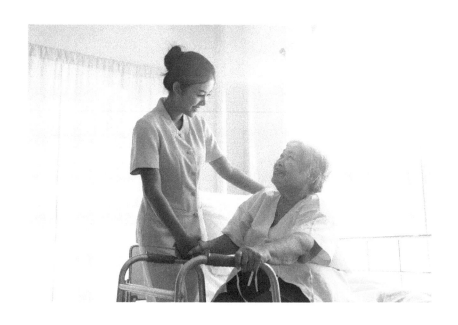

Chapter 12
Presumed consent to organ donation

We render ourselves vulnerable through trust as it puts
in place a certain risk that was not there before.

(Nys, 2016)

Introduction

The UK Act on 'presumed consent' to organ donation
(Department of Health and Social Care, 2020) came into force in
May 2020. This Act may be a dangerous development. This new
law was a quiet development at the height of the coronavirus
pandemic. The time was difficult for those not computer literate
to be able to access online forms to record their wish to 'opt out'.
Such information was difficult to access while libraries were
closed and GPs were not so accessible for face-to-face discussion
during the pandemic.

Despite the government promised public information
campaigns, many people appear to be unaware of the implications
of the Act and how to 'opt out'.

Some 'modern', secular bioethicists and practitioners would
argue that organs are preferably procured fresh from a live patient to
prevent the possibility of organ ischaemia prior to transplantation.
This argument worries most right-thinking people. Such 'progressive'
developments in transplant practice should be prevented by an
internationally agreed, ethical evidence-base for establishing safe
criteria for death confirmation.

Diagnosing death

According to UK NHS guidance on brain death, "brain death
(also known as brain stem death) is when a person on an artificial

life support machine no longer has any brain functions. This means they will not regain consciousness or be able to breathe without support" (NHS, 2022).

Two American neuroscience experts, however, recommend that Clinicians should not allow a dismal prognosis to introduce bias into declaring brain death but should strictly adhere to the clear medicolegal criteria (Burns and Login, 2020). These American neuroscience experts, advocate two critical lessons in patient care: first, the need for rigorous understanding of the means by which brain death is diagnosed and second, the important distinction between a grave prognosis versus brain death (Burns and Login, 2020).

Brain death needs to be medically and legally, strictly defined. In their paper, these two specialists contend that the diagnosis of brain death can only be made, in the absence of intoxication, hypothermia, or certain medical illnesses such as hypothyroidism. A patient with severe hypoxic-ischaemic brain injury may meet the particular neurological features of brain death but concurrent profound hypothyroidism may preclude such a diagnosis.

Universally accepted, ethical criteria for death confirmation and certification are long overdue and a medical imperative. Some countries regard brain stem death as proof of certifiable death, while others regard total brain death as confirming death. Without a true system for certifying death, the attendant, ethical dilemmas for health professionals are apparent.

Brain death

In general, the declaration of brain death usually requires that the cause of brain injury be known, the irreversibility of the injury is certain and important neurological signs of brain function are absent (Scott et al., 2013).

Apnea

The Greek word 'apnea' literally means 'without breath'. There are three types of apnea: obstructive, central and mixed. Of the three types of apnea, obstructive (sleep apnea) is the most common.

The following abstract is from an article in Respiratory Care in 2013: *Apnea Testing During Brain Death Assessment: A Review of Clinical Practice and Published Literature* (Scott et al., 2013):

The diagnosis of brain death is a complex process. Strong knowledge of neurophysiology and an understanding of brain death aetiology must be used to confidently determine brain death. The key findings in brain death are unresponsiveness and absence of brainstem reflexes in the setting of a devastating neurological injury. These findings are coupled with a series of confirmatory tests and the diagnosis of brain death is established based on consensus recommendations. The drive to breathe in the setting of an intense ventilatory stimulus (i.e., respiratory acidosis) is a critical marker of brainstem function. Consequently, apnea testing is an important component of brain death assessment. This procedure requires close monitoring of a patient as all ventilator support is temporarily removed and $PaCO_2$ (partial pressure of carbon dioxide) levels are allowed to rise. A "positive" test is defined by a total absence of respiratory efforts under these conditions. While APNEA testing is not new, it still lacks consensus standardisation regarding the actual procedure, monitored parameters and evidence-based safety measures that may be used to prevent complications.

The Apnea test – a safe test?

Complications associated with apnea testing include hypoxaemia, hypotension, acidosis, hypercapnia (the increase in partial pressure of carbon dioxide ($PaCO_2$) above 45mmhg) increased intracranial pressure, pulmonary hypertension and cardiac arrythmias. Cases of cardiac arrest and pneumothorax have also been reported (Scott et al., 2013).

Such risks have resulted in families understandably refusing apnea testing. It is suggested that informed consent to apnea testing via a surrogate is required as conducting this test to determine whether the patient is dead for the purpose of organ procurement, puts the patient at risk of harm, without consent, for the interests of someone else (Yanke and Rady et al., 2020).

Doppler techniques for testing of brain death

It is argued that patients who cannot have an apnea test because of very low blood pressure or low oxygen levels must have additional radiographic testing, such as radionuclide studies, transcranial Doppler ultrasound, or cerebral angiography, to confirm brain death. The American Academy of Neurology has for considerable time, accepted the use of transcranial Doppler ultrasound to diagnose brain death while acknowledging some limitations (American Academy of Neurology, 1995).

Transcranial Doppler is a sensitive instrument for the diagnosis of brain death. The demonstration of specific blood flow patterns in the anterior and posterior circulation systems can have the limitation of a frequent false finding of no flow, especially when using the transtemporal approach in older women. It was concluded in a study that (where possible), the transorbital Doppler approach is a useful addition for the diagnosis of brain death (Lampl et al., 2002).

The Ischaemic penumbra

Developments in neuroscience are a blessing for many patients who may have suffered what appears to be catastrophic brain injury due to acute stroke. The concept of the ischaemic penumbra was defined over forty years ago by Lindsay Symon and his group and is now an established principle of all acute stroke therapies (Davis and Donnan, 2021). The concept of the ischaemic penumbra was a revolutionary concept which meant that acute stroke should be understood as an evolving process, with definition of cerebral blood flow thresholds for reversible and irreversible cerebral ischaemia. This dynamic process showed progressive cerebral ischaemic damage over an uncertain period of time. Prior to this, the firm dogma was that immediate brain tissue death occurred after stroke onset, with no opportunity for intervention (Astrup et al., 1977).

Lindsay Symon, a professor of neurosurgery at the National Hospital for Neurology and Neurosurgery in Queen Square, in

London, completely overturned this concept. He introduced the term "penumbra" stating that it was "rather like the area around the centre of a candle flame where there is a small bright zone known as the penumbra" (Davis and Donnan, 2021).

Therefore, the possibility of reperfusion treatments, can rescue threatened, critically hypoperfused brain tissue and have been proven to improve clinical outcomes. There is no doubt that the ischaemic penumbra concept will continue to form the basis of therapeutic decisions in acute ischaemic stroke. The digital revolution will take imaging of the penumbra to another level; who knows what the next 40 years will bring! (Davis and Donnan, 2021).

UK Guidelines: Diagnosing brain death

The UK guidelines state the need for diagnosis of brain death to be made by 2 doctors, and at least 1 of them must be a senior doctor. Neither of them can be involved with the hospital's transplant team (NHS, 2022). This NHS guidance is available at: https://www.nhs.uk/conditions/brain-death/and https://www.nhs.uk/conditions/brain-death/diagnosis/

There are known international differences and inconsistencies in various aspects of diagnosing brain death. These may include theory, practice, neurological criteria, lab tests and documentation of brain death. Therefore, universally agreed guidance with ethical criteria for diagnosing brain death for both countries and states is an urgent and long overdue, societal need.

History of medical ethics

From the time of Hippocrates, codes of medical ethics condemned killing by physicians. Together with the biblical prohibition, this age-old rule became part of the medical, ethical and legal opposition to active euthanasia and physician-assisted suicide. Nevertheless, many countries have already broken with this practice by permitting physician-assisted suicide. And once such societies accept killing as an acceptable solution to the expressed desires of a person or their family, it becomes easier to rationalise euthanising patients for their organs as an additional way to ensure effective transplantation – out of compassion for others in need.

Organ Donation (presumed Consent) Act (2020)

Presumed consent is also known as an opt out system and means that unless the deceased has expressed a wish during life, not to be an organ donor then consent will be assumed.

A new system for organ donation that is aimed at saving hundreds of lives, came into UK law on 20 May 2020. This Act will mean all adults in England will be considered potential organ and tissue donors unless they chose to 'opt out' or are in one of the excluded groups.

The following are excluded groups within what is commonly referred to as an 'opt-out' system:

- those under the age of 18
- people who lack the mental capacity to understand the new arrangements and take the necessary action
- visitors to England and those not living here voluntarily
- people who have lived in England for less than 12 months before their death.

The problem of people in need of organ donation

There are more than 6,000 people currently waiting for an organ in the UK. Three people die each day while on the waiting list. It was hoped that the new law will help to reduce the number of people waiting for a life-saving transplant.

Communication problems at the time of the change in the law

Before the changes to the way consent was to be granted, the government's promised public awareness campaign was to make sure people understand the new system and the choices they have. Many people, however, appear unaware of this recently passed Act and its possible implications for the future. It was introduced during the height of the pandemic when GPs were quite inaccessible for helping patients with this issue, Libraries were closed and many older people without computer access or knowledge were unable to complete the online form and needed to be informed of the relevant telephone number to communicate their wish to opt out.

Organ donation laws vary across different countries in the UK (England, Scotland, Wales and Northern Ireland), the Crown dependencies of Jersey, Guernsey and the Isle of Man. People need to acquaint themselves with the individual legal situation for their area and act accordingly so that should they want to opt out, their wishes are registered and family members and friends are aware to help as needed.

Scotland

From 26 March 2021, if people die in circumstances where they could become a donor and have not recorded a donation decision, it may be assumed that they are willing to donate their organs and tissue for transplantation. and this will apply to most adults who are resident in Scotland. Choice is available to people who want to be a donor or not when they die.

The best way to record a donation decision is by registering either an opt-in or opt-out decision on the Organ Donor Register. If people do not record a decision, it may be assumed that they are willing to become a donor. The family will always be asked about people's latest views on donation, to ensure it would not proceed if this was against a person's wishes. It is important that donation decisions are discussed with family and friends so they can support the decision.

Northern Ireland

The current legislation for Northern Ireland is to opt into organ and tissue donation; by joining the NHS Organ Donor Register and sharing the decision with family members. A decision can also be made to record a decision not to be a donor. People can also nominate up to two representatives to make the decision for them. These could be family members, friends, or other trusted people, such as a faith leader.

Following consideration of the issue, in 2020, the health minister said he intends to hold a consultation moving towards introducing a soft opt-out system for organ donation in Northern Ireland. The consultation was expected to begin in late 2020.

Every five years, the department will be required to provide the Northern Ireland Assembly with advice about whether efforts to promote organ donation have been effective and any recommendations it considers appropriate for amending the law to further promote transplantation.

Organ donation – a Christian duty?

Christians generally support organ donation as an altruistic act and accept the process as an individual decision. The Church of England has stated that organ donation is an act of Christian duty (Oliver, 2012).

The Catechism of the Catholic Church states

2296: Organ donation after death is a noble and meritorious act and is to be encouraged as an expression of generous solidarity. While the Catholic Church considers voluntary organ donation as an intrinsic good, Catholics also maintain the right to exercise a decision as to what happens to their body after death, otherwise this undermines the concept of donation as a gift. The body is valued by Christians as the temple of the Holy Spirit (1 Corinthians 6:19) and look forward to a resurrection of the body at the end of time.

(Catholic Bishops Conference of England and Wales, 2020)

Clergy opinion

If people do not record a donation decision (opt in or opt out) it may be assumed that they are willing to become a donor. Catholic Church leaders in Wales have led a united front of Christian opposition to what they called 'ill-judged' proposals for presumed consent rules on organ donation.

Increased organ donation by opt in?

The joint statement from the Welsh churches warns that the belief that the new 'presumed consent' legal status in organ donation would improve the rate of transplantation is not justified by the available evidence. 'Organ donation, surely ought to be a matter of gift and not of duty?' (Morgan, 2012).

It is important for doctors and healthcare providers to be knowledgeable about different theological and cultural views on death and organ donations as nations are becoming more multicultural. Differing opinions can arise depending on whether the death is categorised as brain death or cease of the heartbeat (Oliver et al, 2011). Many different major religious groups and denominations have varying views on organ donation from deceased and live bodies, depending on their ideologies.

Proposed arguments for automatic organ donation

- More than 6,500 people in the UK need a transplant, but a shortage of donors means that around 3,500 transplants are carried out annually.
- Advances in medical science mean that the number of people whose lives could be saved by a transplant is rising more rapidly than the number of willing donors.
- The law as it stands condemns many, some of them children, to an unnecessary death, simply because of the shortage of willing donors, while, as the BMA puts it, bodies are buried or cremated complete with organs that could have been used to save lives.
- Doctors and surgeons can be trusted not to abuse the licence which a change of the law would grant them.
- Objections to a change in the law are sheer sentimentality. A dead body is an inanimate object, incapable of feeling.

Proposed arguments against automatic organ donation

- Few people question the value of transplant operations or the need for more donors. But a programme designed to recruit more donors is preferable to a change in the law.

- The proposed change implies that our bodies belong to the state as soon as we are dead. The assumption is offensive to many people.
- Organ removal without the expressed wish of deceased people could be distressing for their relatives.
- The proposed change in the law can be open to abuse, with the possibility of death being hastened to secure an organ needed by some other patient.
- The safeguard – that is, the right to refuse permission for your organs to be removed– is inadequate. Terminally ill patients or relatives would be made to feel selfish if permission were withheld.
- Families may feel the wishes of their loved ones are more ambiguous compared to opt-in systems, leading to higher risk of family refusal.
- The apparently urgent need for organs can give rise to a push for euthanasia acceptance by society (The Week Staff, 2020).

Obtaining vital organs

The idea of killing someone for the sake of obtaining their organs and transplanting them is gaining enthusiasts (see Chapter 16).

The dead donor rule and imminent death donation

To be considered as 'viable', organs cannot be taken from a cadaver. It is argued, convincingly, that 'brain death' has been invented to harvest viable organs from still-living people. Only when a person's heart stops beating and their breathing ceases for a determinate amount of time can it be said that death has truly occurred. It can be concluded that time is necessary for the brain to heal and recover.

The scarcity of vital organs has caused US government agencies and international medical conferences in 2018 and 2019 to discuss the ethical implications of approving such a policy. Prior to this debate and to protect severely ill patients from being killed for the sake of their organs, the medical field had adopted the 'dead donor rule' which stipulated those donors must meet the legal criteria for death before any vital organ can be taken from their body for transplantation (Goldberg, 2019).

What defines death?

There are different definitions of death. In 1981, the US adopted the Uniform Determination of Death Act (UDDA), which classifies someone as dead either after heart death, that is, irreversible cessation of circulatory or respiratory functions or brain death, that is, irreversible cessation of all functions of the entire brain.

The UDDA Act (1981) has since been adopted by most US states and is intended to provide a comprehensive and medically sound basis for determining death in all situations.

Other countries define death somewhat differently. The UK and India define death solely as the permanent cessation of brainstem function. Israel, Saudi Arabia, South Africa, Japan, Australia and New Zealand follow the whole brain criteria for death. However, they have developed differing tests to determine what constitutes such whole brain death.

Imminent death organ donations (IDD)

Imminent death organ donations (IDD) might be applicable to an individual with devastating neurological injury that is considered irreversible and who is not brain dead. The individual would be unable to participate in medical decision making; therefore, decisions about organ donation would be made by a surrogate or might be addressed by the potential donor's advanced directive.

IDD might also be applied to a patient who has capacity for medical decision making, is dependent on life support, has decided not to accept further life support and indicates the desire to donate organs prior to forgoing life support and death.

Recovery from comas

Patricia White Bull of Albuquerque, New Mexico, woke up, having been unresponsive for sixteen years after suffering a lack of oxygen while giving birth to her son Mark. Two examples of patients who woke up after a 19-year coma are Polish railroad worker, Jan Grzebski, who suffered from a brain tumour and car accident victim, Terry Wallis.

A South African car accident survivor, Ayanda Nqinana, re-awoke after a seven-year coma. On the other hand, Ariel

Sharon, former prime minister of Israel, was stricken with a stroke in 2006 and remained in a coma until his death in 2014. Under Israel's dead donor rule, it would have been unethical and illegal to harvest Ariel Sharon's heart and kidneys during that period.

It is argued that the issue of euthanasia and its proposed extension to death by donation is an important challenge we, as a society, must face. One essential ingredient of this process is to overcome the emerging support for sanctioned killing and to re-anchor contemporary culture in the protection of life rather than its disposal (Goldberg, 2019). The pro-life community needs to be prepared for the issue to arise in the future.

Importance of truth in death certification

In Oregon, where assisted suicide is legal, 'doctors are told to record the patient's underlying disease as the cause of death – as if J.F.K. died of Addison's disease rather than an assassin's bullet' (Cook, 2018).

For all of us, dying is the last and perhaps most significant moment of life. Which is why recording the exact cause of death and ethical means of its true confirmation is a matter that calls for scrupulous accuracy – not just for epidemiological and legal purposes, but also as part of our personal and social history.

Expert medical and nursing opinion

A former transplant chief for the UK government, Professor Chris Rudge, said he was 'horribly opposed' to the proposal that everybody's organs will be automatically considered for donation. He said: 'I think I would opt out because organ donation should be a present and not for the state to assume that they can take my organs without asking me' (Rudge, 2017).

Once a DNACPR order is in place, it is a concern that treatment and care can deteriorate. There have been reports that an American former medical proponent of voluntary organ donation now believes that it is difficult to predict how a decision to donate one's organs will affect one's end of life care, depending on the circumstances and the different protocols for organ donation that are currently possible (Valko, 2012).

Donation after circulatory death (DCD)

This method of obtaining organs refers to the retrieval of organs from those who have died because their heart stopped either naturally or because life support was discontinued and death is diagnosed and confirmed using cardiorespiratory criteria.

Patients for potential organ donation after circulatory death (DCD) can be classified according to the modified Maastricht classification of DCD, which identifies five categories of potential donors and circumstances in which DCD can occur.

The modified Maastricht classification of DCD:

Category I	Dead on arrival at hospital	Uncontrolled
Category II	Unsuccessful resuscitation	Uncontrolled
Category III	Awaiting cardiac arrest	Controlled
Category IV	Cardiac arrest in a brain-stem-dead donor	Controlled
Category V	Unexpected cardiac arrest in a critically ill patient	Uncontrolled

In the intensive care unit, controlled DCD is predominantly from Category III patients as this allows warm ischaemic time to be minimised and organ outcomes optimised. Occasionally, Category III patients are located elsewhere in the hospital emergency departments or general wards. Category IV patients who have already been pronounced dead and are awaiting organ donation to occur but suffer cardiac arrest can still become DCD donors (Dunne and Docherty, 2011).

Worldwide, there is considerable variation in the contributions that DCD makes to deceased organ donation overall. While some countries have no DCD programmes whatsoever, in others such as the UK, Netherlands and Australia, the contributions are significant.

Precipitate practice

At first, there was some criticism of DCD on legal, medical and ethical grounds, especially after a 1997 segment of the TV show *60 Minutes*. This exposed the case of a young gunshot victim whose organs were taken by DCD but the medical examiner who conducted the autopsy said he believed the injury was survivable.

Nevertheless, this new kind of organ donation was deemed ethically acceptable in 2000 by the US Institutes of Medicine while unfortunately also finding opinion is divided on the option of non-heart-beating donation for the patient who is ventilator dependent but conscious and who wants to stop life-sustaining treatment. As of 2015, DCD comprised 8.9% of all transplants in the US, but the procedure is still little-known to the public (Valko, 2017).

In the UK, DCD donation has increased substantially over the last decade from 335 donors in 2009–2010, to 634 in 2019–2020, representing 40% of all deceased organ donors in that year (NHS Blood and Transplant, 2020).

The success of the UK DCD programme can be attributed to the 'resolution' of the apparent legal, ethical and professional obstacles to this model of donation. The underpinning principle of the programme is that donation can on many occasions be legitimately viewed as part of the care that a person might wish to receive at the end of their lives.

How can such a wish be truly ascertained? Whether 'care' is the correct term here is questionable. It should never be applied on the unethical assumption of a patient or a family's wishes.

Policies and guidance

Various publications and professional documents have supported the introduction of controlled DCD programmes into the UK and they should form the basis for the local policies that describe how this type of donation is incorporated into a patient's end of life care. Important national documents relating to DCD include the following professional guidance:

- Consensus statement on DCD from the British Transplantation Society and Intensive Care Society.
- A Code of Practice for the diagnosis and confirmation of death from the Academy of the Medical Royal Colleges.

The guidance provides up-to-date guidance on all aspects of controlled DCD, including:

o   decision-making
o   care before treatment withdrawal
o   criteria for DCD
o   treatment withdrawal and stand down
o   diagnosis of death and post-mortem interventions
o   ethical guidance and legal guidance.

Organ donations after brain death

In the UK, an average of 2.7 transplantable organs are retrieved from DCD donors compared to 3.6 from donation after brain death (DBD) donors. The lower donation potential of DCD is due, in large part, to the ischaemic injury suffered by solid organs in the time interval between treatment withdrawal and cold perfusion, with the liver and pancreas being particularly vulnerable.

In a letter to faith groups, Professor John Forsythe, Medical Director and Dr Dale Gardiner, National Clinical Lead for Organ Donation, of NHS Blood and Transplant, said:

The essential principle we want to reinforce is that a person's faith and beliefs will be respected in discussions with their families about donation, should the opportunity arise – whether or not they have recorded their decision in the register.
https://www.cbcew.org.uk/organ-donation-guidelines-200520/

Family support needs

After writing to NHS Blood and Transplant about organ donation in light of the coronavirus pandemic, Bishop Paul Mason, the Catholic lead bishop for healthcare and mental health, received assurances that practices in supporting families are continuing during the unprecedented time of COVID-19.

- Families of every potential organ donor are to be approached to discuss whether their loved one would have wanted to donate their organs.
- NHS Blood and Transplant also noted that patients who have had COVID-19, or have been exposed to the virus, will not be considered as organ donors.

(Roman Catholic Diocese of Westminster, 2020 –See the link: www.cbcew.org.uk/wp-content/uploads/sites/3/2020/04/ Organ-Donation-Guidelines-Feb-2020.pdf)

Faulty medical science

NHS staff have been told to take "extra caution" when extracting organs after a baby who was declared 'brain-dead' began breathing again. Doctors treating the child at a London hospital conducted two sets of brain stem tests before seeking a second opinion to confirm their diagnosis. Two weeks later, a nurse at the hospital noticed the boy, then four months, was breathing.

The safety alert sent to staff at NHS Blood and Transplant, seen by Sky News, advised them to pay "particular attention to pre-conditions and red flags" in children after the boy began breathing independently.

The child's father has told Sky News that:
extra caution is not good enough.
They did four brain stem tests on him and certified his death.
When I asked whether there was an alternative test, they said no.
https://news.sky.com/story/
nhs-staff-told-to-take-extra-caution-extracting-organs-after-
brain-dead-baby-starts-breathing-12707621
If there's just one test to prove someone is alive or dead,
it should be 100 per cent accurate. They said, it's a miracle.
It's not a miracle, this is faulty medical science.

Code of practice on brain stem testing

The Academy of Royal Medical Colleges, which sets the test, said in August (2022) that it would rewrite the code of practice on brain stem testing after the child's case came to light. It has not offered parents or hospitals advice on what to do in the meantime.

David Jones, a professor of bioethics at St Mary's University, warned there was a risk of organs being extracted from living children:

The doctors could have said 'This child is dead'
and they could have taken his organs,
but they didn't because of an ongoing legal issue,
and because they didn't, they later found out that he wasn't dead.

According to Professor Jones, more and more clinicians are now expressing concern about brain stem testing (Chowdhury, 2022).

The High Court, in June 2022, ruled against the parents of 12-year-old Archie Battersbee, after Barts Health NHS Trust took them to court on the recommendation of doctors who said he was brain-dead.

After a legal battle, lasting weeks, Archie's life support machine was switched off and he died on 6 August 2022 (Chowdhury, 2022).

Conclusion

An American pro-life nurse has suggested that the bottom line is that we need to demand transparency and information before such policies on organ donation are quietly implemented (Valko, 2017). Such policies refer to the promotion of live organ retrieval from the dying/brain-injured but not brain dead, on ventilators and considered hopeless in terms of survival or predicted 'quality of life'.

Dramatic as this may seem, UK healthcare scandals have occurred to the shocked realisation of the public when exposed. Dying and non-dying patients have been deeply sedated, opioid overdosed and deliberately dehydrated for days and weeks, by means of the LCP practice.

'Opting out' of organ donation

A 'compassion' that extinguishes life on account of suffering, practices cruelty against this essential person. Adding in the idea that your organs may save another person's life does not change this perspective. True compassion balances kindness towards suffering with respect for the boundaries and purposes of persons as defined by their Creator (Goldberg, 2019).

Vulnerable people of all ages, need health professionals to stand as advocates for them if they are unsure about their status in relation to organ donation. They may be concerned that they are to be the intended victims of euthanasia for organ harvesting.

All adults in England are automatically organ donors from 20 May 2020, unless they have registered their wish to opt out.

It is possible to opt out of the organ donation scheme by going to the link: https://www.organdonation.nhs.uk/register-your-decision/refuse-to-donate/refuse-donation-form or phoning the helpline on 0300 123 23 23.

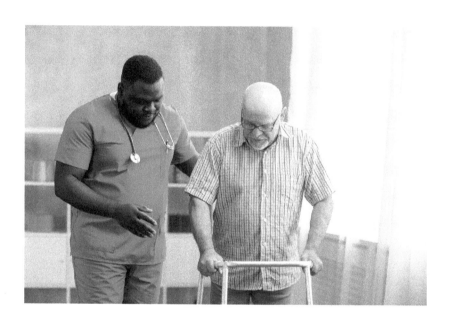

Chapter 13
Assisted suicide

*Preventing suffering and virtually all
difficulty is now paramount.
In such a cultural milieu, eliminating suffering
easily mutates into eliminating the sufferer*

(Levin, 2008)

Introduction

This chapter precedes the next one on euthanasia as the line between
assisted suicide and euthanasia is becoming increasingly fine – and is
becoming almost invisible, where assisted suicide is legalised.

Repeated attempts to legalise assisted suicide in the UK, engender
fear in vulnerable groups who, it is often wrongly assumed, would be
the first to welcome a change in UK law. This is not the case. Opposition
to assisted suicide and the subsequent prospect of euthanasia is one of
the greatest battles over human rights of our time. The threat of a
change in UK law on assisted suicide has been described as 'unnecessary,
ethically dubious and dangerous' (Galloway, 2021).

Beliefs in treatment futility can link with those beliefs that
dignity is contingent purely on physical integrity and independence.
Such beliefs play into the dangerous UK lobby which has been
ongoing for years for assisted suicide. This is a danger to the
elderly and the disabled. Complacent belief that 'safeguards will
protect the vulnerable' is a fantasy as seen in countries and states
where assisted suicide is legal. Legalised assisted suicide will
precede euthanasia. It is wilfully naïve to suggest that pressure,
albeit tacitly, will not be felt by the vulnerable, both from
institutions which want freed-up beds or family members who
cannot wait for a legacy in these economically challenging times.

Lobbyists for assisted suicide, need to bear in mind that their
personal views (even what has been described as selfish views) can
so easily be imposed on both the vulnerable and the majority who

are totally opposed to a change in the law as reflected in the repeated UK failed attempts to date, for legal assisted suicide.

'Death with dignity'

The persisting efforts to change the law on assisted suicide to allow 'death with dignity' can mean that practitioners working in opposition to such a culture are often considered to be lacking in 'compassion'.

The repeated attempts in the UK for assisted suicide pose inherent dangers to the vulnerable and cause concern to all pro-life people. The sad statistic for people's requests, where it is legal in Europe and other countries, is the generally common and consistently reported 'fear of being a burden' rather than the issue of pain.

The Nazi euthanasia programme killed people, whereas legalised assisted suicide, invites people to be killed by their 'carers'. What an immense pressure to place upon the vulnerable and health professionals who did not enter their professions to be expected to help their patients to kill themselves. Their human rights and vocations need consideration.

Patients' real feelings

The topic of assisted suicide (a more honest term than assisted dying) generates debate on a variety of levels – ethical, moral, religious, spiritual, political, cultural, psychological, professional and legal. Medical help for people to end their lives is variously described as: physician-assisted dying, assisted dying, medical aid in dying and assisted suicide.

It is not uncommon for patients with advanced, incurable disease to express a desire to hasten their death. Health professionals often have difficulty responding to such statements and find it challenging to ascertain why these statements are made. They may struggle to determine whether a 'desire to die' statement is about a request for hastened death, a sign of psychosocial distress, or merely a passing comment that is not intended to be heard literally as a death wish (Hudson et al., 2006). All these reasons need sensitive exploration between the Good Samaritans health professional and their patients.

Judeo Christian beliefs

It is argued that from a Jewish perspective that,

A person's own body and soul are not his own possessions
to harm or destroy. Rather they are given by God to
the human being in trust. Since God gives and takes away
life, any form of suicide rejects God's sovereignty. In turn,
protecting and respecting life requires that we follow the
universal ethical values of the Abrahamic faiths
(also known as the Judeo-Christian worldview) and
thus reject contemporary secularism's view that when
suffering renders a person's life burdensome to himself
or to others, we can and may dispose of that life.

(Goldberg, 2019)

Media focus on assisted suicide

Intense media coverage of past and recent UK court cases and high-profile testimonies have helped to project the current debate surrounding the legalisation of assisted suicide to the forefront of the public's consciousness. This focus generates several emotions in all of us as it reminds us of our own mortality and humanity.

Even though medicine evolves in its ability to manage symptoms well at any stage of life in the 21st century, this proposed 'option', where legal, now pertains to all ages and non-terminal conditions in some countries in Europe. Media attention on this topic needs to be balanced by the need for effective care of the dying by well-educated professionals. The specialty of palliative care needs increased focus in the media and campaigns for well-resourced palliative care areas which most people want for themselves and their families.

Effects on health professionals

One group which is generally overlooked in relation to this subject comprises those expected to prescribe and help the patient with taking the drug to end their life. The autonomy of patients appears to trump the rights, beliefs and conscience of opposed health professionals by a possible change in UK law.

Emerging evidence concludes that such a role can be devastating for the medical professional involved. It is inevitable should the law be changed, that such a role will be devolved to nurses. Those involved professionals may believe that such a practice is compassionate, yet other practitioners will perceive such practice as 'false compassion' with its attendant dangers which are explored in this chapter.

A disabled member of the House of Lords, Baroness Campbell of Surbiton has said about assisted suicide: "Assisted dying is practised in Belgium, the Netherlands and elsewhere. Whatever the initial intentions were, decisions to end life in those places are now not taken only by the individual. It is not an autonomous act. The slippery slope is oiled by the vague euphemism of assisted dying" (Campbell, 2015).

Arguments for assisted suicide

The two most common arguments in favour of legalising assisted suicide are respect for patient autonomy and relief of suffering. A third, related, argument, is that assisted suicide is a safe medical practice, requiring assistance from a healthcare professional.

Patient autonomy

This refers to a patient determining which medical interventions to choose or forgo. Beauchamp and Childress, in their well-known textbook, *Principles of Biomedical Ethics*, advanced four fundamental principles as a framework for addressing ethically complex cases: respect for autonomy, beneficence, non-maleficence and justice. Of these principles, autonomy may exert the most influence on medical practice. Patient autonomy may serve as the justification for informed consent; only after a thorough explanation of risks and benefits can the patient have the agency to decide on treatments or participation in medical research. This logic, it is argued, naturally extends to assisted suicide; patients accustomed to making their own healthcare decisions throughout life should also be permitted to control the circumstances of their deaths.

Relief of suffering

At its core, medicine has always aimed to relieve the suffering of patients from illness and disease. In the West, Hippocrates' ancient oath pledged to use treatments to help the sick but not 'administer a poison to anybody when asked to do so' (Loeb Classical Library, 1923). In contrast, advocates of assisted suicide argue that relief of suffering through lethal ingestion is humane and compassionate – if the patient is dying and suffering is refractory. It is argued that some of the most compelling arguments made in favour of assisted suicide come from patients who suffer from life-threatening illnesses.

Safe medical practice

Assisted suicide is praised by advocates for being a safe medical practice – that is, doctors can ensure death in a way that suicide by other means cannot. Aid in dying thus becomes one option among many possibilities for care of the dying. Although individual laws vary, most propose some safeguards to prevent abuses. Some argue that abuse is inevitable.

Safeguards include:

o   The requirement that a patient electing for assisted suicide be informed of all end of life options.
o   Two witnesses to confirm that the patient is autonomously requesting assisted suicide.
o   Patients are free of coercion and able to ingest the lethal medication themselves.

Arguments against assisted suicide

The moral prohibition in discussions against assisted suicide can appear to be lacking yet should be the guiding principle. Common arguments include the 'slippery slope' danger, safeguard limitations, the problem and challenge of suffering and public safety.

The slippery slope

A worrying development in a supposed suicide prevention association is revealed by the non-profit organisation, the American Association of Suicidology.

This Association has even stated that terminally ill people requesting doctor-prescribed death is not really suicide. This accepting attitude has been described as spitting in the face of the hospice care approach, founded by the great medical humanitarian, Dame Cicely Saunders. She believed that suicide prevention was a key hospice service that protected the dignity of her patients (Smith, 2017).

Assisted suicide safeguards

Assisted suicide is a wrong moral concept. Stated safeguards by no means make a change in the law more acceptable or palatable. Any discussion on safeguards pre-supposes that the aim to change current law is legitimate – it is not. Many of the so-called 'safeguards' were rejected as unsafe when they appeared in the late Lord Joffe's Assisted Dying Bill in 2006. Lord Joffe can be commended for his honesty in giving evidence to his own Select Committee: 'This is a first stage. I believe that this Bill initially should be limited, although I would prefer it to be of much wider application' (Joffe, 2006).

False compassion can lead to challenging cases making for bad laws. Any change in the current law would give free rein to eugenics and economically driven or defeatist health professionals and others who would act with impunity. One example is shown by a mother in Quebec who wants to change the law for her four-year-old son to be euthanised because he is disabled.

Assisted suicide, another 'developed' role devolved to nurses?

Assisted suicide, once legalised in the UK, would inevitably require nurses to perform the associated if not actual task as part of the 'developed role' of the nurse.

Nurses are increasingly taking on practice roles, which were previously the sole remit of doctors. This would be another area of ethical discord for those nurses (and doctors) who are opposed to assisted suicide. They would face a battle for their right to conscientious objection to be accommodated.

Nurses are now involved in other countries with the provision and even the drug administration where assisted suicide is legal, such as Belgium, where euthanasia is now allowed also for children who 'want to die'. Whether such children, as with their adult counterparts, are offered ethical, psychological care and counselling is debatable.

Public safety

Even in a free, democratic society there are limits to human freedom and the law must not be changed to accommodate the wishes of a small number of sadly desperate and determined people who wish to impose their goals on all. A small group of people who are, or who are not, oblivious to the momentous effects such a change in the law, need to be aware of the far-reaching, negative consequences. Health professionals who also have conscientious objection to such a law would have pressure inevitably applied to them to comply with a change in the law.

The meaning of suffering

We have a deep-seated need to understand the meaning of suffering – its causes and its purpose – but this does not entitle us to decide suffering lives are better off dead if we cannot come to terms with this aspect of the world. 'Suffering' can be caused not always by (uncontrolled) physical pain but by feelings of abandonment, or of being a burden. These feelings may impact on patients who may feel that society only values the 'quality' or 'productive' life.

Patients who suffer in this way are to be cherished by those charged with looking after them. A professional's prime vocation is to show good will and compassion in caring for their patients' physical, emotional, psychological and spiritual needs (holistic care) in liaison with the relevant others who comprise the multidisciplinary team.

Critical issues in caring for patients' symptoms

My experience is that physical pain and suffering are not necessarily all-encompassing when patients feel loved and valued for themselves. Patient dignity is not contingent on physical condition but on trusting relations between patient and carers. Physical pain can be exacerbated by the anxiety felt by lack of support and understanding of true needs.

The public have long-held expectations of professional expertise in time of need, whether in time of birth, or acute trauma, or in the dying phase. Patients, whatever their state and time of life, do not truly expect their professional carers to be able to abolish symptoms together with their lives.

Contemporary moral discourse

Opposition to changing the law on assisted suicide is due to the ethical and moral concerns and the risk that such changes would pose to public safety and especially the most vulnerable in society.

Alasdair MacIntyre, in his seminal book *After Virtue* (MacIntyre, 1981), observed that contemporary moral discourse is so dysfunctional because it has lapsed into an emotivism in which ethical terminology is used in an incongruent manner, because:

- it is separated from its anchors in the bodies of thought which make it meaningful
- it rests on different and often incommensurable assumptions or narratives; and yet

- it is communicated in public as if it has a universal foundation and meaning.

In such a context, moral discourse is unintelligible because there is no shared system of meaning that can be used to reconcile or adjudicate over moral differences. Therefore, 'compassion' can be used with equal public weight to describe physician-assisted suicide by those who are in favour of it and sharply to critique it by those who are opposed to it.

A key aspect of Alasdair MacIntyre's critique of contemporary moral discourse: that often our moral claims rest on incommensurable visions of what constitutes the good life and without a capacity to deal with the truth or the falsity of these narratives, is that we are doomed to an ultimately hopeless form of moral debate (Fleming, 2019).

The moral status of human beings

A professor of ethics and legal philosophy views human rights as,
... being rooted in the universal interests of human beings, each and every one of whom possesses an equal moral status arising from their common humanity. In other words, in defending human rights, we will need to appeal to the inherent value of being a member of the human species and, in addition, the interests shared by all human beings in things like friendship, knowledge, achievement, play and so on. And we will need to ask whether these considerations generate duties that are owed to each and every human being.

(Tasioulos, 2017)

One Christian ethicist suggests that we should maximise care rather than minimising suffering, which might include eliminating the sufferer (Meilaender, 2017). However, the erosion of human beings' moral status is now being accelerated by beliefs about the economic non-viability of an embryo, the aged, the brain-damaged person and the disabled, despite progress being made on behalf of them all.

A defeatist culture of death?

Strong effort is required to counter the ideology of a defeatist culture of death. A culture of defeatist medicine and nursing can affect the experience for patients and their families who have a need for hope shown in the smallest ways. This need must be known and respected. Patients may recognise that cure may not be a reality but acts of kindness and attention to detail all help lift the spirit and life quality for the patient and family and friends. What affects the patient will affect the family and friends and vice versa.

Depression in advanced illness

Up to half of patients with cancer suffer from symptoms of depression (Rosenstein, 2011). Elderly people also suffer from high rates of depression and suicide (Brown et al., 2016). Because depression often manifests somatically (Tylee and Gandhi, 2005), if patients are not screened, clinicians miss half of all cases of clinical depression (Ansseau et al., 2004). The proponents of holistic care are vindicated by these findings and the need for referral to the appropriate care.

Stephen Phillips, an Indiana medical professor, suggests that sometimes true care is holding someone's hand and suffering right alongside him. It is not taking his life or suggesting that he take his own (Wurster, 2018).

Faith beliefs

The Judeo-Christian worldview is that assisted suicide is against the law of God. All three Abrahamic faiths oppose and condemn assisted suicide. For people to reject the tenets of all three faiths, by acceptance of assisted suicide, those asking for assisted suicide, or those practitioners who are prepared to assist, means that they reject God's enduring commandment, upon which Christian civilisation depends. All the main faiths believe that life is sacred and the following tenets are agreed:

- God the Creator owns every person's life.
- The end of everyone's life is fixed by God and not by the patient, doctor, judge, or Parliament.
- We all are ordered to die a natural death and cannot rush our death.

In addition to those tenets, Christianity holds the following to be true:

- Life is a sacred gift from God (Genesis 2:7).
- When given the choice between life and death, God told Israel to 'choose life' (Deuteronomy 30:19).
- The prohibition against killing innocent people is formalised as part of the Ten Commandments, 'You shall not murder' (Exodus 20:13; Deuteronomy 5:17).
- God has the final say over death (1 Corinthians, 15:26, 54–56; Hebrews 2:9, 14).

For followers of Islam there are many verses in the final Holy Book, *Al Quran*, which emphasise these basic pro-life beliefs about assisted suicide. One such verse is '*In the Name of GOD, the Most Compassionate, the Most Merciful Take not life which Allah has made sacred*' (Chapter 6, verse 151).

In Judaism the clear instruction is given – 'You shall not murder' in Exodus 20:13 and Deuteronomy 5:17.

Medicine and nursing in the 21st century ever seek to increase the percentage of patients achieving a pain-free existence, including in the terminal phase of illness.

The term 'assisted dying' is the term used in the many repeated yet failed attempts in the UK for a change in the law. Who would not want to assist a person with their holistic care needs at the end of life? This is not assisted suicide which should be the term used by those lobbying for a change in law to allow people to kill themselves.

Imposition of minority views on the entire population

It is often overlooked that anyone can take their own life. It seems incomprehensible that those who wish for this approach to their death do not take a long view on behalf of the people who will be inevitably most affected by the law being changed. This would include the vulnerable elderly and the disabled, who would be caused fear and distress by possible pressure being applied to them. Many of those in these vulnerable groups are already feeling an insidious fear of being a burden to health services and their families. This fear is exacerbated by those lobbyists who never appear to acknowledge it on their behalf or the fact that safeguards are proving to be no protection in many areas where assisted suicide is legal.

A disabled person's perspective

Baroness Jane Campbell said in her contribution to the debate on the Falconer Bill (2014) on assisted dying:

Terminally ill and disabled people are in a worse position today than was the case five years ago. National economic instability means that public support services are under more pressure than ever. That has hardened public attitudes towards progressive illnesses, old age and disability. Words such as "burden", "scrounger" and "demographic time bomb" come to mind and hate crime figures in relation to vulnerable people have increased dramatically. This is a dangerous time to consider facilitating assistance with suicide for those who most need our help and support. It is not only dangerous for those who may see suicide as their only option but can be tempting for those who would benefit from their absence.

(Campbell, 2014)

Risk to the vulnerable

The economic situation today is considerably worse than at the time of the Falconer Bill in 2014. Financial abuse of the elderly is now recognised as an increasing form of abuse in the UK which is suffered by thousands of elderly people.

The views of the healthcare professions

The proposals for change to allow assisted suicide, together with its inevitable expansion, are totally unacceptable in the eyes of many nurses and doctors. The many impacts on health professionals are now emerging from studies in Holland where assisted suicide has been legal since 2001.

Most people who are approaching the end of their lives in the UK do not ask a health professional to hasten their death, but a minority of individuals do express a readiness or desire to die. Most patients expressing such sentiments do not go further by asking a nurse to hasten their death. However, it can be difficult where the RCN and the BMA have both taken a neutral stand on assisted suicide. On such a monumental issue, there is no neutral stand possible.

A nursing perspective

Opinions of healthcare professionals and my own experience of palliative care, requires that our experiences be not overlooked in the deliberations for assisted suicide to become law. I have so often experienced the inner strength and compensatory forbearance afforded to so many patients at the most vulnerable time of their lives. They show hope and courage so often at time of death and often for the sake of their loved ones.

The positive narratives of contentment by people at the end of life are superseded, so often, by the lobbyists who can create a climate of fear among the public. This can cause them to believe that the skill and dedication for effective symptom control is sadly lacking. This is not the case. I have been told by several patients that this time of their life, was 'the happiest'.

A bitter legacy

The abuses of the LCP, viewed in retrospect by the relatives of patients placed on it have coloured their attitude to their future care needs and many voice concern that they would prefer assisted suicide to witnessed deaths of relatives. It seemed to them that death following sedation and hydration were the prevailing norm for all at the end of life. This is a bitter legacy of the LCP for people who have had such a sadly negative view on 'palliative care' as they understood it for their family member. LCP practices did not and still do not offer true palliative care and people need to understand this. Where practice remains incomprehensible to relatives, mistrust will arise.

It has been known that relatives would sadly need to refer to the internet to find out what type of latest 'care' involved dehydration of patients when such ongoing practice was not explained.

When someone asks to die

The RCN have issued guidance for nurses who may be placed in a difficult position by a patient requesting assisted suicide: 'When someone asks for your assistance to die' (RCN, 2018). An extensive range of information, audio and video resources on how to conduct difficult conversations can also be found online at the RCN's dedicated end of life care website at: https://www.rcn.org.uk/clinical-topics/End of life-care.

The Royal College of Nursing Assisted Suicide Survey (RCN, 2009)

The RCN is neutral on assisted suicide for people with a terminal illness and this position has been held since 2009, based on a minimal response by members to the RCN survey. The Royal College has dropped its previous opposition to assisted suicide and now neither supports nor opposes a change in the law. This is an untenable position. Nursing's vocation to care will be destroyed should assisted suicide be approved by the membership. The RCN will be watching closely the voting results of the medical colleges on this contentious topic.

The British Medical Association

The BMA, in February 2020, ran one of the biggest surveys of medical opinion on this issue. The survey highlighted those doctors who were in favour, but were not willing, however, to carry out assisted suicide in practice. This would be another source of conscientious objection for pro life doctors as with abortion.

A year of change

On 28 September 2020, the BMA restated its position on assisted dying, asserting that the BMA believes no form of assisted suicide should be made legal within the UK. One year later, on 14 September 2021, the BMA formally adopted 'a neutral position' on physician-assisted dying at the BMA's annual representative meeting (ARM). It narrowly passed a motion to move from the stance of opposing a change in the law to allow physician-assisted suicide and instead to adopt a position of neutrality. Some 49% of representatives (149) voted for the motion, 48% (145) voted against and eight abstained.

A doctor's opinion:

One clinician referring to the pandemic, commenting on yet another attempt to change the law argued that terrible things have happened to people at the fringes of life over the last twenty months. He went on to say this needs acknowledgement and reflection. Now is not the time for assisted dying. Now is the time for us all, doctors and society, to talk about what makes a good death (Randall, 2021).

A possible UK law change for assisted suicide, could mean the destruction of ethical medicine and even medicine itself, as no doctor should accept the role of allowing patients to kill themselves, no matter how carefully couched as 'assisted dying' to make it more palatable.

The Royal College of Physicians

The Royal College of Physicians (RCP) clarifies that it does not support a change in the law to permit assisted dying at the present time following their survey of members in 2019, which revealed that

43.4% of respondents said that the RCP should be opposed to a change in the law on assisted dying, 31.6% said the RCP should support a change in the law and 25% said the RCP should be neutral. Should the RCP find itself in a position of supporting assisted suicide, ethical medicine's demise will be finalised (RCP, 2019).

Based on these results, the RCP Council adopted a position of neutrality on 21 March 2019. 'Neutrality' was defined as neither supporting nor opposing a change in the law, to try to represent the breadth of views within its membership. Regrettably, this position has been interpreted by some as suggesting that the college is either indifferent to legal change or is supportive of a change in the law.

The Kennedy Institute of Bioethics

Dr Daniel Sulmasy, the acting director of the USA Kennedy Institute of Bioethics, has written that moving from opposition to neutrality is not ethically neutral, but a substantive shift from prohibited, to optional. In other words, lack of opposition is tacit approval (White, 2019).

The American Medical Association

In a move which has global repercussions, in 2020, the American Medical Association (AMA) voted to reaffirm its opposition to physician-assisted suicide. The AMA's official position is that legalised assisted suicide is contrary to the physician's role as healer, puts vulnerable patients at risk and would be difficult or impossible to control. The AMA defines physician-assisted suicide as follows:

> Physician-assisted suicide occurs when a physician facilitates a patient's death by providing the necessary means and/or information to enable the patient to perform the life-ending act (e.g., the physician provides sleeping pills and information about the lethal dose, while aware that the patient may commit suicide).

> (AMA, 2020)

Death preferable to life?

The AMA adds that 'it is understandable, though tragic, that some patients in extreme duress – such as those suffering from a terminal, painful, debilitating illness – may come to decide that death is preferable to life. However, permitting physicians to engage in assisted suicide would ultimately cause more harm than good.

Physician-assisted suicide is fundamentally incompatible with the physician's role as healer, would be difficult or impossible to control and would pose serious societal risks. Instead of engaging in assisted suicide, physicians must aggressively respond to the needs of patients at the end of life (AMA, 2020).

The American College of Physicians

In specific reference to physician-assisted suicide, the American College of Physicians (ACP) has affirmed that 'the medical profession should not be neutral regarding matters of medical ethics' (ACP, 2017). The college has stated that it is crucial that a responsible physician perspective be heard as societal decisions are made.

The American College of Physicians acknowledges the range of views on, the depth of feelings about and the complexity of the issue of physician-assisted suicide, but the focus at the end of life should be on efforts to prevent or ease suffering and on the often, unaddressed needs of patients and families. As a society, we need to work to improve hospice and palliative care, including awareness and access.

(ACP, 2017)

Knowledge of palliative care

A recent study found 90% of US adults do not know what palliative care is, but when told its definition, more than 90%

said they would want it for themselves or family members if severely ill (Ende, 2017).

Patients look to their carers to affirm their lives, not offer them death as a defeatist, cheap and easy option. My experience when working in a palliative care unit did not include patient demands for assisted suicide. There was only one request in my experience and the patient was fully aware of the law and the implications for the nurse in breaking the law and would never have wanted to put a professional at risk of prosecution. I remember the same patient's comment at the end of my conversation with her: 'I didn't mean it, you know'.

Effective practitioner-patient relationships allow expression of patient fears, needs and achievement of peace without the need for assisted suicide. This is the reality of nursing experience.

Views of palliative care clinicians

Amy Proffitt, a physician and executive secretary of the UK Association of Palliative Medicine has stated that there is a core question for physicians who are contemplating their vote for or against assisted suicide. She suggested the following question should be asked, 'If the law were changed, would I be willing to supply or administer: (Canada's law includes this) a massive dose of sedative +/- a muscle relaxant to patients with the deliberate intent of bringing about their death?' (Proffitt, 2019).

Baroness Finlay of Llandaff, the palliative care specialist and former president of the BMA, who was at the forefront of the fight against the failed Meacher Bill, has said in relation to the bill:

Are the lives of those who are dying less deserving of efforts to improve their quality, even if prognosis is short? We are told the numbers would be small, yet other legislatures have shown such deaths increase year on year, often with the law's boundaries becoming ever slacker, rising rates of suicides and yet their palliative care remains patchy and inadequate. As observed previously – such legislation would change the moral landscape.

(Finlay, 2021a)

The Baroness added:

The safeguards were effectively meaningless. What appear at first to be safeguards are nothing of the sort, but instead are vague and empty assurances that will provide, at best, only a symbolic function. They present an unworkable ideal which will be virtually impossible to codify and which will be frequently and easily circumvented, misinterpreted, ignored, overlooked and rejected before they are replaced or expanded, as has been witnessed in every other jurisdiction which imagined that assisted suicide or euthanasia could be controlled or contained.

(Caldwell, 2021a)

The National Council for Palliative Care (NCPC) has produced a series of publications designed to inspire confidence and help health and social care professionals start and continue important conversations with people living with a range of conditions. You can find out more at www.ncpc.org.uk/difficult_conversations.

Another doctor's opinion

A UK physician wrote to the British Medical Journal in 2005 about how legalising assisted suicide is unnecessary. This was at a time when there was, yet another attempt at changing the law: If strong opposition is expressed by the medical profession, it is because we are, in-dividually and corporately, profoundly concerned that hastening the death of patients is both wrong and unnecessary. Wrong because deliberately causing death is an immoral act and unnecessary, because we now have the skills and technology to allow people to be comfortable, even as they approach inevitable death. Hastening the death of patients is a neat, sterile and attractive solution to the mess and uncertainty of dying. But it is deeply dangerous, because it is based on the obliteration of, rather than care for, the individual person.

(Hain, 2005)

331

Europe – universal human rights?

The human rights of both patients and professionals alike, in relation to assisted suicide, can be addressed and apparently protected, by the European Convention on Human Rights – Article 2 of the European Court of Human Rights (ECHR): 'a terminally ill or dying person's wish to die, cannot constitute a legal justification to carry out actions intended to bring about death' (ECHR, 2009). These words can apply equally to the terminally ill and the non-dying patient.

Now the UN Human Rights Committee has drafted a memorandum, in 2018, which stated controversially that: abortion and physician-assisted suicide should be universal human rights (Carr, 2018). Should such new perceptions of universal human rights prevail to include the right to kill, the 'right to life' would also condone a 'right to death'.

Apart from the obvious contradiction and dereliction of states' duties to protect their citizens, the respect for human life would only be guaranteed for those persons already born and in good health. Human rights are not the property of ideologies but rather of a humanity that neither forgets nor turns its back on natural law and the Creator.

The UN must recognise the need for effective palliative care in this time of recognised advances in knowledge and skill in this field of care which was pioneered in Britain through the work of Dame Cicely Saunders. Her objection to voluntary euthanasia was that it is: 'a flat denial of God's power and wisdom and above all, of His love' (Raglan, 1969).

The UK All-Party Parliamentary Group on Dying Well

The UK All-Party Parliamentary Group (APPG) on Dying Well opposes a change in the law on assisted dying and euthanasia and argues that high-quality palliative care is instead the solution to end of life issues. Mr Danny Kruger, MP, a member of this group, spoke at a meeting of the group on 16 June 2021. He highlighted the fact that more than one in 25 deaths in the Netherlands are now recorded as euthanasia or assisted dying and that a mere 5% of UK doctors working in end of life care wish to see a change in the law.

Risks vs benefits

Katherine Sleeman, the Laing Galazka Professor of Palliative Care at King's College London, argued at the same meeting against a change in the law. She told the meeting, 'The risk of harm of changing the law outweighs the risk of harm if we leave the law as it is.' She added: 'I am deeply concerned that our societal conversation is being driven by hyperbole and fear, not by evidence and information and it's wrong and dangerous to frame this as a choice between suffering and suicide' (Right to Life News, 2021).

Matt Hancock, the former Minister for Health, attended the same meeting and confirmed that the government is 'not recommending' the introduction of assisted suicide to the UK. During the meeting, he also endorsed setting up a 'What Works' centre to gather evidence on the quality of end of life care in the UK. Mr Hancock said: 'I think it is important that any debate that we have is nested in a wider debate about how we support people better towards the end of their lives' (Right to Life News, 2021).

Europe – the Netherlands and Belgium

Both countries legalised assisted suicide in 2001 and 2002, respectively, but only when the patient's medical condition warranted it. However, safeguards have been breached on many occasions. Common reasons for this 'compassionate' option are now reported as: feeling tired of life or getting old and in 2023, the Dutch government announced its intention to permit euthanasia for children. Belgium has preceded Holland's latest decision on paediatric euthanasia, so the warnings about the slippery slope must be taken seriously – not wilfully ignored.

Assisted suicide – Holland

Countries around the world are making it easier to choose the time and the manner of death. Doctors in Holland, however, the world's euthanasia capital, are starting to worry about the consequences, e.g., the insurance companies that are refusing to pay for treatment but willing to pay for euthanasia.

Theo Boer, between 2005 and 2014, was a member of one of the five Dutch regional boards set up to review every act of euthanasia in Holland where assisted suicide has been legalised (and to report any suspicious cases to prosecutors). He concluded, 'We have put in motion something that we now have discovered has more consequences than we ever imagined… if you think you can have assisted suicide without euthanasia, this is a fantasy' (De Bellaigue, 2019).

Dutch palliative care

Experience in Holland, where euthanasia is widespread, reveals that efforts to kill patients often go wrong and that palliative care, which can enable patients to live through very grave illness in a dignified manner with control of pain and other symptoms, is far less widely available there than here in Britain where the modern hospice movement began (Goldberg, 2019).

Dutch nurses have explained to me that they came to Britain to learn about the specialty of palliative care as it is virtually non-existent in Holland, adding that, 'people have the injection at home'.

Belgium

Children in Belgium have been killed because they were terminally ill, or babies have been killed due to their prospects of an 'intolerable life'. In total, 10% of new-borns are euthanised by Flemish doctors, for whom 'there is no hope of a bearable future', no doubt in agreement with their parents (Cook, 2021).

Activists in countries like the UK and Sweden will perhaps use this novel reasoning to again push for assisted suicide (Cook, 2020). The eugenic basis for such a relentless drive must not be underestimated.

Germany

Germany recently lowered the criteria for assisted suicide to merely 'a person's choice' and, if people are declared mentally incompetent, such a choice can be made for them by someone else: relatives, doctors, or legal authorities. In other words, this is simply a new, legal fiction for eliminating 'undesirable' or 'deplorable' or 'too expensive' human beings.

This change in German law alarmingly establishes euthanasia as a basic human right. In Germany, any reason will be sufficient: fear of illness or old age, romantic disappointments, professional failure, or just the feeling that life is no longer interesting. The 'right to die' movement, especially in Western Europe, will be proud of this development which defies faith, hope and charity. It is legalised murder.

In the wording of the defeated UK Meacher Assisted Dying Bill (2021), to be eligible for assisted suicide, it was not necessary for the person to give any reason as to why they wished to end their life. They simply had to demonstrate a 'settled wish'. So, the proposed UK legislation was based on the presumption that the suicide of a person with limited life expectancy should be supported and facilitated whatever the motivation, if the person has legal capacity and is 'uncoerced' (Wyatt, 2021).

Learning from the past?

Germany's recent acceptance of assisted suicide in 2020 reminds us of the Nazi euthanasia programme. This is well described by a UK pro-life writer:

Germany's highest court has repealed a ban on commercial assisted dying clinics, introduced in 2015, paving the way for doctors and Dignitas-style organisations to supply lethal drugs to seriously ill patients. Relatives or doctors who helped a patient to die were already exempt from punishment. While concern has been expressed about the resurgence of Nazism in Germany, memories seem to have failed when it comes to recalling the Nazi euthanasia programme for the sick and disabled. The 'right to die' campaign would argue that while the latter was compulsory, this is 'voluntary', but how much power does a disabled and/or elderly person have when they depend on others for their very lives? Until now, it has been expected that the strong would care for the weak, but if those who are meant to care, stop caring, the weak might decide that they would be better off dead. The Nazis also portrayed killing the sick as a merciful act, but not even the Nazis thought of shifting responsibility to the victims by getting them to ask for it.

(Farmer, 2020)

Other countries

- Jersey approves principle of legalising assisted suicide by 2023.
- Guernsey and the Isle of Man have initiated debates for a change in their laws.
- Austria and Spain have recently legalised euthanasia. Both countries were hitherto known as Christian/Catholic countries.
- New Mexica (USA) Assisted suicide came into law in June 2021.
- Portugal – Parliament voted on 12 May 2023 to allow medically assisted suicide in limited cases. The legislation states that a person requesting assisted death should be "in a situation of great intensity of suffering, with definitive injury of extreme gravity or serious and incurable disease". A doctor can also euthanize a patient when "medically assisted suicide is impossible due to a physical disability of the patient". Portugal, considered as a Catholic country has passed this new law, which was passed by a strong majority. It overturns earlier vetoes from Catholic President, Marcelo Rebelo de Sousa (Brockhaus, 2023).
- Italy – The referendum to decriminalise assisted suicide was blocked by the Constitutional court in 2022. The proposed Bill would make assisted suicide legal for patients who suffer from an irreversible illness with an 'unfortunate prognosis' that causes 'absolutely intolerable physical and psychological suffering' (Euronews, 2022).

- Canada – The Canadian government is threatening hospices that their funding will be withdrawn if they refuse to enable patient suicide. Is this to be expected? Should the UK cross the line of safety and allow such a terrible legal consequence and diminishing of palliative care as has happened in those countries where such care is becoming 'superfluous' to requirements?
- Australia – In Australia, voluntary assisted dying (VAD) laws have been passed in Australia's six states: Victoria, Western Australia, Tasmania, South Australia, Queensland and New South Wales (where it will come into effect in November 2023, after an 18-month implementation period), Victoria and Western Australia's VAD laws have commenced operation. VAD in Tasmania, and South Australia was passed in 2022 and Queensland in 2023 (End of Life Law in Australia, 2021).
- New Zealand – The law changed in 2021. This permits doctors to prescribe drugs for self-administration and, in cases where an individual is physically unable to take the drug, the doctor can administer the drugs. This allowance is understandably concerning for the future of vulnerable patients and corruptible practitioners.
- Columbia, Latvia, France and Ireland – These countries have all recently blocked a bill for assisted suicide, even though the current French president has made clear his own wish for choosing the time of his own death.

Irrespective of the numbers of countries who have changed their laws, they are not a positive example to follow as a 'compassionate' stand, as such a change is morally wrong. Any country thinking of changing the law to be in step with 'current' and 'compassionate' thinking is deluded. Such a direction also devalues and diminishes palliative care as a compassionate answer to the needs of the ill and dying. Advocates for this 'civilised' ending of life need to remember how abortion, once legalised, bears no relation to what was envisaged by the initial 'strict' criteria. People wilfully ignore what happens once law is changed which used to afford protection for the vulnerable.

Suicide rate increase

Suicide rates in the UK have fallen in recent decades. Contrast this with Oregon, where the overall suicide rate (excluding assisted suicide) has risen by 17% since 'assisted dying' was legalised. Oregon's suicide rate remains one of the highest in the United States (Finlay, 2021a).

Human frailty

Any right-thinking person knows that a suggestion that a change in the law will only strictly apply to a small minority is a fantasy. History has shown that 'safeguards' in law are very soon considered as mere impediments to be overcome, then later, become meaningless. Those who ignore this truth wilfully deny current USA and European reality, the history of the Abortion Act of 1967 and the fallibility and frailty of human nature. No matter how many countries change their law, this does not alter the long-held prohibition on killing.

Acknowledging the fallibility of human beings is a step in the right direction when legal changes are being discussed which currently should protect the vulnerable, whose lives will inevitably be under threat by this relentless drive for assisted suicide.

The fundamental obligations of Parliament to the vulnerable

A democratically elected Parliament exists to protect the citizens from threats to life and limb from within and without, to make laws for the common good and to protect the fundamental human right to life of all citizens.

The relentless lobby for assisted suicide

The UK proponents of assisted suicide never appear to give up on lobbying for a change in the law, despite numerous failed attempts in the UK. Assisted suicide provides for the lawful killings of innocent human beings in certain circumstances.

Such a law would greatly impair the capacity of Parliament to carry out its duty to impartially protect the right to life of all citizens no matter how weak, vulnerable, or impaired those lives may be.

Parliament and government have a duty to protect the vulnerable, not to put them in jeopardy. We must not be afraid to argue that there is nothing compassionate about putting the vulnerable at risk. This is a matter of public safety and we must not allow it to be spun otherwise. Parliament's role is to defend the vulnerable, not to open a Pandora's box with the consequences we see in countries and states where assisted suicide is legalised.

Public safety

Some parliamentarians may agree in principle that we should permit others to help people to die, but there is no way around the argument that allowing the practice would put vulnerable people at risk as Belgium, Germany, Holland and Oregon have shown. This risk continues to be denied by those proposing a change in the law who declare that 'the time has come for a change' – but for whom and with what consequences? One logical outcome would be the anticipated pressure on the vulnerable to accept this destructive agenda. Parliamentarians must maintain the public safety angle.

Public confidence

Legalised assisted suicide would smooth the path to legalising euthanasia. And it would also erode the confidence that people have in Parliament by questioning the reliability of Parliament as the defender of the universally recognised inalienable right to life.

British parliamentarians have rightly rejected the legalisation of assisted suicide in Britain numerous times out of concern for public safety. Repeated extensive enquiries have concluded that a change in the law is not necessary.

An issue of conscience, rather than a decision for government

The UK government announced in 2021 that it had no plans to review the law on assisted suicide or to issue a call for evidence. In response to a parliamentary question, the government announced that any change to the law in this area must be for individual parliamentarians to consider as an issue of conscience, rather than a decision for government.

The announcement came after a question from assisted suicide supporter, Andrew Mitchell, MP. Assisted suicide campaigners have been putting pressure on the government to undertake a review of the current law on assisted suicide. The government's response at the beginning of 2021 is consistent with the continued parliamentary rejection of assisted suicide legislation.

The rejection of yet another attempt for a change in the UK law on assisted suicide (The Marris Bill in 2015) was a bad blow for those who are relentlessly fighting for a change in the law. This defeat happened against a background of the obvious will of the people who inundated their parliamentarians at the time, requesting they vote against such a proposed change. Many MPs changed their voting intention due to their constituents' huge mail increase on the issue and voted against a change in the law. This miracle occurred despite the apparent public will for a change in the law, according to the opinion polls which so often are proved to be wrong.

The public's view: opinion polls

A British Social Attitudes survey, in 2007, found 80% of the public said they wanted the law changed to give terminally ill patients the right to die with a doctor's help. In the same survey, 45% supported giving patients with non-terminal illnesses the option of euthanasia. 'A majority' was opposed to relatives being involved in a patient's death (Clery et al., 2007).

People frequently request euthanasia when they are emotionally and/or psychologically distraught. Assisted suicide is overwhelmingly requested and granted based on misguided 'compassionate' concerns such as burdening family and caregivers. It is prompted by fears of the loss of autonomy, need for dependence, possible loss of control over bodily functions and inability to participate in enjoyable activities. How many are offered psychological help and social support in line with holistic and compassionate care?

The fact that a reported 80% of people had agreed with a change in the law needs careful analysis during the time of Lord Falconer's Assisted Dying Bill (2014). Any poll on assisted suicide which has been commissioned by the biased campaign group 'Dignity in Dying' (formerly the Voluntary Euthanasia Society) cannot be taken seriously.

It is necessary to better inform both professional and public debate. Looking at opinion polls, we need to look carefully at the fact that a reported 70% of people agree with a change in the law. A House of Lords Select Committee Report suggested that opinion polls purporting to show that a large majority of people would favour a change in the law are misleading. This is because they are based on a simplistic format for answers to questions without any explanatory context. In a Gallup poll conducted in 2013, 70% of the participants agreed with the proposition to, 'End the patient's life by some painless means' but only 51% were ready to agree to 'Assist the patient to commit suicide' (Saad, 2013).

Whatever the views of the public on this issue, doctors and nurses do not enter the professions to kill people. Corruption, indoctrination and pressure need to be guarded against.

Parliamentary debate on the defeated Marris Bill (2015)

Opinion polls were again confounded when in 2015, there was a shock result for the cause of assisted suicide, with the unexpected, crushing defeat of the Marris Bill, which saw 118 who voted for a change, while 330 voted against a change in the law. Some prescient questions were asked of Rob Marris during the debate by various MPs.

Susan Elan Jones (Clwyd South) (Lab) asked the bill's promoter, Rob Marris, 'Can my hon. Friend tell the House why he thinks that so many disability organisations and the BMA are opposed to the Bill? (Elan Jones, 2015).

John Pugh (1995) (Southport) (Liberal Democrat) asked: 'Will the hon. Gentleman clarify something that has been bothering me? He has called this Bill the Assisted Dying Bill but there is not a person in this room who would not assist the dying. In the interest of clarity, why did he not call it the assisted suicide Bill?' (Pugh, 2015).

Helen Jones (2015) (Warrington North) (Lab) said: 'The Bill is founded on the belief that it is possible to predict the time of death accurately up to six months. In fact, most doctors would say that that is impossible. It is certainly impossible to predict death beyond a week or two. Is that not the case?' (Jones, 2015).

Rob Marris (2015), in response to the question from Helen Jones, said, 'My hon. Friend, like me, is a solicitor and she will know that professionals commonly give advice on a balance of probabilities. That is the same for medical professionals. On the gross statistics, when errors in prognosis occur for the terminally ill, it is usually an overestimate of life expectancy' (Marris, 2015).

Six years on from the defeated Marris Bill, (2015) yet another, defeated assisted suicide bill, the Meacher Bill, was debated in the Lords in 2021. The following spoke in the Parliamentary debate against the UK Meacher Bill in October 2021.

Lord Robert Winston (2021):

It raises the most important moral question and needs clarity without euphemism. "Assisted dying" could equally be applied to palliative care, so the Bill's title does not represent what is really intended. The word "euthanasia" – from the Greek "eu", meaning well or good and "thanatos", meaning death – is what we are actually talking about.

The Archbishop of Canterbury (2021):

All of us here are united in wanting compassion and dignity for those coming to the end of their lives, but it does not serve compassion if, by granting the wishes of one

closest to me, I expose others to danger and it does not serve
dignity if, in granting the wishes of one closest to me,
I devalue the status and safety of others. I hope your Lordships
will reflect and, while recognising the good intentions we all
share, resist the change the Bill seeks to make.

Baroness Hayman (2021):

The most reverend Primate accepted that there is no unanimity of
view among people of faith, doctors, lawyers and members of my
Select Committee. There is not; there are differences of opinion and
they are compassionately and ethically held. But the public know
what they think on this issue. They have been consistent on the
issue and I believe we should respect that and support the Bill.

Assisted suicide audits

No one should be unaware of European audits and audits in
states, such as Oregon, where assisted suicide is legal, which reveal
that rather than pain, the 'fear of being a burden' underlies many
people's chief reason for requesting assisted suicide. The worst
pain, it seems, experienced by ill or dying people is the fear of
being a burden to their loved ones or carers. Do we now compound
this fear by offering the abolishment of the patients' lives in the
increasing numbers as seen in European countries?

Many of these patients have never been assessed by a
psychiatrist for treatable clinical depression. In view of the alarming,
encroaching assisted suicide laws and the established common
reason for requesting assisted death – fear of being a burden – the
need for nurses to act as the Good Samaritan and provide holistic
care to vulnerable patients is ever more pressing a duty.

The slippery slope – a fallacy?

The term 'slippery slope' implies passive change over time; what we are
seeing in Belgium is more accurately termed 'incremental extension',

the steady intentional escalation of numbers with a gradual widening of the categories of patients to be included (Care not Killing, 2012).

During 2016 and 2017, three children in Belgium were given euthanasia and the media reaction was indifferent. Apparently, this has barely been reported outside Christian and pro-life circles. Pro-life people who warn against weakening the legal protection offered to all human life are often accused of believing in the 'slippery slope fallacy'. But the Belgian experience, since euthanasia was introduced (in 2002), suggests that logical slippery slopes do exist (Gooch, 2018).

There is euthanasia in countries like the Netherlands, Belgium, Switzerland. There are nurses who help with execution of prisoners in the US. Even pre-natal screening for disabilities can be an ethical dilemma for nurses and doctors.

In 30 years, the Netherlands has moved from euthanasia of people who are terminally ill, to euthanasia of those who are chronically ill; from euthanasia for physical illness, to euthanasia for mental illness; from euthanasia for mental illness, to euthanasia for psychological distress or mental suffering – and now to euthanasia simply if a person is over the age of 70 and 'tired of living' (Pereira, 2011).

Assisted suicide does not solve suffering nor improve care

The Oregon Death with Dignity Act (1997) legalised euthanasia by allowing terminally ill Oregonians to end their lives through the voluntary self-administration of lethal medications, expressly prescribed by a physician for that purpose.

Despite including the word 'dignity', 'a survey found that physicians who prescribe the lethal drugs for assisted suicide were present at only 21.7% of reported deaths and so could not deal with any complications arising from their use' (Cole and Duddington, 2021b).

Oregon has reported the following complications, in 2020, which have inevitable, psychological consequences for all involved and need acknowledgement:

- Over half of patients who underwent assisted suicide took more than three-quarters of an hour to die; some more than four days and 6% had complications.
- The eight patients who reawakened after receiving their drugs did not repeat the experience.

(Finlay, 2021b)

Despite best intentions for the dying, it is inevitable that they will suffer rather than benefit from legalised assisted suicide as evidenced elsewhere. Some argue that palliative care cannot meet all needs. This should not mean that patients should be deprived of the excellent expertise on offer.

Denial of palliative care

Baroness Finlay reminded the Lords in her speech that the (failed) Meacher Bill (2021) does not focus on the need for bridging gaps in palliative care. She also reported troubling statistics in Belgium, where assisted suicide is legal and two-thirds of all dying people do not access specialist palliative care (Finlay, 2021b).

Hospice defunding

There is evidence of hospice defunding in Canada of some hospices wishing to maintain ethical standards and not promote legalised assisted suicide. Research from Canada reveals the negative impact that assisted suicide has had on palliative care treatment, adversely affecting such care. Both the patients and the palliative care providers found this distressing (Matthews et al., 2020).

Baroness Hollins with GP and also psychiatry experience, spoke against the Meacher Bill in the House of Lords. She quoted a Canadian doctor, Leonie Herx, who has said that administering death is cheaper and easier than providing good care (Hollins, 2021).

This result may be followed by other countries and states where assisted suicide is legal. This would be a travesty of human rights and the destruction of the palliative care advances made over the years.

Psychological basis for requests for death

Twenty-five years ago, just prior to Oregon State's pioneering legislation on assisted suicide, 12% of patients in hospitals and care homes reported feeling that they were a 'burden' on their relatives – by 2018, it was 68% (Le Fanu, 2021). Yet, assisted suicide in Oregon, is considered and repeatedly described as a success by pro-euthanasia campaigners.

Symptom relief and loving care

In the 21st century, symptom relief can be sophisticated and, in most cases, can achieve proper palliation. Today, suffering can be ameliorated in almost all cases and yet the cause of 'death with dignity' is promoted more energetically than suicide prevention. No one of any age or degree of illness is granted a pain-free existence. To suffer is part of the human condition. We see practical love operating frequently in times of trauma, to make bearable the suffering of those having experienced loss, natural disasters, torture, persecution, injustice, or bereavement, in other words, in all forms of suffering, whether mental or physical. What makes suffering bearable is the constant invaluable support by family and friends and of course, the carers, in their loving concern, support and practical care for pain, wounds and misery.

The WHO has demonstrated that access to pain-relieving drugs, along with a simple educational programme, can achieve relief in most patients. Specialists in various parts of the world estimate these basic approaches can control 85 to 96% of cases. The remaining cases require more careful attention and the use of multiple drugs and therapies to achieve complete relief (Scott, 1995).

Skills for life quality, not death

Not every situation involving end of life issues means wrestling with big ethical dilemmas. Many times, there are simple considerations or strategies that used to be commonly employed until the introduction of the so-called 'Right to die' movement.

Patients with end-stage disease are a constant challenge to the vocational skills of their professional health carers.

In my experience of many years in nursing, patients look to their carers to affirm their lives, not offer them assisted suicide as a defeatist, cheap and easy option. Those close to patients in the clinical setting should be considered for their experience of what patients genuinely need and want. These practitioners should be listened to, rather than ignored, instead for the voice of the vociferous lobby groups who generally have no clinical experience.

A defeatist option

It is reasonable to assert that such lobbying for the defeatist option of assisted suicide can engender fear in the public and a belief that skills to care for them are sadly lacking. Moreover, consistent statistics reveal, where assisted suicide is legal, that the top reason for asking for assisted suicide is fear of being a burden, not troublesome symptoms.

An experienced nurse comments from America: 'Accurate information, common sense and a good understanding of ethical principles can cut through the 'right-to-die' fog and make a person's last stage of life as good as possible both for the person and his or her family' (Valko, 2007).

Dangers of minority beliefs imposed on the majority

Personal reasons often are an undercurrent in the lives of those who sadly become interested in the law change due to their own particular health prospects which appear to be dwindling. Life is to be cherished. What we should all campaign for is a better effort in care for all people in need, whether dying or not.

Health professionals need to understand what the implications of movements such as the assisted suicide (minority) lobby means for the elderly, the disabled and the majority of the population who do not want a change in the law as evidenced by the numerous failed attempts to legalise assisted suicide in the UK.

Some European countries may be going down the road to perdition of assisted suicide. No advocated safeguards and (misguided) compassionate arguments, however, can counter the monumental change for UK society should the change in the law be achieved by the minority supposedly speaking for the majority.

Despair

The 'right to die' movement and 'end of life' discussions are more about despair rather than hope or true justice. People deserve the best in healthcare and that includes the right to humane care, trust in their caring team and a natural lifespan. Apart from the fact we cannot truly know how the patient feels or whether they might recover, there is the problem that we all change our minds. Such patients may be vulnerable to the decisions that they could have taken some time before in an advance directive. This might be used against them. They may be reliant on others who may be unwilling to offer a chance for any treatment to aid in their survival.

Lobbying for 'dignity'

The lobbying for a change in the law is so often promoted by 'Dignity in Dying'. This organisation repeatedly supports those most vulnerable who wish for a change in the law in line with their own personal circumstances. A change to the current UK protective law would ultimately affect vulnerable people on a national scale, based on the wish of a few sad, desperate and determined individuals. Dignity in the face of death cannot be given from the outside; it derives from the dignity of soul in the human being. Dignity, moreover, is not contingent on physical condition alone. We must promote and ensure patient dignity to eliminate the fear of its perceived loss.

Debunking the death with dignity myth

A blogger logically explores the dignity concept and the blog is entitled 'Death with Dignity':

'Assisted suicide sounds merciful. It sounds peaceful. If I were terminally ill, I would not want to die a painful death, either. I have no doubt that advocates of death with dignity (physician assisted suicide) have good intentions, but beneath the peaceful face of the 'death with dignity' movement is a spiritually dark concept that has practical implications.

'What 'death with dignity' advocates forget is that no matter how much suffering the patient is going through, even if they are suffering without hope of survival, these terminally ill patients are still just as valuable and worthy of life as they were before they were suffering' (Dawson, 2017).

We cannot control every aspect of our lives and to believe otherwise is a form of pride. Those lobbying for a radical change in UK law should acquaint themselves with the vocation and training of health professionals which is aimed at cherishing and saving lives. Many health professionals see legalised assisted suicide as a failure in care for vulnerable people.

Patient affirmation

The most common reason for mortality of young men in the UK is suicide (CALM, 2020). Legalised assisted suicide in the UK would be a public message that society endorses this sad statistic.

A noted American psychiatrist suggests that 'patients look at healthcare providers as they would a mirror, seeking a positive image of themselves and their continued sense of worth. In turn, healthcare providers need to be aware that their attitudes and assumptions will shape those all-important reflections' (Chochinov, 2007).

Recommendations outlined as a guide to promote empathy among clinicians is termed 'the A, B, C and D of dignity-conserving care' (Chochinov, 2007).

The importance of the four parts of the dignity-conserving care guide – A, for attitude, B for behaviour, C for compassion and D for dialogue – is emphasised in communicating empathy, compassion and support for patients. This guide on empathy has its origins in palliative care but Chochinov suggests that it can be applied across all of medicine. Based on empirical evidence, the guide explains how kindness, humanity and respect are core values of medicine, but which are often thought of as the 'niceties of care', only offered to patients if time and circumstances allow.

Dignity-conserving care

Irene Higginson, a palliative care doctor, and Sue Hall, a psychologist at King's College London, suggest that perhaps changing attitudes needs to pervade all medical school teaching, they suggest that Chochinov's 'ABCD' approach to conserving dignity, should be the first mnemonic that we teach all professionals entering health and social care (Higginson and Hall, 2007).

Effective drugs?

It is acknowledged that drugs given in the Swiss 'Dignitas' clinic do not always work in the way some patients might imagine. Who, then, is responsible for intervening to achieve the wished-for death?

Latest UK moves for assisted suicide: England and Wales

Baroness Meacher, an independent member of the House of Lords and chair of the assisted suicide advocacy group 'Dignity in Dying', on 26 May 2021, proposed a private member's bill to legalise assisted suicide in England and Wales, rephrased as 'aid in dying' by its supporters. No doubt, with the best of intentions, the Baroness wished for choice to be enabled for mentally competent adults in the final six months of a terminal illness, with each request to be assessed by two doctors and a judge.

Vulnerability compounded by a possible change in the law

In the UK, financial abuse by family members has typically been the most common abuse reported to the helpline 'Hourglass'. This is the charity which is dedicated to ending harm, exploitation and abuse of older people. The charity reports that a staggering one million people over the age of 65 are victims of abuse each year in the UK (Hunt, 2021).

The UK Meacher Bill, if it had succeeded, would make the anticipated deluge of abuse of the vulnerable so much more likely.

Scotland

Liam McArthur MSP plans to introduce an "Assisted Dying for Terminally Ill Adults (Scotland) Bill" in early 2023. This would give people who have lived for 12 months in Scotland, access to life-ending drugs to take themselves if:

Two doctors are satisfied that they meet safeguards, including being mentally competent.

Previous attempts to legalise assisted suicide in Scotland have failed.

The proposal envisages assisted suicide for persons:

1. Aged 16 or over (the age of majority in Scotland)
2. Resident in Scotland for at least 12 months
3. Deemed to be "terminally ill", which Mr McArthur understands to mean "a registered medical practitioner has diagnosed them as having a progressive disease, which can reasonably be expected to cause their death".

Care Not Killing

'Our Duty of Care' is a group of UK healthcare workers who oppose the intentional killing of patients by assisted suicide or euthanasia. They are a campaign group that is financed and administered by the Care Not Killing Alliance. It is supported by a wide range of healthcare professionals and has campaigned during the membership polls run by the Royal College of Physicians, Royal College of General Practitioners and British Medical Association to maintain medical opposition to assisted suicide.

Preparing the way?

Dr Gordon MacDonald, CEO of 'Our Duty of Care', notes that in 2019, campaigners for a Scottish assisted suicide law were "coached" by a prominent member of the Canadian euthanasia lobby. Dr Ellen Wiebe, a practitioner of Canada's MAiD (Medical assistance in Dying), attended the Annual General Meeting at Holyrood of the Cross-Party Group (CPG) on End of Life Choices as the Group's special guest.

The point of Dr Wiebe's visit to Scotland was to advise Scottish parliamentarians on how to frame euthanasia law "… so that Scotland and the UK can learn from them [Canadian practitioners] before the legislation changes".

Minutes of the CPG's AGM show the meeting was packed with supporters of Friends at the End (FATE) and Dignity in Dying (DiD)— groups committed to changing the law on assisting suicide.

That same year (2019), Professor Jocelyn Downie, a legal expert on Canada's MAiD and euthanasia law, was the guest speaker at a 'Friends at the End' Scotland event at the Scottish Parliament.

Public Consultation concerns

On 8 September, 2022, Mr McArthur's office published a summary of responses to a public consultation from both organisations and private individuals about a change in the law for assisted suicide.

'Our Duty of Care' CEO, Dr MacDonald, reports that Mr McArthur's office has claimed that 76% of the 13,957 individual responses received were in favour of his proposal. But worryingly, this was only after at least 3,352 responses from supporters linked to the Right to Life campaign group had been discounted. Over 17,000 individual responses were received, and only about 61% were supportive of a change in the law. So, the figure of 76% not only does not reflect the actual responses received, but it is also heavily weighted in favour by the activists who wish to see the law changed to allow assisted suicide.

The campaign groups wanting a change in the law were also active in mobilising their supporters to respond to the consultation.

If the law changes in Scotland, this will add fresh momentum to the campaign to push through similar legislation at Westminster, thereby impacting many more people who are vulnerable in England and Wales too (Macdonald, 2022a).

Mental Health issues

Kevin Sutherland, a 31-year-old, from Edinburgh, who was diagnosed with Borderline Personality Disorder (BPD) nine years ago, has launched a petition calling on Liam McArthur MSP to extend the criteria for assisted suicide in his proposed Bill to: "[...] include those suffering with incurable mental health issues".

Mr Sutherland says that he:

"[...] would like Scotland to come in line with the progressive policies of other countries and the ECHR.

He is referring here specifically to Belgium, where Mr Sutherland says, he plans to travel to end his life.

Mr Sutherland's perception of the 'progressive policies of other countries' in relation to assisted suicide should be reconsidered in light of the truth of the tragic repercussions of these regressive and heartless policies.

Belgium formally legalised euthanasia in 2002, and allows patients to apply to be killed who are deemed to be in a "futile medical condition of constant and unbearable physical or mental suffering that cannot be alleviated".

Belgian cases have included instances where patients have been euthanised for psychiatric conditions, including depression.

Mr Sutherland's petition is currently receiving wide coverage, including from Scotland's leading tabloid, the Daily Record (MacDonald, 2022b).

Economics

Economic consideration can be the sinister underbelly of the attempts to allow patients 'compassion' and 'dignity' by doctor-assisted suicide. The nurses' code of professional conduct (NMC,

2018) states that nurses must adhere to the laws of the country in which they practise. Hope remains that nurse managers and nursing representatives will support and protect nurses who refuse to comply with any change in law that compromises their conscience and who wish to provide continuing, safe, humane care to their patients until their natural end.

Views of UK bishops

Catholic English bishop Mark Davies of Shrewsbury warned that Baroness Meacher's 2021 bill on assisted suicide, if successful, would cross a 'moral line'. He added:
The language employed in seeking this seismic change in the law is one of compassion, knowing that no one is opposed to the relief of human suffering. However, the fact this legislation is being proposed in Parliament by the chair of what was the Voluntary Euthanasia Society should leave us in no doubt as to 'the goal of medical killing of the sick and aged.

(Davies, 2021a)

The following words from Mark Davies and John Sherrington, Catholic bishops of England and Wales, summarise what many believe will happen, should there be a UK change in the law on assisted suicide:
If Parliament were ever persuaded to legalise Assisted Suicide, we should be in no doubt as to the moral line that would be crossed. A line that has never been legally crossed in our care of the sick and elderly since the foundation of our society.

(Davies, 2021b)

Life is a gift to be valued and cherished until its last breath, through natural death, which opens into the promise of eternal life.

(Sherrington, 2021)

Those who cannot bear to deal with the suffering and disability of those whom they love all too easily may reduce vulnerable people, who may or may not be dying, to 'objects' to be managed. Detachment is an understandable defence, but this withdrawal of contact, affection and care is probably the greatest single cause of the suffering of patients by the dehumanisation of dying.

The proposals for assisted suicide are at odds with the ethos of Christianity, which is to uphold the value of human life, at its end as at its beginning. What these bills would do, if enacted, is present vulnerable people with an intolerable choice. Those who feel they are a burden will opt to end their lives to spare their families and society the 'expense and trouble' of their care. Many people with disabilities or conditions such as dementia would, if presented with this terrible choice, opt for death for altruistic reasons. Many of whom, however, are vociferous in their opposition to a change in the law. As Cardinal Hume once put it, 'the right to die can become the duty to die'. No human being should be put in this position (Catholic Herald, 2021).

Conclusion

Dangers to the disabled

Dr Miro Griffiths, an editor for the International Journal of Disability and Social Justice and Leverhulme Research Fellow at the University of Leeds Centre for Disability Studies, explains that assisted suicide and euthanasia interventions would alter how health and care provision is offered to disabled people and those with illnesses and health conditions in society. Griffiths argues that rather than prioritise support for disabled people to participate in communities, debates will take place as to whether an individual's death should be accelerated via state and medical opinion. Dr Griffiths also observes, 'This is one of the reasons why the Meacher Bill is dangerous – it flirts with the idea that some lives are not worth living' (Caldwell, 2021b).

Corruption of the vocation to heal

Many health professionals who would refuse the implementation of such a dangerous and unnecessary change in the law would, no doubt, experience persecution for a lack of so-called 'compassion'. Any change in the law would corrupt the mission and training of nurses and doctors who would arbitrarily be expected to help people kill themselves, despite supposed conscientious objection provision. This is not true nursing or medicine.

Euthanasia and assisted suicide are always the wrong choice: the medical personnel and the other healthcare workers – faithful to the task always to be at the service of life and to assist it up until the very end – cannot give themselves to any euthanistic practice, irrespective of the request of the interested party and much less that of the family. Since there is no right to dispose of one's life arbitrarily, no healthcare worker can be compelled to execute a non-existent right (Pontifical Council for Pastoral Assistance to Health Care Workers, 2017, section 169, p.121).

Effects of assisted suicide on doctors

The impact on doctors is less frequently brought into discussion but in Belgium, where physician-assisted suicide and euthanasia have been legal for nearly 20 years, many specialists are beginning to actively consider the rise of a new 'survivor syndrome' among medics.

Doctor-assisted death is a practice which is impossible to contain or control anywhere and now it is creating emotional and mental health problems among those people exposed to it. The phenomenon emerged as a key concern of contributors to a book called 'Euthanasia: Searching for the Full Story: Experiences and In-sights of Belgian Doctors and Nurses', published in the same month as the Meacher Bill was introduced into Parliament (Caldwell, 2021c).

One contributor, François Trufin, a hospital emergency nurse, said that more often than not, I have been a direct or indirect witness to the deep distress that doctors experience when they perform euthanasia. One filled with tears as he confessed that some nights he wakes up in a sweat, seeing the faces of the very people he has euthanised in front of him. Can there be anything harder to bear? Who could guess that behind the confident and experienced doctor, an honest and sincere man endures such suffering? (Trufin, 2021).

Legalising assisted suicide for the terminally ill is a stepping-stone to legalising euthanasia. In both cases, the intention is the same: if patients in law have the right to ask for a lethal prescription to take the drug themselves, why not for a lethal injection, particularly if they are physically unable to take the drugs, or having taken them, are suffering a complicated, difficult death?

Assisted suicide is 'euthanasia by the back door'. If there can be any dignity in dying, it must be by the continuation of trusted, humane treatment and holistic care until the natural end of life.

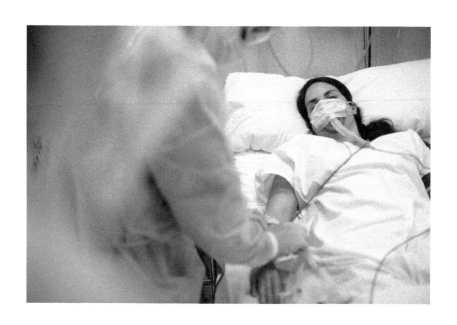

Chapter 14
Euthanasia

Those who cannot remember the past are condemned to repeat it. Those who do not know history's mistakes are doomed to repeat them.

(Santayana, 1905)

Introduction

Any experience of attempting patient advocacy against a culture of eugenic beliefs, unethical practice and defeatist patient care, is never forgotten. Managerial and peer support is vital for nurses who try to adhere to the code of conduct against a culture of death.

Definitions

- The word 'euthanasia' comes from the Greek; '*eu*' and '*thanatos*' meaning, literally, 'a good death'. It is the practice of intentionally ending life to relieve pain and suffering (Stanford University Encyclopaedia of Philosophy, 2018b).
- The British House of Lords Select Committee on medical ethics defines euthanasia as 'a deliberate intervention undertaken with the express intention of ending a life, to relieve intractable suffering' (Harris, 2001).

Today, euthanasia is generally accepted as 'mercy killing' which can be a deceptive and questionable term.

'Mercy killing'

The very expression 'mercy killing' is an oxymoron that alarms the conscience of anyone with a background in the Abrahamic faiths and in the universal ethics incorporated within those faiths.

From a biblical perspective, no active intervention may be undertaken to terminate the life of a dying person and this principle is at the heart of our social order's moral commitment to respect life (Goldberg, 2019).

Eugenics and 'health' ideologies

Opinions and discussions about the pro-death culture we are seeing in some European countries and elsewhere, as being reminiscent of Nazi Germany, are met with disbelief, disdain, or horror and sometimes threats of litigation by promoters of assisted suicide. We have seen eugenic ideology before. Such an ideology must be rejected as dangerous, particularly for the most vulnerable people who require the most protection.

The British Eugenics Society (the Galton Institute)

In 1907, the Eugenics Educational Society (it became the Eugenics Society after 1926), was founded in Britain on the initiative of a polymath, Francis Galton (1822–1911). It included issues and interests such as social Darwinism and eugenics. Galton became the society's first president and served until his death.

The goal of the society was one of furthering eugenic teaching and understanding in the home, in the school and elsewhere (Chitty, 2007). In other words, it focused on education and popularisation of eugenics. It was a small organisation, and its membership was made up of middle-class professionals (physicians, scientists, writers, prominent politicians and Marie Stopes). Even though the society was small, it enjoyed a degree of influence due to its prominent members.

Palatable names

Following World War II, eugenic ideologies and policies were considered as discredited by many due to their association with Nazi Germany. Yet, the British Eugenics Society was slow to catch up and only changed its name to the Galton Institute in 1989 (Bland and Hall, 2010). The Galton Institute name was perhaps thought to be a more palatable term for public consumption.

Nazi Germany's euthanasia programme

The German euthanasia programme which preceded the Jewish holocaust relied upon compliant practitioners to carry out the orders given. At the end of World War II, many doctors were tried for war crimes. Some were executed, some imprisoned and many walked free. Much research has been done on what the doctors did, but little research has been done on the role of nurses. One fact is certain, we have a precedent set for us by the tragedies on many levels by the Nazi practices employed on vulnerable people. We ignore this history at our peril.

'Lives unworthy of life'

The claims of the propaganda machine were that the patients for extermination (children and adults) were economically non-viable, were living lives 'not worthy of life' and were 'useless eaters', common terms used by the Nazi regime. The propaganda campaign caused the population to believe that such killing was 'mercy' killing. But also, that such people were a burden on the state and a threat to the Aryan race (children were taught at school about the cost of caring for these people).

Nurse involvement in the Nazi euthanasia programme

Vast numbers of nurses were involved in carrying out the doctors' orders, helping with the experiments on prisoners in concentration camps. With the doctors, nurses were part of the Nazi 'death selection' panels. Examination of the doctors' major involvement is well known in the post-World War II period. It took until the 1980s for the involvement of nurses to be studied.

Remembering history: nurse freedom within the Nazi euthanasia programme

The Nazi regime provides a precedent for nurses today. Education programmes for nurses must include such momentous, historical issues involving nurses in such an evil ideology. A good start would be to recommend a book written about the nursing involvement in widespread euthanasia, edited by Susan Benedict and Linda Shields: *Nurses and Midwives in Nazi Germany: The Euthanasia Programs* (Benedict and Shields, 2014). They published a collection of essays asking how, notwithstanding their role as care givers, nurses became killers. Shields says she is often asked why she continues with her research, given that these crimes were committed such a long time ago, but she says the ethical questions they raise are still relevant.

It would be easy to make several assumptions about the nurses' motivation for complying with the demands of the Nazi regime. Firstly, they were too terrified about the consequences of refusing orders as they were not given any choice and that the propaganda machine was so powerful that most nurses believed in its claims. These assumptions are wrong.

Nazi respect or nurse conscientious objectors?

Nurses were given a choice whether to be complicit in the euthanasia programme or to be part of the 'death selection panels' for children and adults. Those who chose to refuse were not, consequently, sent to the gas chambers for defying orders. They were merely moved from the practice areas where they were working as some did have the courage of their convictions, for conscientious objection and strength in numbers.

There is no record of any nurse being punished for refusing to participate in the Nazi death policy for patients with psychiatric illness, alcoholism, epilepsy, mental incapacity, physical or learning disability, or birth 'defect'. Such 'defects' ranged from Down's syndrome to cleft palate. The numbers of patients to have been killed, and hospitals emptied as a result, for use as barracks, was owed to the complicity of many nurses and midwives, who actively killed their patients in the Nazi euthanasia programme. They complied with the doctors' orders to give the intravenous drug overdoses or deliberately leave infants outside in the cold weather to die of hypothermia.

The book by Benedict and Shields is about the ethics of nursing and midwifery and how these were abrogated during the Nazi era. Nurses and midwives actively killed their patients, many of whom were disabled children and infants and patients with mental (and other) illnesses or intellectual disabilities. The book gives the facts as well as theoretical perspectives as a lens through which these crimes can be viewed. It also provides a way to teach this history to nursing and midwifery students, and, for the first time, explains the role of one of the world's most historically prominent midwifery leaders in the Nazi crimes.

Some nurses said that they were simply following orders. Others openly admitted their belief that they were doing the right thing for the patients – that they were providing a service to society by putting them out of their misery. They believed that killing was a legitimate part of the caring role. Others were perfectly free to refuse and be moved to another care setting.

Following such barbarity, three concepts must predominate in care of vulnerable people: conscience, codes of conduct and an anti-eugenic and pro-life ethos. Even nurses in Nazi Germany had a choice as to how they managed the orders given that were against their conscience and some followed their conscience.

Questions for practitioners today

The nurses who agreed with the ideology, murdered patients of their own free will. Two questions arise for us in the post-Nazi era:

- Why did the nurses kill?
- How could they do it, when the focus of nursing is to care, not to kill?

Nurses in the 21st century, working in ethically difficult situations which will compromise their conscience, must remember that they always have a choice as there is protection in the form of conscience and the code and required compassion as nurses.

A psychiatrist, Leo Alexander, wrote the Nuremberg Code of research ethics after World War II, following his studying of the actions of German SS troops and concentration camp guards. He noted that they were on the whole, meek and overpolite fellows who committed inhuman crimes because they found themselves suspect by their superior. Alexander also wrote that science under dictatorship, becomes subordinated to the guiding philosophy of the dictatorship (Alexander, 1949).

Rights of health professionals to resist euthanasia

Those advocates for assisted suicide should remember that doctors and nurses were trained to protect life and its quality. Many will refuse to collude with a change in the law. Nurses who will be expected to be involved in the practice, if legalised in this country, cannot abandon the long-held principles of '*primum non nocere*': first do no harm. Health professionals should not be corrupted by the propaganda about the 'compassionate' decision for ailing patients. It is false compassion. They must remember why they entered the profession, which was to defend the lives of patients and help them to see light in their care, not the darkness of abandonment to a self-destructive culture of death.

Dignity in death and life are debatable concepts

Euthanasia devalues the lives of those who are seriously ill or disabled by saying that such lives are not worth living – that the negative feelings of people suffering these problems are quite appropriate and that they are right to want to die. In contrast, if we hear about a suicide of a young healthy person who was jilted by a girlfriend/boyfriend, or whose career prospects were poor, euthanasia proponents don't (usually) say that we should pay doctors to help these people to kill themselves.

Experience in Holland, where euthanasia is widespread, reveals that efforts to kill patients often go wrong, with protracted dying and that palliative care (which can enable patients to live through very grave illness in a dignified manner with control of pain and other symptoms) is far less widely available there than here in Britain, where the modern hospice movement began. It is a mistake to think that, on the one hand, euthanasia is dignified and painless and equally, to imply that living with disability or grave illness is inevitably not dignified and is painful. Euthanasia plans can be imposed against the will of patients while many vulnerable or disabled people who love life, fear the prospect of a law offering them or inevitably suggesting death as the compassionate option, even by their loved ones.

First do no harm

At a symposium, several years ago, a Dutch physician was asked how he feels when he kills a patient. He replied, the first time it was difficult... believe that the Dutch experience should provide a dramatic warning to physicians the world over. We should not abandon the long-standing honourable medical tradition of not deliberately terminating human life (Glick, 2004).

Belgium

It has been reported that thousands of elderly people in Belgium have been killed by their doctors under the country's euthanasia law, despite them not giving permission.

It is claimed that around one in sixty deaths that happened under family doctor care, involved someone who has never requested euthanasia. The research also showed that more than half of the patients killed without giving their consent were over the age of 80 years while two thirds of them were in hospital but not suffering from terminal illness (Care not Killing, 2012).

Sanctity of life

There is today a political and philosophical objection to euthanasia that says that our individual right to autonomy against the state must be balanced against the need to make the sanctity of life an important, implicit value of the state, whose role in protecting the public is understood.

Working against a dangerous ideology

One personally dismaying experience in my career, was working with a medical member of the Galton Institute (Eugenic Society). The clinician's membership was unknown to me at the time. I could not understand the cavalier approach to the dying. This was manifest in terms of questionable drug dosages and impatience with 'protracted' dying as it could be viewed by the doctor. The experience was scarring for me, yet I learned the importance of vigilance about questionable medical orders, the right to refuse and the need to act as the patient's advocate and experienced how hard the role can be, despite peer support but little managerial backup. The role of patient advocate needs to be respected by all involved in care responsibility not just those on the frontline. Much of my time was spent in constant discussion and debate on the treatment decisions being made, which in my professional opinion would not offer the patient benefit, but harm, if obeyed.

The power exerted over the team was considerable. I could not and would not reconcile my philosophy of care with that of the clinician. This experience taught me that safeguarding of patients from staff members with eugenic sympathies is not what is taught in nurse training school. It could be argued that this need is becoming more apparent and urgent today.

Economics and euthanasia

Australian ethicist Daniel Fleming presents a novel socioeconomic critique of euthanasia rhetoric, analysing the global campaign for assisted dying from the perspective of contemporary economic theory. He argues that the push to legalise euthanasia is symptomatic of an ideology known as neo-liberalism (Fleming, 2019).

Neo-liberalism

While the precise meaning of the term is debated, neo-liberalism is usually used to denote an approach to economic and social policy – popular in the late 20th century – which would profoundly augment consumer choice and market freedom. It has been criticised for reducing the human person to a self-regulating, economic actor with no connection to community or history (Symons, 2019).

Fleming argues that this mentality is reflected in the way in which people use terms like 'compassion' in the euthanasia debate. Compassion, in the context of arguments for euthanasia, is just a byword for a desire to promote the autonomy of individuals at the end of life – as if the way in which we die was just one more market choice. Fleming writes:

> *According to the neo liberal narrative, physical suffering is less a concern than the suffering incurred by the dependency that fragility and illness entails and its consequent loss of autonomy, self-regulation and self-surveillance. To be compassionate according to the neoliberal narrative, is to suffer with these particular concerns. The commitment following such suffering is to open up hitherto unavailable options for the exercise of autonomy, in order to reinstate what has been lost, even to the extent of that ultimate expression of individual choice: to end one's life.*
>
> (Fleming, 2019)

Fleming further argues that neoliberalism predominantly serves the preferences of the socially privileged which is reflected in the data related to who accesses assisted suicide in Oregon. Placing this framework in contrast to different narratives, including the Hippocratic and Christian ethics of compassion, reveals the stark contrast here and the substantial concerns that arise when neoliberalism is used to claim that assisted suicide is compassionate.

Virtues and vices

Liberalism can be seen to extol the virtue of faith as opinion, whereas faith is a knowledge of something real and objective. It is not a feeling or an opinion.

Aristotle defines moral virtue as a disposition to behave in the right manner and to stand between the extremes of deficiency and excess, which are vices (Stanford Encyclopaedia of Philosophy, 2018a). True Christianity means a state of obedience and faith.

Obedience is a virtue and a habit that teaches us to be humble. Faith is a theological virtue that compels obedience. Without considering and respecting both the virtues of faith and obedience together, we are in danger of insisting on neither of them.

The contagion of euthanasia vs true compassion

Arthur Goldberg, the co-director of the American-based Jewish Institute for Global Awareness, in the following extract, observes the dangers of both euthanasia and organ donation.

> The movement to liberalise euthanasia through withdrawal of life-sustaining medical treatment and regimes in which euthanasia prevails, create a contagion of killing, which travels far beyond the "limits" initially intended by its proponents.
>
> Humans do not live in isolation. The more a culture sends messages that some lives are less valuable than others, the more some people will internalise messages to end their lives or possibly view themselves as heroes by providing their life-sustaining organs to save another. The psychological contagion of suicide is unleashed by euthanasia and assisted suicide laws. Condoning suicide in one circumstance implicitly condones it across the board. The wrong of suicide is no longer absolute: Death is made a reasonable – even the expected – response to pain, misfortune and sadness.
>
> (Goldberg, 2019)

A nurse's experience of fighting against a culture of death

A nurse friend recounts her experience of fighting for her mother's life against the harsh decision being made about arbitrary withdrawal of treatment, despite having a lasting power of attorney and despite the recommended demise of the discredited LCP in 2014. She had experienced a similar battle to ensure that her father was not also starved and dehydrated to death as planned by the medical team. She had a negative result from the doctor in charge of his care despite this being a reasonable request which in the end, after her pleading, was respected. Relatives should not have to undergo such stress in trying to protect their relatives from a culture of death.

My mum, after surviving COVID-19 against all the odds, did really well considering her frailties and chronic lung problems. Having come through that with the grace of God, her hospital doctor told me that we need to not consider hydrating her if she falls ill again. He said we must think of her quality of life! I am afraid he asked the wrong person. I said I do not want her to dehydrate or starve to death and that the LCP was outlawed a few years ago for not factoring in fluids. He fell silent and said no more. She has since gone into hospital for dehydration and a chest infection and responded well to IV antibiotics and fluids.

My mother was asked about resuscitation in my presence and she told them my daughter will know what to do. So, when discussing this issue with the doctor, I said I didn't want to agree to a 'do not resuscitate order' as I was worried treatments wouldn't be given. The doctor said she can take it out of my hands as she can make the decision legally and medically and didn't need my agreement. About a week later a letter came in the post and the doctor stated that she had asked my mum again, when I wasn't present and had said she didn't want to be resuscitated (very convenient)!

I put in writing that Mum has dementia and as her power of attorney, I didn't agree to it for reasons that I was worried that treatments around it would be omitted. I thought they could at least read it in her notes. The doctor put in writing that mum would still have all her treatments but as I had feared, that proved to be incorrect two years down the line.

It's this desire to bring about death that is so obsessive and driven.

Down's syndrome

Dominic Lawson, a well-known journalist and father of a girl with Down's syndrome, rails against the notion that people 'suffer from' Down's syndrome, 'an expression designed to reassure people that termination is the caring option'. He narrates the results of a survey of mothers of children with Down's syndrome. Roughly half of the 1,231 surveyed mothers of children with Down's syndrome born over the past 20 years spoke of the insidious pressure to have the 'tests' even when they had indicated they did not want to. And if the tests did prove positive for Down's, the pressure to terminate was persistent. He concludes: '… and how hypocritical it is for a society that claims to have rejected eugenics not only to promote it within the NHS, but to do so through fear and ignorance. Above all, it does not understand love' (Lawson, 2020).

Propaganda today

Do nurses and doctors, today, believe in propaganda about allowing patients to die as being in the 'best interests' of those with varying degrees of dementia, chronic illness, or disability, to be placed on an 'end of life' (death) 'care' pathway? In Nazi Germany, death became a 'medical cure' for certain people and some nurses and doctors owed their allegiance to the propaganda and the state above that of individual patients.

False compassion

The cause of euthanasia is more than 'false compassion', it is economically driven and those of its proponents who worship at the altar of economic efficiency espouse a cause not dissimilar to the ideology of Nazi Germany, disregarding the threat of unfettered assisted suicide in Europe.

Catholic teaching on euthanasia

Before addressing the issue of euthanasia, we must first remember that the Catholic Church holds as sacred both the dignity of each individual person and the gift of life. Therefore, the following principles are morally binding:

1. First, to make any attempt on the life of or to kill an innocent person is an evil action.

2. Second, each person is bound to lead his life in accord with God's plan and with an openness to His will, looking to life's fulfilment in heaven.

'Samaritanus Bonus' (The Good Samaritan), a newly published letter by the Congregation for the Doctrine of the Faith, reiterates the condemnation of any form of euthanasia and assisted suicide and advocates support for families and healthcare workers. 'Euthanasia is a crime against human life, incurable does not mean end of care' (Congregation for the Doctrine of the Faith, 2020a).

Religious opponents of assisted suicide disagree with euthanasia because they believe that the right to decide when a person dies belongs to God. Euthanasia abandons people at their most vulnerable. Rather than providing compassion and holistic support for people in their suffering, assisted suicide or euthanasia presents a callous and insensitive 'alternative'. The responsibility for such an 'alternative' would be devolved to nurses, corrupting their vocation by being expected to act as agents of the state, conforming to the doctor's euthanasia orders, replicating the Nazi crimes.

The Catholic Church has an unwavering position on euthanasia. Pope Pius XII, who witnessed and condemned the eugenics and euthanasia programmes of the Nazis, was the first to clearly explicate this moral problem and provide guidance.

Intentionally committing suicide is a murder of oneself and considered a rejection of God's plan. For these reasons, the Second Vatican Council condemned 'all offences against life itself, such as murder, genocide, abortion, euthanasia and wilful suicide' (Second Vatican Council, 1965). 'Euthanasia is a grave violation of the law of God since it is the deliberate and morally unacceptable killing of a human person' (Pope St John Paul II, 1995a).

The Catholic Catechism provides a succinct explanation of Catholic teaching on this subject:

2258 Human life is sacred because from its beginning it involves the creative action of God and it remains forever in a special relationship with the Creator, who is its sole end. God alone is the Lord of life from its beginning until its end: no one can under any circumstance claim for himself the right directly to destroy an innocent human being (Congregation for the Doctrine of the Faith, 1997).

Conclusion

The Catholic Church's teaching on the end of life care is reproposed in 'Samaritanus Bonus' (Good Samaritan):

> It is gravely unjust to enact laws that legalise euthanasia or justify and support suicide, invoking the false right to choose a death improperly characterised as respectable only because it is chosen. The person is to be taken care of and surrounded with affection until the end. To say someone is incurable is not synonymous with "uncareable".
> (Congregation for the Doctrine of the Faith, 2020b)

Where there is life there is hope

'[From] century to century . . . the Church has re-enacted the Gospel parable of the Good Samaritan, revealing and communicating her healing love and the consolation of Jesus Christ' (Pope St John Paul II, 2000).

'Unfinished business' is an imperative for many dying patients and manifests in different ways. It is suggested that:

> *Hope requires a sense of connection to the future. Hope is the oxygen of the human spirit. Without it our spirit dies, with it we can overcome even seemingly insurmountable obstacles. Dying people cannot have long-term hopes, but they can be given mini-hopes that make life worth living – that reignite their will to live. Common examples are of a person not dying until after their first grandchild is born or a beloved grandchild is married or graduates from university or an old friend from faraway is coming to visit. It is not uncommon to hear palliative care professionals say that many terminally ill people seem to choose when to die a natural death.*

(Somerville, 2021)

Many patients appreciate discovering the latest innovations in trials and new treatment. My clinical experience, over my years in nursing, is of patients wanting to avail themselves of latest treatments even when in a stage of advanced illness. Developments in medicine are ever evolving and patients are more interested in such opportunities, in my experience, than in assisted suicide.

Writer Christopher De Bellaigue has warned after his investigations in the Netherlands and Belgium: 'Euthanasia won't be an occasion for empathy, ethics or compassion but a bludgeon, swinging through people's lives, whose handiwork can't be undone' (De Bellaigue, 2019). We need to counteract the prevailing attitude that it is better to be dead than disabled and that people in need are burdens to themselves and others.

Are respect, honour and dignity afforded by changing the law?

The French writer and poet Houellebecq, among
his other talents, argues:
The honour of a civilization is not exactly nothing. But really
something else is at stake, from the anthropological point of view.
It is a question of life and death. And on this point, I am going to
have to be very explicit: when a country – a society, a civilization
– gets to the point of euthanasia, it loses, in my eyes, all right to
respect. It becomes henceforth, not only legitimate, but desirable,
to destroy it; so that something else – another country, another
society, another civilization – might have a chance to arise.

(Houellebecq, 2021)

True dignity is inherent in us all, as is the virtue of hope and both concepts are not contingent on physical condition or removed by dependence on others by need of required, safe and true care. A sense of entitlement needs to be checked when it impacts on those health professionals who wish to hold onto their principles of compassionate and practical care for those most vulnerable to a culture of death.

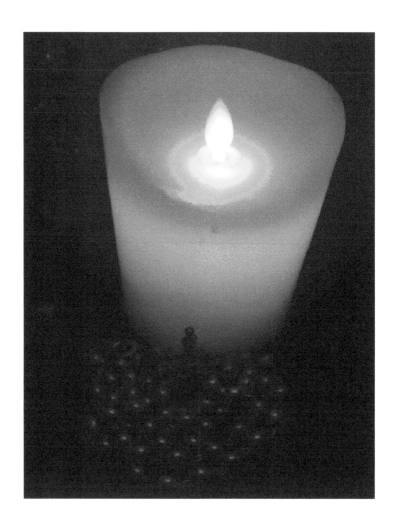

Chapter 15
Care of the dying patient: holistic needs

Dear Lord
In my sorrow, give me assurance that you suffer
with me,
and that eventually we shall be together
in complete happiness

(Julian of Norwich)

Introduction

In the Bodleian Library's collection are several editions, copies, and versions of a popular fifteenth-century work called *Ars Moriendi* (The Art of Dying). This tract was intended to bring Christian comfort and practical instruction to the dying man and his family, and all later versions relate to two Latin texts dating from 1415 (the 'long version') and c.1450 (the 'short version'). The popularity of these works was no doubt in part, due to the widespread incidence of fatal diseases throughout the period.

The long version was written by an anonymous Dominican friar, probably commissioned by the German Council of Constance (1414-1418). It incorporates six chapters, the first four of which encourage the dying Christian with hope, steer him from temptation, remind him of Christ's love, and exhort him to imitate Christ. The final two chapters instruct friends and family with proper bedside behaviour and appropriate prayers for the dying.

Compassionate care of the dying is an achievable aim in the UK, where the modern hospice movement originated. Deliberate acceleration of death has no place in good medical and nursing care. Palliative care is a specialty where holistic care is vital to ensure every patient's needs are assessed and met. This ensures individualised care, rather than a 'blanket' approach to care of the dying. Considerations for care of the dying:

- Palliative and terminal care is appropriate for the person when their health deteriorates to an irreversible state.

- Introduce palliative care based on patient need, as prognosis can be a subjective judgement.
- Caring for the dying is a special privilege in serving humanity, accompanying people to the natural completion of life.
- Treatment and care priorities must include symptom relief as part of individualised, holistic care to allow patients to live as comfortably and as fully as possible.

When palliative care is required, patients need to be helped to realise from the Good Samaritan nurse, the confidence in the wonderful array of treatments for symptom control to allow for a peaceful, natural death, together with the holistic approach to healing of the mind and spirit before death. This is part of the duty of care, rather than a care culture of over reliance on unnecessary drug therapy, such as sedation without hydration.

Palliative care definitions

It is vital to understand the concept of palliative care and be agreed on the definition. '*Palliare*' is Latin, meaning 'to cloak' – from a holistic care perspective, we cloak the symptoms that may be present.

Holistic palliative care

The WHO has defined the concept of palliative care in holistic terms as: 'An approach which improves the quality of life of patients and their families facing life threatening illness, through the prevention, impeccable assessment and treatment of pain and other problems, physical, psychosocial and spiritual (WHO, 2011).

The Palliative Care Bill (2020)

Baroness Ilora Finlay, an expert professor in palliative care, has introduced the 'Access to Palliative Care and Treatment of Children Bill' [HL, 2020].

Within the Palliative Care Bill, palliative care has
been defined in a holistic way as:
Care which is delivered to seek to improve the quality of life of
persons with life-limiting illness or approaching the end of life,

through the prevention and relief of suffering by means of early identification, assessment, treatment and management of pain and other problems whether physical, psychological, social, or spiritual.

(Finlay, 2020)

The aim of the bill is to make provision for NHS service commissioners to ensure that persons for whom they have responsibility for commissioning physical and mental health services have access to specialist and generalist palliative care and support services; to enable hospices to access pharmaceutical services on the same basis as other services commissioned by a clinical commissioning group; and to make provision for treatment of children with a life-limiting illness.

Palliative care, a special privilege

Care for the dying is a special privilege in the stewardship of creation because it is serving the life of the human person. Serving life in palliative care means accompanying it to its natural completion with the patient who needs to believe in the skill and dedication of their health team, whether in hospital, hospice, or home. The maxim *primum non nocere* (first do no harm) of traditional medical ethics has guided medicine and nursing for centuries.

Palliative care includes many elements:

- Individual, ethical, moral, legal, practical, social and spiritual.
- Prognosis – a difficult and often subjective judgement. Prognosis is made more difficult if the patient is suffering from chronic conditions such as heart and lung diseases.
- Evidence-based practice is essential (as with any other speciality).

Evidence-based practice should incorporate integration of best research evidence with clinical expertise and patient values.

The hospice movement

Cicely Saunders was the founder of the UK modern hospice movement. She revolutionised the care of the dying, by promoting the hospice movement as the optimum standard in palliative care. She did not consider the challenge of caring for dying people as an impossible burden, requiring assisted suicide as an 'option' in palliative care. The progress in palliative care has improved ever since. The hospice movement was created to provide palliative care for any patient.

The evolution of palliative care

The following is the abstract from a paper by Cicely Saunders about palliative care:

> An encounter with one patient in 1948 was the catalyst for the Hospice Movement. The challenge to undertake appropriate pain and symptom control together with experience in further listening to patients in the small number of homes especially planned for dying people, finally came together during the 1960s as the impetus for the first modern hospice which opened in 1967. Since then, palliative care has been developing worldwide and has shown that the basic principles demonstrated in those early years can be interpreted in various cultures and with different levels of resources.
>
> Symptom control by a multi-professional team backed by research and education of both professionals and public has spread both into home care and into general hospitals. The family is seen as the unit of care as it finds its own potential, searches for meaning and makes the achievements possible at the end of life.
>
> (Saunders, 2000)

Prognosis

- Palliative care should be introduced based on the patient's needs, rather than relying on prognosis, which is generally a subjective judgement.

- The NICE guidance on care of the dying adult (2015) recommends diagnosing who is dying without providing any objective ways to do this.
- Questions about prognosis are to be encouraged from the patient and the family members.
- It is, however, notoriously difficult to give a completely accurate prognosis. This particularly applies if the patient has a medical condition, for example, due to chronic heart and/or lung disease.

Aim of palliative care

One of the primary purposes of care for the dying patient is the relief of pain and suffering. Effective management of pain and other symptoms, in all forms, is therefore, critical in the appropriate treatment and care of the dying. This aim underlines the need for holistic approaches, aimed at maintaining optimum mental and physical function.

Ethical palliative care

In good clinical practice, an awareness of the condition and true prognosis for the patient may lead to a change in the focus of treatment from cure to palliative care.

Ethical issues in palliative care often arise because of concerns about how much and what kind of care makes sense for someone with a limited life expectancy. There may be conflict between clinicians, nurses, other healthcare team members, patients and family members about what constitutes appropriate care, particularly as patients approach death.

A lesson can be learned from the discriminatory and ageist practices of the intrinsically flawed LCP. Health professionals should seek to preserve life quality and not destroy it. We are not the arbiter of anyone's death or life. Health professionals must not participate in any act directly aimed at shortening or suppressing life.

Concerns of the LCP Review panel

- Lack of respect and compassion for patients.
- Lack of patient informed consent.

- Lack of effective communication with the dying person and relatives.
- Lack of required hydration for many patients.

(DH, 2013)

Informed consent

Informed consent is a fundamental principle of medicine and matters of consent are especially serious when dealing with a dying patient. This was a reported lack in many cases in relation to the LCP as documented by the LCP review.

It is a fundamental patient right and applies in all fields of treatment and care and is included as an important expectation of the nursing code of conduct:

- (1.5) respect and uphold people's human rights
- (2.3) encourage and empower people to share in decisions about their treatment and care
- (2.4) respect the level to which people receiving care want to be involved in decisions about their own health, well-being and care
- (4.2) make sure that you get properly informed consent and document it before carrying out any action.

(NMC, 2018)

Precious time

It is particularly important to ascertain consent in palliative care before the patient may lose capacity, due to deterioration

The NICE guidance on care of the dying adult (created in 2015 to replace the LCP), does not give complete reassurance that informed consent to treatment will be obtained from the patient, where possible. This is especially needed where a proposal might involve sedation which must always be clinically justified, among the team, to the patient and to the family.

Patients' rights to information

Patients warrant education from practitioners, all of whom must be aware of legal developments which may impact on professional ethics. One of the healthcare provider's first duties to a patient is to inspire hope through the development of a therapeutic relationship and the provision of appropriate and accurate health education and information. This may help patients to understand that their rights to autonomy must confer real benefit, not harm.

Communication

Issues such as the complexities of CPR and advanced directives need sensitive discussion with patients by the doctors and nurses as part of effective communication with their patients. Concerns raised in the review of the LCP related to poor communication with the dying person and their relatives, including surrounding the issue of hydration.

Effective communication is fundamental to good clinical practice and in line with patients' rights. Health professionals caring for a patient in danger of death from illness, accident, or complication of advanced age should provide the patient with appropriate information to help with understanding of the condition. This gives patients the opportunity to discuss the situation with family members, as wished, unless the patient is lacking capacity.

A study conducted just over twenty years ago, highlighted the need for the initiation of training programmes for physicians oriented toward enhancing communication skills when caring for dying patients and their families. Such training programmes should focus on teaching physicians to talk about dying, to listen to patients and family members and to be sensitive to when patients are ready to talk about dying. The ambiguity that exists between the need to be honest and the desire to maintain hope is a challenge for physicians and a critical area for future research (Wenrich et al, 2001).

Regular communication with dying patients is essential. The need for nursing advocacy and questioning practice in line with the code of conduct must be at the forefront of the mind when caring for dying patients. The nurses' code of conduct expects nurses to 'make sure that those receiving care, are treated with respect, that their rights are upheld and that any discriminatory attitudes and behaviours towards those receiving care are challenged' (NMC, 2018).

The review panel of the LCP emphasised the importance of maintaining a record of clinician communication with patients and family including the following:

- Face-to-face conversation and explanation (dated) that the patient is now dying.
- How death might be expected to occur, using language, which is clear, direct and unambiguous.
- When the 'end of life' care plan was first discussed with the patient and the relatives or carer.

(DH, 2013)

Documentation of conversations between the senior clinician and family

If the family or carers do not accept the judgement that the patient is dying, the clinician explains and documents **the basis** for that judgement and documents that the relatives or carers had the **opportunity** to ask questions.

(DH, 2013)

The GMC, in its latest guidance, recommends that the doctor: 'explore **options** including the patient's right to seek a second opinion' (GMC, 2022a).

Such medical conduct may have prevented the arbitrary placement of patients on the LCP by junior doctors and some nurses.

Listening as companionship, an essential part of communication

The following suggestions have been made by a retired Palliative Care specialist who has written books about communicating with the dying: 'With the end in Mind' and 'Listen'.

Good listening means that companionship is paramount. Often this requires:

- Questions more than statements
- Silence often more than talking (be quiet but stay present)
- Curiosity more than certainty
- Acceptance of complexity, distress and uncertainty.

Forget about what to say- just understand the other person's perspective.

- Listen
- Reflect
- Understand

Check understanding as you go. Summarise after questions and review own assumptions

Being curious is essential as it allows the person to tell more and saying it out loud helps them to make sense of their experience. Be a companion. We may have to fix a time when proper attention can be given for one-to-one discussion or with the person's relatives (Mannix, 2022).

Hope

This virtue is a vital element in healing and can be considered as an important, invisible virtue even though the possibility of a cure may be remote. Human beings need encouragement in practising this virtue as it is a positive orientation to life rather than despair. Patients need faith and hope in their carers' skill and experience and their readiness to always meet any challenge, regarding symptom prevention and control.

Complete openness?

The danger of crushing a patient's hope can outweigh the usual imperative to tell all, doctors argue in a new commentary that has touched off a debate on honesty. By suggesting the danger of crushing a patient's hope can outweigh the usual imperative to tell all, some doctors have subtly challenged the prevailing wisdom. They suggest there are times when complete openness may not be what patients want, when soft-pedalling the grim nature of an illness might be preferable to full disclosure. This new commentary has started a debate on honesty during the sensitive times of the physician-patient relationship.

Before exercising 'therapeutic privilege' to withhold information, though, physicians need to determine how much knowledge the patient desires and be guided by those wishes. 'It's very disconcerting to a medical professional; we really feel it's not ours to withhold information. [But] some people don't feel that that knowledge will help them in any way... Forcing people to know what they don't want to know can be harmful' (Blackwell, 2014).

Nevertheless, the concept of attending to unfinished business is especially important and it can be a wide-ranging concept for some people, nearing the end of their lives, requiring timely action, as necessary, following sensitive communication.

Holistic care

This is an active and total approach to care, from the point of diagnosis and prognosis, respecting the person's life, death and beyond. It embraces physical, psychological, emotional, social and spiritual elements and focuses on the enhancement of quality of life for the person and support for the whole family.

Holistic care involves interacting and integrating care with the assistance of the chaplains, social workers, family members and friends to allow the patient to accept death and live out life until its natural end. It includes the management of distressing symptoms, provision of short breaks, care at the end of life and bereavement support. This all requires the involvement of all relevant members of the multidisciplinary team.

Florence Nightingale – advocate for holistic care

The WHO designated the year 2020 as the 'Year of the Nurse and Midwife' and extended this designation into 2021. This is in honour of the 200th birth anniversary of Florence Nightingale, who is considered as a healthcare pioneer, an early statistician and the founder of modern, holistic nursing.

Florence Nightingale taught nurses to focus on the principles of holism: unity, wellness and the interrelationship of human beings and their environment. Holistic Nursing is not merely something we do. It is also an attitude, a philosophy and a way of being that requires nurses to integrate self-care, self-responsibility, spirituality and reflection in their lives. This often leads the nurse to greater awareness of the interconnectedness of self, others, nature, spirit and relationship with the global community.

Holistic needs assessment

*The NMC expects nurses to be able to,
...in partnership with the person, the carers and their
families, make holistic, person-centred and systematic
assessments of physical, emotional, psychological, social,
cultural and spiritual needs, including risk and develop a
comprehensive, personalised plan of nursing care.*

(NMC, 2010)

Holistic needs assessments are detailed in Chapter 4 and are promoted by the Macmillan charity. (See the link: https://www.macmillan.org.uk/healthcare-professionals/innovation-in-cancer-care/holistic-needs-assessment)

The gift of medicine and nursing

If we only see death as a medical failure, then we fail to understand that the real gift of medicine and nursing is not just a science but a wisdom: how to live life, of which dying is a part. That requires a sense of the wholeness of the person and the wholeness of a life, thus genuine care will have time for the multifaceted reality of dying.

Proportionate vs disproportionate treatment

The health team has a moral obligation to use ordinary or proportionate means of preserving a patient's life. Proportionate means are those that in the judgement of the health team and the patient offer a reasonable hope of benefit and do not entail excessive burden. The Catholic Church teaches that there is no moral obligation to use disproportionate means and that the patient has a right to refuse them.

The actual validity of the traditional teaching on ordinary and extraordinary means of the preservation of life has been confirmed by the Magisterium of the Church during the 20th century, in the context of the complex moral dilemmas presented by the practice of contemporary medicine. The magisterial documents emphasize the importance of understanding and applying this doctrine in light of the unconditional respect that all human life merits — from conception to natural death — by reason of its ontological dignity (given as much by its origin as by its destiny) (Tabouada, 2008).

While patients may forego treatments that are disproportionate or considered extraordinary means, there is always an obligation to provide ordinary care that is due to the sick person by good nursing care and any relevant proportionate treatment where obviously required. An example is the appropriate use of antibiotics where tissue pain due to infection may improve.

Wisdom and conscience

Compassionate practitioners provide ethical treatment as part of their duty of care. They do not persist in treatment, which is evidently futile, which would confer no patient benefit and perhaps cause harm. A sensitive, informed conscience is our guide, aided by ethical guidance such as the new manual for healthcare workers, issued by the National Catholic Bioethics Centre (2017). This centre has upheld the dignity of the human person in health care and biomedical research for fifty years

Patient autonomy

Many professionals sincerely respect patient autonomy, but cost factors will always be there in the background. Should concepts such as managed care settings/managed death and the GSF be uncritically accepted?

It is argued that autonomy is a misused word. It can be valuable in the context of medical ethics by emphasising the importance of the patient rather than any process, but it can also be a pretext for selfishness, for none of us are completely autonomous: we depend on each other. Moreover, an overemphasis on autonomy in the context of euthanasia places the doctor in the position of a servant to do the patient's will, unable to exercise any independent, professional judgement (Cole and Duddington, 2021b).

Do patients fully understand when they sign up to an advanced directive via the MCA? How can they know whether the care they receive will be truly compassionate and effective as a result? Will they know that assisted food and fluid is considered as medical treatment?

Physical needs

Symptom control

Nadine Dorries, MP and former nurse, spoke against the Assisted Dying (Marris) Bill and talked about the beauty of palliative care: 'no one needs to die a painful death. The combination of drugs that are administered to people in their final days ensures that they do not suffer pain' (Dorries, 2015).

Patients in the advanced stage of a life-threatening illness typically experience multiple symptoms, the most common of which are pain, depression, anxiety, confusion, fatigue, breathlessness, insomnia, nausea, constipation, diarrhoea and anorexia. In all circumstances, health professionals must be knowledgeable (as with any other specialty) to provide basic, humane care and relieve all symptoms (with the assistance of specialist expertise where needed) and prevent other distress such as hunger and thirst.

Nutrition and hydration

A retired geriatrician and author of books on medical ethics, including the dangers of dehydration, notes that if food and water is regarded as a basic human need, rather than 'treatment', doctors might pay more attention to hydration and nutrition in terminal care (Craig, 2004). Hydration should never be withheld or withdrawn, with the sole purpose of causing the death of the patient. Such unlawful and unethical practice was condemned by the panel charged with the independent review of the LCP which was discredited and recommended for withdrawal in 2014.

The LCP review panel also stated that doctors and nurses should be held to account by their regulatory bodies, as deliberate denial of fluids is unacceptable and unethical. This happened for years without evidence of the impact on thirst sensation as questions tended not to be asked.

Clinically-assisted nutrition and hydration

Debate appears to centre around whether prolonging life can be attributed to assisted hydration. This debate should rather focus on the concept of thirst in line with planning for quality life for the dying patient. This stance is more humane than concerns about unnecessarily prolonging life. Thirst should not be a compounding factor for the dying patient, who may be unable to voice such a sensation. It should be considered as a preventable and treatable problem.

Associated symptoms of dehydration

The importance of treating thirst and dehydration in all patients must be understood. It is especially important not to forget those patients at the end of life, when those particular signs and symptoms may be missed or ignored (Bubna-Kasteliz, 2017).

Patients have reported feeling terrible thirst and other effects when being denied hydration. Additionally, the following dehydration-associated symptoms cannot be dismissed as just unfortunate:

- Restlessness, confusion, agitation.
- Lowered pain threshold (Bear et al, 2016).
- Opioid neurotoxicity (Magnussen and Mulder, 2001).
- Delirium (Lawlor, 2002).

Patients can be sedated or confused so that they cannot manage end of life thirst by taking any oral hydration. Mouth care is fundamental to nursing care but cannot alleviate thirst. Offering oral fluids may be dangerous or ineffectual when dehydration is established. Therefore, where patients are critically dehydrated, they may be unable to take oral fluids so will need assisted and monitored hydration.

Patients need their individual requirements to be assessed and their preferences addressed on admission to hospital, by means of a fluid-assessment chart. Alternative methods of hydration should also be considered. Education and training on the importance of hydration remain key. These minor changes could improve patient hydration and independence, thus preventing avoidable harm (Johnstone et al., 2015).

The team leader

The senior clinician must lead the palliative care team (DH, 2013). Medical problems do still exist in palliative care, e.g., unstable diabetes so it is important to liaise with relevant specialists, including, for example, the nutritionist and speech therapist. This is an example of good medical practice in accessing other expertise where need is identified (GMC, 2022a).

Assisted hydration, when required, absorbable, practicable and carefully monitored, will not harm patients and should be included as part of fundamental and humane care. The LCP review panel recommendation in relation to hydration needs was that practitioners will monitor and review rate and volume (DH, 2013). The GMC latest guidance on hydration and nutrition when caring for the dying includes the following principle:

> 111. If you are concerned that a patient is not receiving adequate nutrition or hydration by mouth, even with support, you must carry out an assessment of their condition and their individual requirements. You must assess their needs for nutrition and hydration separately and consider what forms of clinically-assisted nutrition or hydration may be required to meet their needs.
>
> (GMC, 2022b)

Nutrition and hydration are distinct elements and should be approached as such

For I was hungry, and you gave me something to eat, I was thirsty, and you gave me something to drink.

(Matthew, 25: 31–40)

*There should be a duty on all staff to ensure that patients
who are able to eat and drink should be supported
to do so [unless they choose not to].
Failure to support oral hydration and nutrition when still possible
and desired should be regarded as professional misconduct.*

(DH, 2013)

Hydration

*When patients are thought to be dying, that does
not mean that fluids become futile.*

(Finlay, 2008)

The NICE guidance, titled *Care of Dying Adults in the Last Days
of Life* (NICE, 2015), emphasises the need to maintain hydration
in dying patients to minimise symptomatic dehydration or
delirium.

A former neuroscience specialist, who was one of the first
clinicians to raise concerns about the LCP, voiced concern about
this guidance which also confusingly states that death is unlikely
to be hastened by withholding hydration. It is incredible that
supposed LCP replacement guidance by NICE is 'a disaster of
misinformation, distortion and ambiguity' (Pullicino, 2015). Staff
effort should focus on life quality, rather than concerns about
potential extension of life.

Safe oral hydration

Safe swallowing assessment is essential for patients who are
in a weakened state, including patients requiring post stroke
support. The Speech Therapist is an essential member of the
multidisciplinary team at this time to teach patients, staff and
relatives, the importance and usefulness of thickened fluids.
Excellent thickening products are available and commonly used
and can be acceptable to patients. This can be a measure to ensure

swallowing safety. Where this method to help in oral hydration is no longer possible, then other routes for safe hydration need to be explored.

The subcutaneous (s/c) route

Although the s/c route can be erratic in absorption, it may be easy to manage in home settings. The nurse should consider it unethical not to promote assisted fluids for helpless, ill patients. Health professionals need to question themselves about where does palliative care end and euthanasia begin? We live in the days where 21st-century palliative care can offer so much more than before, including at home.

The s/c route has distinct advantages over the i/v route in the elderly confused and at the end of life. The s/c route is easier to use when the patient is dehydrated with collapsed or thrombosed veins, or if i/v cannulae keep being pulled out. For instance, a s/c Teflon or Vialon s/c catheter can be kept out of a patient's sight, while still being accessible, by placing it into the skin behind the shoulder. There is no risk from inadvertent air bubbles or delay in replacing empty bags and it is therefore useful when rehydrating a patient at home or in a nursing home (Bubna-Kasteliz and Bodagh, 1993). Vigilance is also required to ensure that the simple s/c route is not used to ease patients into an 'end of life' care routine when i/v fluids can be used.

Rates of Infusion

'Nutrition and hydration provided by tube or drip are regarded in law as medical treatment and should be treated in the same way as other medical interventions' (Airedale NHS Trust v Bland, 1993). This, judgement, related to the Tony Bland decision at the time, can be refuted, since life-sustaining food and fluids are basic needs of everyone.

The benefits and potential disadvantages of assisted hydration should be explained. There should be a clear timeframe for review after about 48 hours; by then the patient may be able to drink more or not, which may be because the patient is dying. Several studies of adverse effects from s/c fluid have found them to be infrequent and are easily avoided (Dalal and Bruera, 2004). It is also important to make families aware that such fluids will need to be slowed or re-sited if they cause obvious complications such as signs of fluid overload, skin swelling, discomfort, or signs of pulmonary oedema.

Fluid monitoring

Competent medical and nursing practitioners, either in the hospital or community settings, should be able to manage such simple infusions without difficulty, by monitoring hydration, titrating to need and physical signs and the response of the patient. This can ensure, in most cases, the comfort, ethical and safe care of the dying or non-dying patient in need of assisted hydration.

Various modes of providing clinically-assisted hydration may be explored and depending on the healthcare setting, should be appropriately used. Competent practitioners will monitor patients' hydration needs accordingly. The monitoring and adjusting of drug doses are also well-established practices when ensuring effective pain and other symptom relief.

Guidance on the s/c route is available via the following link: https://www.palliativedrugs.com/download/180214_Subcutaneous_hydration_in_palliative_care_v2.4_Final.pdf

Pain and use of opioids

The cause for pain needs to be investigated and relevant drugs employed. This can minimise the known complications of opioid drugs.

Opioid toxicity

The European Association of Palliative Care (EAPC) research network has developed recommendations for treating opioid-induced adverse effects (Cherny et al., 2001).

Long-term use of opioids can lead to accumulation of its toxic metabolites, leading to various adverse events, known as opioid toxicity. This condition is often missed and misdiagnosed in clinical practice and hence seldom managed appropriately (Ostwal et al., 2017).

Opioid-induced toxicity should be regularly assessed and aggressively treated to improve the quality of life of the patient and to decrease distress in both patient and their caregivers (Ostwal et al., 2017). A change and/or rotation of opioids would allow for clearance of metabolites while maintaining or improving pain control in patients on chronic opioid treatment for cancer pain who develop symptoms of toxicity (de Stoutz et al., 1995).

Individualised pain relief

It should be known whether pain relief should be targeting nerve pain or inflammation, to be able to offer the appropriate analgesic agent, such as nerve pain agents where pain is nerve-based. Escalation of analgesic opioid drugs for pain is not always wise when the pain may be neuropathic in origin. Therefore, opioids are not always first line to use for neuropathic pain.

Neuropathic pain

Effective pain relief should be specific in targeting neuropathic pain. The role of low dose tricyclic antidepressants (TCAs) in the treatment of neuropathic pain is now well established with best documented evidence (Saarto and Wiffen, 2007). Amitriptyline is a type of drug called a tricyclic antidepressant. These drugs were originally developed to treat anxiety and depression, but when taken at a low dose they can reduce or stop pain. A low-dose antidepressant, it is well known can help patients with nerve pain, whereas opioids may not be suitable.

Anticonvulsants

These have been evaluated and used effectively in neuropathic pain.

Tissue pain

Antibiotics can provide relief of pain in infected tissue.

Anxiety reduction

My experience in palliative care was that aiming to reduce patient anxiety can greatly reduce the experience of pain. This aim was not necessarily dependent on drug therapy.

Breathing problems

Shortness of breath or the feeling that breathing is difficult is a common experience at the end of life. Measures which can be used to help ease a patient's breathing include:

- Raising the patient's position in bed/chair.
- Opening a window, without causing a draught.
- Using a humidifier or using a fan to circulate air in the room.
- Holding a small fan about six inches from the central part of the face so that the cooling effect felt around the sides of the nose and top lip can reduce the sensation of breathlessness. The benefit should be felt within a few minutes (Guys and St Thomas NHS Trust, 2015).
- Using morphine, or other medications such as diazepam to help relieve the sense of breathlessness.
- Giving oxygen, if required on a continuing basis requires nebulisation to prevent drying of the mouth and nasal mucosa.

The elderly person

Due to the older person's particular sensitivity to drugs, it is recommended that evidence for both non-pharmacological and pharmacological interventions is known and evidence-based for symptom management (Palliative Care Clinical Studies Collaborative, 2014).

Many frail older people have died without needing an opiate and often required no medication at all. Combination of unnecessary doses of opioids and sedation together with dehydration, will kill the strongest patient.

Constipation

One of the common side effects of opioid medication is constipation, which some patients have reported as worse than the original pain. This must be prevented by the appropriate agent. Non-drug treatments, such as increasing fluid and dietary fibre intake can be helpful.

Preventive monotherapy with stool softeners alone may be ineffective and use of a scheduled stimulant laxative often is required. Co-prescription is required of either a softener and/or stimulant e.g., magnesium sulphate/senna is cheaper and most efficient rather than psyllium or glycol derivatives which are expensive and require adequate water ingestion (1,000 to 1,500 mL per day) (Swegle & Logemann, 2006).

Though often used, syringe drivers are not always obligatory

The Neuberger LCP Review Panel heard reports of patients being given drugs by a syringe driver so quickly that they rapidly became drowsy and so were unable to ask for, or safely take, something to eat or drink (DH, 2013). Maintain medications orally for as long as possible, ensuring they are 'rationalised' – particularly sedation.

Syringe drivers and the elderly

Kinley and Hockley (2010) undertook a baseline review of the medication of 48 nursing home residents in their last month of life and found that, of the eleven residents who had a syringe driver in the last days of life, eight of the syringe drivers were in place for less than one-and-a-half days.

Control of symptoms in older people may be more appropriately managed using bolus/buccal/sublingual medication or rectal suppositories in the last days of life (Webb, 2017).

Questions to ask

- Has the person been taking oral analgesics?
- Are any of their other medicines essential for their comfort?

- Is the person agitated?
- Does the person sound chesty or have retained secretions?

The doctrine of 'double effect'

There has been significant disagreement about the precise formulation of this principle, it generally states that, in cases where a contemplated action has both good effects and bad effects, the action is permissible only if it is not wrong and if it does not require that one directly intends the evil result. It has many obvious applications to morally complex cases in which one cannot achieve a particular desired good result without also bringing about some clear evil. The principle of double effect, once largely confined to discussions by Catholic moral theologians, in recent years has figured prominently in the discussion of both ethical theory and applied ethics by a broad range of contemporary philosophers.

A study by palliative care specialists was prompted by public and professional concern that the use of opioids for symptom control might shorten life. A retrospective analysis was conducted of the pattern of opioid use in the last week of life in 238 consecutive patients who died in a palliative care unit. Median doses of opioid were low (26.4 mg) in the last 24 hours of life. Patients who received opioid increases at the end of life did not show shorter survival than those who received no increases. The researchers concluded that the doctrine of double effect, therefore, need not be invoked to provide symptom control at the end of life (Thorns and Sykes, 2000).

The topic is controversial and yet it is argued that

> it is important to emphasize that there is no debate among specialists in palliative care and pain control on this issue. There is a broad consensus that when used appropriately, respiratory depression from opioid analgesics is a rarely occurring side effect. The belief that palliative care hastens death is counter to the experience of physicians with the most experience in this area. The mistaken belief

that analgesia will have the side effect of hastening death
may have the unfortunate effect of leading physicians,
patients and the patients' families to under-treat pain because
they are apprehensive about causing this alleged side effect

(Fohr, 1998).

More studies may draw similar conclusions, that double effect plays no role in justifying the use of opioid drugs for pain relief in the context of palliative care. However, when combined with unnecessary sedation, both opioid and sedation drugs will need challenging.

Tolerance

Long term opioid use leads to tolerance. Opioid tolerance is characterised by a reduced responsiveness to an opioid such as morphine which can result in a need for higher and more frequent doses to achieve the same analgesic effect.

Hyperalgesia

This state can occur when opioid-based medications are taken for an extended period. Opioid-induced hyperalgesia can mean that opioids change how the body handles pain signals making pain feel much more intense. It is one of the key reasons why pain experts do not advocate long term use of opioid medications or premature and inappropriate commencement. Should such a complication arise, prescribers can lower the dose of the medication and gradually stop it. The cause of the reported pain must be known for the most suitable drug regime.

Use of sedation

Widespread practice of the discredited LCP was the use of terminal and 'blanket' sedation and often inappropriate use of opioids.

'Blanket' sedation – holistic care?

Sedation, as part of required treatment, may be needed for patients who are: terminally agitated, delusional, or psychotic and becoming a danger to themselves or others. Sedation drug regimes, without hydration, give patients no chance of return from the point of oblivion. Such practice goes against health professionals' mandate to provide ethical, individualised and humane, holistic care. Spiritual needs cannot be met if patients are routinely and inappropriately sedated to death. The importance of spiritual care applies whether patients are imminently dying or not. Therefore, there is a need for caution with sedation, particularly in line with this spiritual aspect of holistic care required by patients as an expectation of the code of conduct.

Midazolam

The risk of serious side effects such as slow/shallow breathing and severe drowsiness/dizziness may be increased if midazolam is taken with other drugs that may also cause drowsiness or breathing problems such as opioid drugs. This was a common combination in the use of the LCP. This sedative drug is considered a high alert medication because of the risk of respiratory depression and respiratory arrest when used without appropriate resuscitative equipment or qualified personnel for patient monitoring and management.

Patients in need of palliative care warrant first-class, not second-class, care. Staff should be knowledgeable and competent in the use of resuscitative equipment and appropriate antidotes (flumazenil for midazolam, naloxone for opioids).

Sedation and dehydration

Who knows whether patients are quietly suffering while sedated and unable to express pain of hunger and thirst? The research on such practice is not possible, so such practice remains non-evidence based. It is recognised that opioids given to dehydrated patients are diminished in their analgesic properties and produce opioid neurotoxic side effects. Opioid-induced toxicity should be regularly assessed and aggressively treated to improve the quality of life of the patient and decrease distress in both patient and caregivers (Ostwal et al., 2017).

The provision of fluids to prevent dehydration is the sensible, kind approach to treatment and care of the dying who may infrequently require sedation.

Avoidance of sedation

Palliative care specialists have argued that, with careful assessment of reversible factors and alternative management for problems like delirium, some of the need for sedation may be avoided (Thorns and Sykes, 2000). The ethical and legal risks of sedation would be greatly reduced if palliative carers took a more active approach to hydration and quite simply provided hydration for a matter of days until life ends naturally (Craig, 2002).

Other drug support

Noisy respiratory secretions

These can occur in the dying patient and can be upsetting to the relatives. Careful patient repositioning can be helpful. Compared to atropine, glycopyrrolate has reduced cardiovascular and ocular effects. It diminishes the volume and free acidity of gastric secretions and controls excessive pharyngeal, tracheal and bronchial secretions. In common with other antimuscarinic drugs, caution is advised in patients with prostate enlargement, paralytic ileus, pyloric stenosis and closed angle glaucoma. 'Buscopan' can reduce secretions but must be given early to have an effect.

The route of administration can be intramuscular or intravenous. Patients will be more comfortable at home by the insertion of an indwelling cannula to the arm so that regular administration is possible by the district nurse/rapid response team, day, or night.

The imminently dying

The Catholic, moral tradition does not tell us that we are obliged to do everything we can to preserve life, whatever the cost. Dying patients requiring palliative care will not benefit from burdensome and non-effective treatments in the clear circumstances of the dying process.

The phase of dying

The process of dying is the result of the body eventually becoming overwhelmed with the burden of the disease. Though potential thirst can be distressing for relatives to imagine, much comfort can be provided by explanation about the dying process and ensuring understanding of reasonable measures that can still be employed, such as safe oral intake and s/c fluid as needed and moistening the mouth. This regular and important nursing practice, however, does not substitute for comfort of clinically assisted fluids when appropriate.

Staff education

The LCP review panel in 2013 recommended that in relation to nutrition and hydration, the importance of staff education was to be given emphasis.

The review panel recommended that all staff in contact with patients should be trained in the appropriate use of hydration and nutrition at the end of life and how to discuss this with patients, their relatives and carers.

Specialist services, professional associations and the Royal Colleges should run and evaluate programmes of education, training and audit about how to discuss and decide with patients and relatives or carers how to manage hydration at the end of life (DH, 2013).

Maintaining hydration at the end of life is both controversial and emotive. There was significant media coverage surrounding the LCP and relatives' concerns about people dying from dehydration and suffering with distressing symptoms due to inadequate fluid intake. Suspicion was also raised that fluids were withheld and even denied to dying persons to hasten death (DH, 2013).

Palliative care in accident and emergency departments (A and E)

There is growing literature about ways to best use palliative care services in accident and emergency departments (Quest et al., 2013). The palliative care nurse can provide support for the A&E staff, often overwhelmed by:

- medical emergencies, sudden deaths
- failed efforts at resuscitation
- trauma care
- victims of crime
- an increasing population of vulnerable, complex patients, accessing the A&E department as their only source point for care in chronic disease.

Oncology emergencies

The palliative care nurse specialist will be able to help to manage for example, such acute oncology emergencies as haemorrhage, bone marrow depression, sepsis and spinal cord compression.

The nurse specialist in palliative care can support the A&E staff in giving news of a death by explaining what has happened, assessing the family members' immediate coping, and physical, spiritual and psychological needs and assisting in making decisions about care and transition of the body.

Ethical decision-making

Open discussion, collaborative decision-making and consistent review in practice are crucial for avoiding moral distress for those involved during treatment cessation. Consensus in decision-making is key to minimising ethical discord and personal beliefs and experience are crucial factors (McLeod, 2014). However, termination of required assisted hydration and nutrition when a patient is not obviously in the dying phase, in palliative care, is unethical.

Psychological/emotional care

Patient distress

Along with the five vital signs of temperature, respiration, heart rate, blood pressure and pain, the sixth vital sign in cancer care is regarded as 'distress'. It is important for health professionals to include emotional distress as a factor when assessing the well-being of patients with cancer. It could also be useful for assessing the emotional status of patients with non-cancer conditions.

Many patients can experience a feeling of being a burden, either to their family or the carers. This is now established as commonly, the chief reason for requests for assisted suicide in countries where assisted suicide is legalised. It is important to understand that those patients asking for assisted suicide are more commonly in mental pain, rather than physical pain. This fact is a recognised and constant statistic. Health professionals who ignore this statistic and leave mental pain unaddressed can be regarded as being neglectful.

Depression in advanced illness

Where depression and anxiety are suspected, or exhibited, the team members have a duty to seek appropriate help for the patient to allow thorough assessment and appropriate treatment and care.

Nurses cannot diagnose depression but are to be alert to possible signs and act on their suspicions by ensuring required assessments for suspected depression. This approach is holistic, ethical, compassionate and rational. Where there is no further active treatment possible for physical illness, health professionals must be alert to distress in patients who may benefit by treatment of their psychological needs. Despite a period needed for antidepressants to achieve optimum effect, this is not always a prohibition for patients whose time remaining on earth can so often be ill defined.

Spiritual care

The dying experience is unique for everyone. For many individuals, death is not considered as an end to life. It is simply a passage to another dimension, called heaven, the spiritual world, another plane of existence, or nirvana. Florence Nightingale considered that the needs of the spirit are as critical to health as those individual organs which make up the body. Thus, spiritual care can be a natural part of holistic care (Hutchison, 1997).

To further clarify what is understood by spiritual care and following extensive review of the literature, Govier (2000) summarised the concept as the 'five Rs of spirituality':

- reason
- reflection
- religion
- relationships
- restoration

Reason and reflection

The nurse who takes a sincere and active role and recognises that the physical, psychological/emotional, social, cultural, and spiritual realms are all interconnected, is in a position to help those who may be suffering, to reflect upon and find meaning in their experiences.

Religion

Patients' beliefs demand the respect of the nurse who seeks to listen to and respect the views, values and practices of patients, without always agreeing with them or imposing their own views.

Relationships

A longing to relate to oneself, others and a deity/higher being (may be expressed via service, love, trust, hope, and/or creativity) and the appreciation of the environment.

Restoration

Certain life events can be detrimental, resulting in spiritual distress. Attention to spiritual care, as part of holistic needs may positively influence and restore patient wellbeing.

Spiritual distress

This is considered to be an approved nursing diagnosis which has been defined as a disruption in the life principle that pervades a person's entire being and that integrates and transcends one's biological and psychological nature (McFarland and McFarlane, 1997).

As knowledge of issues involved in death and dying increases and positive attitudes are promoted, the spiritual care and support for people who are dying will improve. In 2010, the RCN commissioned an online survey on spirituality and spiritual care in nursing practice. Nurses taking part in the survey considered the following factors to be important:

- education and guidance about spiritual care
- clarification about personal and professional boundaries
- support in dealing with spiritual issues.

(RCN, 2010)

One of the RCN survey respondents summarised the role of the nurse in relation to spiritual needs of patients as,

I believe that spiritual care is not only an essential component of nursing practice but often the arbiter of how a patient responds to their illness and life experiences.
It would appear, that when people encounter certain life events like serious trauma and illness, fundamental spiritual issues often emerge that question their very existence.

(RCN, 2010)

Such need for spiritual support as part of expected, holistic care by nurses may be denied patients if the healthcare team are solely concerned with the need for extreme sedation in the last stage of life. Such inappropriate practice, as so often occurred with the LCP, is a grave disservice and serious breach of the duty of holistic care that we owe to patients. Spiritual well-being is a concept well recognised for its importance by the nursing profession and the

NHS and is incorporated in NHS guidance for professionals and patients (INHS inform, 2020).

Spiritual awareness involves care to alert the patient and family to the spiritual dimensions of human life. Spirituality and the intrapsychic strength of the ageing individual can provide a source of help when coping with stressful life events. This can take the form of intrinsic religiosity: prayer, a sense of meaning and purpose and transcendence (Fehring et al., 1997).

Cultural sensitivity

Health professionals should help patients to prepare for death according to their religious beliefs and strive to put at their disposal the comforting rituals and sacraments of their individual religion. It is good practice for nurses to have an awareness of cultural sensitivity and flexibility and accept and understand practices may differ in the care of patients during their illness and after death.

Last rites

This term is more commonly replaced by the term 'sacrament of the sick'. This is a comforting sacrament for Roman Catholics who are extremely ill or near death. Its purpose is sanctification and remission of sins. Catholic teaching is that it enables remission of sins. it should, therefore, be offered to all Catholics who are dying as an essential source of sanctifying grace as we prepare for our final journey to eternal life (UK Catholic Nurses and Catholic Medical Associations, 2021).

Companionship as comfort

The book by Leo Tolstoy about the death of Ivan Ilyich is essential reading for those considering palliative care as a career. It shows the character, Gerasim, who can both comfort and heal the dying man, Ivan. When he supports Ivan's legs, Gerasim bridges the gap, both physically and spiritually, between Ivan and the world. It is not a coincidence that Ivan first realises the error of his past life while staring at Gerasim's face. Gerasim is a truly spiritual character. He exemplifies the right way to live and his contact with Ivan eases the man along the road to spiritual health.

Tolstoy shows the importance of companionship to provide comfort, through sensitive human contact for someone dying, feeling alone and in need of empathy:

> *It was a comfort when Gerasim sat with him sometimes the whole night through. Gerasim was the only one who did not lie; everything he did showed that he alone, understood what was happening and saw no need to conceal and so, the relationship was a comfort to him.*

(Farmakidis, 2005)

The most important assistance to dying patients is the 'loving presence' at the bedside. This makes the patient feel comforted. The terminally ill patient needs human accompaniment which health professionals must bring to bear on their relationship with the patient. The dying person should not be dismissed as incurable and abandoned to his own family, but the patient and whole family unit should be assisted by the loving care of the members of the health team.

The role of the Chaplain

Chaplains may be ministers of religion, or nurses, or lay people. Definitions of dying need to be carefully explored and understood. Where such labels are applied to patients, practitioners must always be prepared to question whether they are truly appropriate, mindful of the difficulties in diagnosing 'dying'.

Sometimes chaplains are called to a patient (who is obviously not dying) to give the patient the last rites. Such patients have been deemed to be 'at end of life' when this is not always the case. Some patients would be horrified that this label has been applied, unbeknown to them. Chaplains have an important role within the team and are entitled to ask questions and voice opinions about the general welfare of patients they may minister to, in addition to their spiritual needs. Nurse chaplains are in a particularly good position to liaise with the team members to build up trust for the patient and family's benefit and understanding of the true situation.

Unfinished business

Opportunities are treasured by most patients whether or not they may be dying for completion of 'unfinished business'. Wherever possible, the onus of meeting the need for addressing this important completion issue is on those healthcare professionals who are responsible for patient treatment and holistic care. Do social services need to be involved? Unfinished business does not only apply to financial affairs; does the patient need emotional/social/spiritual support or support in making amends? Does the patient need reconciliation with the prognosis or with someone distanced that they need to see again? Is the patient depressed, or perhaps concerned about their pet?

The concept of 'unfinished business' is important to be addressed and is a truly relevant concept for many patients who are reaching the end of their lives and for their families. The aim of those who care for dying patients is not to speed them towards death. Contrary to such an ethos, health professionals are very well placed as companions for the dying patient. Professionals must develop their skills to acknowledge sensitively, with patients, the inevitability of death. This allows professionals and patients to concentrate on improving the quality of their lives, put their affairs in order and, wherever possible, say goodbye before it is too late.

Financial/practical/social needs

The following can all be considered part of the holistic approach to care for patients to discuss what is really worrying them:

- Preferred place of care? Discussions are important with a realistic mode of discussion for what may or may not be possible.
- Does a will need to be made?
- People with cancer are considered disabled under the Disability Discrimination Act (1998) and the Equality Act (2010) protects the disabled.
- Patients with less than six months to live are eligible for non means tested benefits. See more information about benefits via the link: https://www.mariecurie.org.uk/help/support/benefits-entitlements/benefits-social-care-system/what-benefits-can-i-claim#are
- The Cinnamon Trust can help elderly patients with arrangements for their pet's welfare and rehoming in the event of their death.

Team working in palliative care

Palliative care is the province of those with specialist expertise. Other specialists must not be professionally in conflict. However, their respective expertise may on occasion be needed for a perhaps complex case.

A study by Bliss et al. in 2000, identified the features underlying successful interprofessional working in palliative care. These included:

- The importance of team members sharing a common language.
- This does not necessarily relate to the need for the same shared language to communicate with each other, some individuals' philosophies of care may differ.
- The need for individuals in teams to be prepared to work together and not to feel under threat from other professional groups.

The study concluded that collaborative relationships could exist, which include shared planning, shared decision-making, shared responsibility and non-hierarchical relationships (Bliss et al., 2000).

A specialist palliative care nurse, however, cites plenty of evidence that these conditions are not achieved in practice (Corner, 2003). Corner's study revealed a lack of understanding of what palliative care is and that individual practitioners were not understanding of other professional groups, or at what point in the illness such care should commence, or even who should own the specialty.

The team leader

It should be noted that although this specialty is the province of palliative care specialists, this should not mean the denial to patients of the expertise of other specialist practitioners, who may provide benefit for the patient's particular problems which do not stop because the patient is receiving palliative care, such as unstable diabetes. Relevant specialist domains, however, should not be conflicted in terms of patient benefit. The LCP review panel recommended that a senior clinician lead the palliative care team (DH, 2013).

Palliative care promotion

The duty of concerned people is to lobby for appropriate funding for both training of staff in palliative care and for staffing to be improved.

Those responsible for medical and nursing curricula need to consider the time allocated for education on this important specialty.

Care assistants and volunteers, with appropriate training and safe monitoring, can be invaluable members of the care team.

The overall responsibility for palliative care should not be devolved to unsupervised junior doctors. The responsibility for patient care is within the province of the consultant or general practitioner.

Audit

This should be a regular part of best practice in palliative care. It should involve examining medical treatment, nursing care, spiritual support and any concerns of relatives and carers.

Specialist services, professional associations and the Royal Colleges should run and evaluate programmes including education, training and audit about end of life hydration and how to discuss this with patients, relatives, or carers (DH, 2013).

Conclusion

While many individuals may see palliative care as a simple or a straightforward concept, healthcare professionals know that there are many different issues and challenges associated with the specialty and that as a concept, it is not black and white or straightforward. There are individual, ethical, moral, practical, local, logistical and spiritual elements that are central to ensuring that palliative care is not only person-centred, but effective, dignified, safe and compassionate (Tallo, 2016).

Palliative care is an issue of significant importance within our society with many clinicians and academics alike arguing that there should be more investment from the government, charities and other bodies to ensure the delivery of safe, effective and high-quality palliative care across the UK.

Health and Care Act (2022)

Lord Kamall's amendment (Clause 16) to the Health and Care Bill meant that a new legal duty will be placed on Integrated Care Boards to commission palliative care (including specialist palliative care) as they consider appropriate for meeting the reasonable requirements of the people for whom they have responsibility. The Health and Care Act (2022) introduced new legislative measures that aim to make it easier for health and care organisations to deliver joined-up care for people who rely on multiple different services.

Dying people will be given an explicit legal right to healthcare for the first time in NHS history, requiring every part of England to provide specialist palliative care which it is envisioned will provide equity in palliative care provision for people of all ages, including children and young people.

This is a progressive development which should help discourage the tragic drive for assisted suicide, seen as a 'solution' to certain challenges, including perceived deficits in palliative care.

The end of the road

None of us in the end can stand in the way of death. Committed Christians and those of other faiths see that death, as well as a sad farewell, is a gateway to a new and promised life. Thus, as we care for the dying, acceptance of that dying is centrally important to the care we give with empathy, compassion, justice and hope.

The RCN has programmes promoting individualised care including spiritual needs via the following links:

- https://www.rcn.org.uk/clinical-topics/End-of-life-care
- https://rcni.com/keywords/spiritual-care

A helpful reference book, The New Charter for Health Care Workers (Dying: pp. 105-122) can be accessed via the following link: file:///C:/Users/User/AppData/Local/Microsoft/Windows/INetCache/Content.Outlook/Y23VSDO4/431501363-The-New-Charter-for-Health-Care-Workers.pdf

There is no dispute that the NHS is under strain, particularly since the advent of COVID-19. However, rather than defeatist staff attitudes to the challenges of palliative care or a 'tick-box' mentality, patients warrant optimum, holistic management and care by committed professionals. It is not an insurmountable challenge.

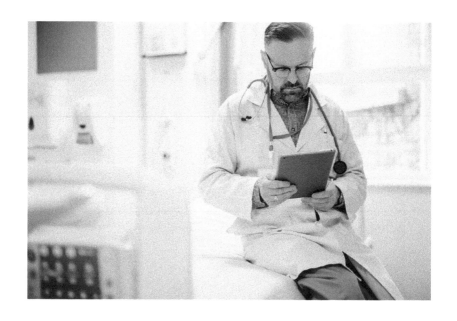

Chapter 16
Medical Futility

Thou shalt love thy neighbour as thyself.

(Matthew 22:3)

Introduction

The English word, 'care' derives from the Anglo-Saxon word *'carian'*, which meant 'putting oneself out for another'. 'Vocation' comes from the Latin word *'vocare'* meaning a calling - regarded as worthy and requiring dedication.

The definition of futile treatment is variable

It appears that there is no single definition of what constitutes futile care. The term is used by health care providers as they counsel patients and family members regarding what is appropriate care at the end of life (Fulp, 2007).

Futile treatment has been defined as 'treatment evaluated by the healthcare team, the family, or both, as being non-beneficial or harmful to a dying patient' (Barnhart et al, 2004).

While end of life and palliative care measures are difficult subjects to address, decision-making for patients and family members becomes more complicated when there is a lack of understanding of when care is appropriate or when it is futile in nature. The debate and media coverage surrounding the cases when futile care was deemed as the realistic option (see Chapter 8) has brought this issue to the forefront of concerns in medicine and nursing.

The purpose of an independent study was to begin to develop and apply a definition of futile care and to discover if there are commonalities when a situation is thought to be futile. The study (Fulp, 2007), included an in-depth review of the current literature, both research-based and opinion articles to explore this issue. The goal of the study was to better define futile care in terms so that health care practitioners and patients can understand and use in clinical settings. Implications for nursing would include better communications and to improve care offered to patients in a variety of clinical settings, as patients at the end of life are seen in all clinical settings and among all age groups.

By reviewing the literature on certain circumstances of the application of what is thought to be futile, a better working definition of futile care can be developed and patients and family members will hopefully become more informed decision makers. The study concluded with recommendations for nursing practice, research, education and health policy (Fulp, 2007).

Medical futility is a vague concept which is often surrounded by confusion. Conflicts persist regarding how to determine what futile means in particular circumstances. The explosion of medical technology and the intense media focus on real-life cases (promoting public outcry and dissenting views) only serve to foster this perplexity (Angelucci, 2006).

The Good Samaritan's example in the Lord's famous parable is today in danger of being replaced with the following question in too many cases: is this a 'futile' life not warranting 'futile' treatment, care and costs?

'Futile care'

This is an emerging and increasingly fraught concept. It might be more correctly termed 'futile treatment', which inescapably morphs into care, then perceived as 'futile'. Futile treatment and care concepts include questions of ethics, justice and autonomy for patients, doctors, nurses and patients' families. Treatment and prognosis are the province of doctors and nurses provide care. It would be wrong, however, to suggest that doctors do not 'care' for their patients.

Futile care: old vs new concepts

Ethical questions are debated by bioethicists (often with no medical qualification or clinical experience). The reality of what may be considered as 'futile' treatment and care can cause ethical difficulty for many healthcare professionals.

The old concept of futile care

Traditionally, this concept was considered as giving inappropriate/ineffective or intrusive treatment to the dying person.

The new version of futile care

This is based upon the beliefs of secular, 'modern' bioethicists that some patients have 'a duty' to die because the quality of their life is not worth the 'costly' finite medical resources.

It must be understood that often cost is not a barrier to good care and appropriate treatment. Decisions on expenditure may be based on discriminatory judgements. Further treatment, other than 'comfort' care, can be deemed 'futile', regardless of the desires of the patient or family. Families today, can be told by some doctors that the state of their loved one is hopeless and that all treatment should be withheld or withdrawn to allow them to die. This may happen within hours, days, or weeks of a person suffering a brain injury, stroke, or critical illness. Additionally, some families may not want to fight for their relative's possible recovery. So, the patient's survival and rehabilitation chances are slim. They are then reliant on a Good Samaritan practitioner who is prepared to offer them a fighting chance to survive.

Modern' bioethics: theory and practice

There are two concepts to be considered:

1. Quality of life

    Bioethicists, doctors and nurses judge the worth of a patient's life, according to mental and physical capacity.
    If a life is judged of such 'low' quality, it is considered not worth extending.

2. Economics

Limited resources can be an especially potent concept in increasingly strained medical systems.

Money may be saved not by providing services but by primarily controlling costs being motivated by concerns over 'social justice', which simply means the community is assumed to take precedence over the individual patient.

Utilitarianism/consequentialism

This ethical theory goes back to Greek philosophers, the most renowned being Epicurus. This is the tradition in ethical philosophy that holds that actions are right or wrong depending on the extent to which they promote happiness or prevent pain or are for the benefit of the majority. It is a doctrine that an action is right as far as it promotes happiness and that the benefit of the greatest number should be the guiding principle of conduct.

It can be argued that a utilitarian model can compromise the required nursing focus on individualised care. We see this in the failed project of the LCP where 'blanket' practices were common. Where still practised with vulnerable patients, lessons have not been learned and accountability will be demanded.

A change in spiritual outlook?

A change from a spiritual outlook to a more materialistic, cost-driven and ultimately dehumanising one is where the notion of healing, albeit sometimes without 'cure', in the accepted sense of the word is discredited. Are such ethical beliefs reflective of utilitarianism, eugenics, and the Nazi ideology of useless eaters?

'Defeatist' care ethic

Nurses must recognise the new secular and dangerous ethic of 'compassionate death'. A 'futile care' philosophy can ensure the death of those patients deemed, incorrectly, to be 'dying'. The result can be forced withdrawal of treatment from patients and their protesting families are informed that they perhaps are not accepting the 'right' option.

Quality-adjusted life years (QALYS)

It is true that healthcare technology is increasingly expensive and healthcare spending becomes a bigger burden on taxpayers. The price of health requires a pre-calculation as to whether a new medicine or treatment is worth the cost. While making such determinations may seem unseemly, some countries, including Britain, are explicitly using the cost-effectiveness of treatments in deciding what drugs can be made available to patients in need.

The price of health: quality-adjusted life years

Economists are sometimes accused of knowing the price of everything and the value of nothing, but perhaps the most difficult question requiring them to answer may be the price of health. To make the process more explicit, economists want to compare the cost-effectiveness of different treatments in a single measurement, one that the doctors and policy makers will trust enough to use.

Once they know how to rank the 'costs' of various diseases, economists can determine the worthiness of a particular treatment. To do so, they use the 'quality-adjusted life year' (QALY) measure. This is a measurement of disease burden which encompasses the quality and quantity of life lived. It is used by health professionals to determine the value of health outcomes. QALYs have been used for decades in healthcare allocation decision-making.

'Well-being-adjusted life year'

The UK Medical Research Council and others are exploring improvements to, or replacements for, QALYs. Among the possibilities are extending the data used to calculate QALYs (e.g., by using different survey instruments); 'using well-being to value outcomes' (e.g., by developing a 'well-being-adjusted life year';

and using value outcomes in monetary terms) (Brazier and Tsuchiya, 2015).

Who decides on life quality?

Decision-making bodies that use QALYs always consider other factors, such as clinical benefit, the rarity and severity of the disease in question, ethical considerations and the feasibility of an intervention. Important conceptual issues will also remain. An example is the question of whose preferences should form the basis of the quality-of-life weights used to construct QALYs: those of patients or members of the general population? Another concern is that QALYs are not 'patient-centric'.

Some research supports this contention; QALYs may not reflect certain goals and priorities individuals have in treatment decisions, such as their effect on family circumstances (e.g., desiring a therapy because it may increase the chance of attending an upcoming family wedding) (Doshi et al., 2018).

Limits to QALYs

QALYs do not inherently distinguish between a lengthy period spent in a moderately diminished health state and a shorter period spent in a more severe health state. Additional concerns about QALYs are directed at the idea of an authority, such as policy makers or economists, placing numbers on what people are 'worth'.

Elderly care discrimination

Michael Mandlestam, in his book of 2011, *How we Treat the Sick: Neglect and Abuse in Our Health Services*, suggests that there is a suspicion or danger that the way the health service is beginning to be run (or not run) for the elderly is based, at least in the eyes of central government and NHS trust executives, on a variation of this principle of utility, albeit unspoken. Namely, that older people with significant health needs will have to put up with deplorable levels of service, including suffering, pain, degradation and death for the good of everyone else. He also argues that it is far from clear who 'everybody else' is, especially as we all get old (Mandlestam, 2011).

A professor, who cared for the elderly, suggests that even if such a policy were to be made transparent, it would be morally unacceptable, as this creates a class of elderly, whose lives and well-being are not considered worth spending money on (Grimley-Evans, 1997). Therefore, current 'end of life' care plans need scrutiny in terms of patient safeguarding (see Chapter 4).

Striving officiously to keep alive

Ethical practitioners will not persist in treatment, which is evidently futile, which would confer no patient benefit and perhaps cause harm. Appropriate treatment and care can always be truly compassionate, holistic and do no harm, at all stages of life. A healthcare ethos which is overly focused on the futility of treatment and even care itself, is generated by false compassion. Such a defeatist ethos is dangerous and unworthy of those whose calling is to provide compassionate treatment for their patients.

Professional insecurity due to uncertainty

Concerns are expressed that the contemporary focus of healthcare ethics diminishes the importance of emotion in both moral judgement and action in clinical practice (Scott, 2000). Additionally, the evidence suggests that professionalisation and organisational structure can inhibit the ability to be sensitive to the moral aspect of clinical practice.

Professionals may find their long-held beliefs and values undermined, which threatens them, creating the insecurity resulting from uncertainty. It has been argued that increasing nurses' level of professionalism, can provide a positive contribution to the ethical decision-making level (Cerit and Dinc, 2013).

Exploration is required on what it means to attempt to engage in a 'post-emotional society' and what impact this dulling of the emotions has had on professions that locate 'care' as a central concept.

Post-emotional society, moral and ethical sensitivity

The capacity for interpreting an ethical dilemma was introduced to science as 'moral sensitivity'. This concept was defined and portrayed as the perception that something one might do or is doing, can affect the welfare of someone else, either directly or indirectly (by violating a general practice or community-held social standard) (Rest, 1982).

Ethical sensitivity

The concept of moral sensitivity was later operationalised as 'ethical sensitivity' (Rest, 1982). This was to reflect its linkage to codes of conduct. It is currently a low-level, emerging scientific concept, lacking comprehensiveness and clarity, yet should be considered as a positive and mandatory concept for professional practice (Weaver, 2007). Ethical sensitivity needs to be fostered by mentors and educators in teaching programmes for all healthcare staff. It links closely to the concept of conscience.

Controversial theories endanger patients

Two authors of a new paper (Shaw and Morton, 2020) which has recently been reported in the *Journal of Clinical Ethics,* claim that permitting assisted dying would substantially benefit both those seeking assisted suicide and the public. In their highly controversial paper, David Shaw, an ethicist from the Universities of Basel and Maastricht, and Alec Morton, a health economist of the University of Strathclyde in Scotland, both argue that granting terminally ill patients help to die would save money and potentially release organs for transplant.

These two Scottish academics pose three economic arguments:

- The cost to terminally ill patients of a poor quality of life.
- The cost of care that could be better used elsewhere.
- Potential benefits to organ donation.

Their report has been condemned by both opponents and supporters of assisted suicide. The authors stress that they do not intend their arguments to be used as the basis on which to change present UK legislation, which does not permit people to help another to die even if motivated by compassion. In their paper *Counting the cost of denying assisted dying*, the two authors write:

> *By combining quality of life and mortality into one metric, they enable quantification of the medical gains and losses and relative financial costs of a vast diversity of treatments and interventions, in turn enabling these different treatments to be compared against each other and funding decisions to be made.*

(Shaw and Morton, 2020)

Dr David Shaw, the lead author, argues:

> *Some people might suggest that it is callous to consider assisted dying from the perspective of resource management; these are real people with real lives. This criticism is misplaced. Part of the motivation for our argument is precisely that these are real people with real lives who wish to avoid suffering.*

Assisted dying (assisted suicide)

The first argument proposed by the authors in favour of assisted dying is that it enables consenting patients to avoid negative QALYS.

Secondly, they argue that resources consumed by patients who are denied assisted dying could instead be used to provide additional QALYs for patients elsewhere who wish to continue living and improve their quality of life.

Thirdly, they say that organ donation may provide an additional source of QALYs in this context.

The authors also argue that 'together, the avoidance of negative QALYs and gain in positive QALYs, suggests that permitting assisted dying would substantially benefit both the small population that seeks assisted suicide and the larger general population' (Shaw and Morton, 2020).

The authors argue that denying assisted suicide is a 'lose-lose' situation for all patients. They suggest that:

> Organ donation could also benefit because there are several reasons why donation after assisted dying is better from a clinical and economic perspective.

> First, if patients are denied assisted dying, organ function will gradually deteriorate until they die naturally, meaning that transplantation is less likely to be successful. Second, patients who choose assisted dying must go through a lengthy process and organ donation can be easily integrated into that process, non-coercively, decreasing the risk that family members will attempt to overrule donation, which often occurs when a patient dies in a way that is not planned.

> The legal arrangements for assisted dying vary widely from country to country and if the UK were to legalise assisted dying (presumably in the form of assisted suicide) the calculations here could be made more precise based on the specifics of the approach under consideration. Nevertheless, our paper shows in general that denying dying plausibly imposes great costs on both patients who wish to die and those who do not. Our argument is not that legalisation of assisted dying should be primarily based on economic arguments; these are supplemental facts that should not be neglected. Legalising assisted dying in the UK is likely to yield a substantial increase in QALYs across the patient population as a whole.

> (Shaw and Morton, 2020)

Dr Gordon MacDonald, of the lobby group 'Care Not Killing', which opposes assisted suicide, said, in response to these chilling proposals:

> *This report is highly disturbing. It highlights the dangers of legalising euthanasia. Very quickly the argument moves from that of personal autonomy to doctors and nurses*

making value judgements about the quality of other people's
lives while seeking to save money and tackle so-called
"bed blocking" in health services.

(MacDonald, 2020)

Vitalism

It is argued that the idea of keeping terminally ill patients alive, who are living in constant pain, is a perversion of a life, a conscious torment of an innocent person. This comment suggests that pro-life health professionals take a 'vitalist' position – that all people should be kept alive indefinitely by all means. This is a caricature of a pro-life approach – although one that is often put forward by critics and sometimes picked up by journalists.

True compassion

Unless compassion is combined with the desire to tackle
suffering and support those who are afflicted, it leads
to the cancellation of life in order to eliminate pain, thereby
distorting the ethical status of medical science.
True compassion, on the contrary, encourages every reasonable
effort for the patient's recovery. At the same time, it helps draw the
line when it is clear that no further treatment will serve this purpose.

(Pope St John Paul II, 2004b)

It is wrong to say that a life of suffering is a 'perversion of a life'. This view demeans those whose lives entail great suffering – either for a certain time, or for their whole life.

Individualised vs 'futile care'

A consideration of the whole person – their whole humanity and their intrinsic dignity and worth – is compassionate, rather than focusing on what may be considered as 'mere bodily existence'.

Dieticians have an increasing influence with vulnerable patients who need their support in terms of allowing 'a fighting chance' for quality life and survival. Nurses need to work closely with this member of the multidisciplinary team, in their role as the Good Samaritan.

Conclusion

Numerous reports of patients in a MCS who have heard what is going on around them, can also recover with non-defeatist treatment and rehabilitation.

Continuing care

A DNACPR order may be in place, but antibiotics may be appropriate. Simple nursing care is essential, designed to minimise infection and to support and benefit patients' physical, mental and spiritual wellbeing.

Providing CANH, where clinically indicated (ordinary care), feasible and practicable, should be part of compassionate, effective, evidence-based and positive treatment and care.

The 'poor'

In the Scriptures, the phrases 'people who are poor' and 'the little ones' commonly refer to those who, through no fault of their own, are powerless in society. Structures of oppression condemn them to economic, social and political poverty.

Jesus identifies with the actions of the Good Samaritan. His primary concern in His ministry is to be with those who are marginalised in society. By His actions and words, Jesus frequently repeats this message: 'I was hungry, and you gave me food. I was a stranger and you made me welcome' (Mt. 25:35). Jesus becomes so closely identified with people who are poor that when we refuse them justice, we are refusing Him.

Our neighbours

The ultimate test of our concern for human dignity will be the priority we give to people who are especially disadvantaged, people whom society considers worthless, as having nothing to offer society, as second-class citizens.

The past, ongoing and relatively recent healthcare scandals, and some comments of 'progressive' secular bioethicists, are becoming known and of great concern to both health professionals and the public.

Patients must be able to trust their health team to help them with their needs with good will, providing attentive, compassionate and appropriate care. Treatment, and even care, wrongly deemed as 'futile' can become the prevailing norm and practitioners can feel powerless against it. Staff can be haunted thereafter, with the realisation that their patients were not given the best possible treatment or none.

The NHS is for those in need of real help. It receives billions of pounds each year. What oversight and accountability exists for the use of such apparently needed, massive and ever increasing amounts?

It is argued that if the NHS worked as it should, given the amount of money pumped into it, then no one would need private insurance. One reason it doesn't work as it should is the objection of vested interests to the idea of charges or co-payments and other reforms that might improve the service for everyone but are blocked on ideological grounds (The Daily Telegraph, 2023).

The concept of hospital is historically understood as a haven, a safe place. Hospitals have always been institutions providing medical or surgical treatment or nursing care for sick or injured people. The word 'hospital' comes from the Latin 'hospes' signifying a stranger or foreigner, hence a guest.

Our patients are guests who may be needy, aged, infirm or young. All of whom warrant the utmost respect offered to them, whether they are for cure or not. Discriminatory attitudes to their perceived 'value' does a disservice not only to them but to the professions and to the parable of the Good Samaritan.

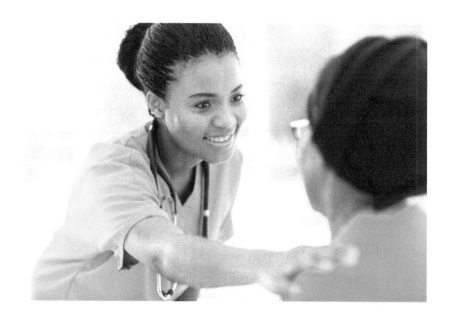

Chapter 17
Staff support

We are not ourselves, when nature, being oppress'd,
commands the mind to suffer with the body.

(Shakespeare's King Lear, Act II, Scene 4)

Introduction

The role of the Good Samaritan must extend to both our patients and our colleagues in keeping with the human imperative to care for others.

There are several areas to consider when identifying the pressures that are inherent in the caring professions, which can present the following conflicting demands:

- Attempts to maintain historical standards in a changing health culture of a 'marketplace'.
- Public and patient expectations.
- Demands from government and professional directives and managerial dictates.
- The professionals' own expectations of maintaining both high and consistent levels of care delivery.
- Lack of awareness and understanding of our own needs and those of colleagues.
- An inability to recognise the effects of pressures.

Self-care

The following words were published in the early 19th century and come from a four-act lyrical drama based on a Greek mythological play. They can apply to those who have lost heart in their ability to care for themselves which can be relevant for us all:

You have suffered sorrow and humiliation. You have lost your wits and have gone astray; and like an unskilled doctor,

fallen ill, you lose heart and cannot discover by
which remedies to cure your own disease.

(Shelley, 1820)

Healthcare pressures

People need to have experienced the pressures of healthcare to understand why there is a staff shortage crisis. According to NHS figures there are about one in ten posts being vacant in the NHS at the end of June 2022, the highest proportion on record. Factors include stress, sickness, early retirement and practitioners often choosing to work part-time, even without the usual associated factors such as family commitments.

In biblical times, it was common among the Jewish culture to use the phrase: 'Physician, heal thyself'. This had a nuanced meaning. They believed that before physicians could cure the disease that others were experiencing, they must first heal themselves. It is the idea that you cannot fill the cup of others unless your cup is full, too. This fullness is not necessarily associated with material wealth but a spirit of strength and health to cope with what life presents to each of us.

It is argued that we know that big houses, fast cars, private schooling and expensive gadgets do not make you happy (Turner, 2019). Goals, however, are reasonable for material goods as financial contentment is a right of all.

Work related stress defined

The HSE describes work-related stress as:
The adverse reaction people have to excessive pressure
or other types of demands placed upon them at work.
Work-related stress is one of the biggest health hazards in the
workplace. Stress is difficult to identify, but it can be
caused by excessive workloads or pressure placed on employees...
The law requires employers to carry out risk assessments to
identify hazards, including stress.

(HSE, 2021)

Heroes and heroines

There are many good doctors and nurses in the NHS and private care sectors. Some have given up their lives to the care of their patients during the COVID-19 pandemic. Many have received counselling for post-traumatic stress disorder and many have either taken sick leave or remain off work. The physical and mental health of nurses is under scrutiny due to the COVID-19 crisis. Many will need to be monitored due to recognised, ongoing post-traumatic stress disorder.

COVID-19 and critical care work stress

The COVID pandemic revealed even more publicly what a precious vocation it is to care for people most in need. Health professionals have risen to the occasion, despite the significant impact on mental and physical health. The pandemic was at its height in May 2020, when NHS Digital reported that more than 500,000 days of sick leave were taken by NHS staff due to mental health issues (NHS Digital, 2020).

Nikki Credland, Chair of the British Association of Critical Care Nurses, has reported that a significant amount of critical care staff experienced 'mental issues' due to what they have witnessed during the pandemic. Intensive care nurses have been sectioned under the Mental Health Act due to the psychological trauma that they experienced during the first wave of the pandemic.

Admitting stress

There have been many debates on workforce shortages within health and care settings and yet there remain unanswered questions on the changes needed to remedy these pressures.

More than 3,000 nurses have responded to a survey conducted by the RCN that revealed the increasing pressure felt by those in the profession. Respondents reported going on sick leave due to stress and taking antidepressants. Out of the 3,103 nurses and healthcare assistants who responded, 80% said the quality of patient care had declined since 2012 and they were more stressed now than they were at that time.

About 50% said they had seen patients suffer due to services being cut and had felt under pressure to save money. More than 50% said they only sometimes or never had time to deliver safe care. The RCN survey concluded that nurses are at an increased risk of burnout related to ongoing stress and job dissatisfaction (RCN, 2019).

Pre-pandemic stress levels

Prior to the COVID-19 pandemic, stress was a huge, reported factor among nurses as part of sickness rates. An exclusive Nursing Standard survey in conjunction with the Sunday Mirror newspaper revealed that stress is responsible for 40% of sickness rates in the nursing profession in the UK. Almost 60% of nurses feel stressed all, or most of the time (Dean, 2017).

Emotional exhaustion

One study of newly qualified and inexperienced nurses revealed they are at particular risk of suffering emotional exhaustion and burnout in unsupportive, practice environments. Almost every fifth nurse reported extremely high levels of burnout at some point during their first three years after graduation. Changes in burnout levels were accompanied by concurrent changes in depressive symptoms and intention to leave the profession. This study also showed that negative development of burnout was predicted by not feeling well-prepared for a nursing job, lacking study interest, elevated levels of performance-based self-esteem and depressive mood in the final year of education (Rudman and Gustavsson, 2011).

The cost of nursing stress

'Cost' in the caring profession relates to more than financial outlay. Unresolved, constant stress and sickness needs attention in terms of staff absence. Such focus can mean a possible reduction in nurses' attrition rates due to pro-active attention to physical and mental health issues.

Copp (1986), in her paper, *The nurse as advocate for vulnerable persons* concentrated on 'vulnerable persons' who are dependent on the nurse as their advocate in various care settings. Nurse patient advocacy often means potential and actual stress of that role for the nurse. Copp identifies the concept of 'feeling the heat'. This, she describes, is when a nurse is caught in the middle of complex, social interactions that usually include highly charged emotional exchanges. Such a formula has the potential to excite chemical reactions of such a magnitude as to cause ill health to the nurse.

It is distressing for nurses to feel that satisfactory care for patients is not always an achievable aim due to the work demands and the resource constraints.

Stress and burnout

It has been argued that during conflict and stress, the focus of interactions shifts to preserve the individual's dignity and self-esteem by withdrawal or avoidance (Drinka et al., 1996).

Maslach and Jackson (1981) defined burnout as a psychological syndrome, involving physical depletion, feelings of helplessness, negative self-concept and negative attitudes towards work, life and others. Stress and burnout have been described as having their origins in different sources, some of them individual factors and some of them situational factors.

Individual factors include:

- age and experience
- self-esteem levels
- personal resilience
- job satisfaction.

Situational factors include:

- regular exposure to pain and distress
- conflicting information about what the organisation expects from staff

- what the organisation places value in
- poor feedback systems or lack of recognition or praise for individual acts of compassion and care
- lack of time and simultaneous pressure to meet targets.

(Cornwell and Goodrich, 2009).

Nurse reasoning

Omery (1985 and 1986), identified two groups of nurses working in Adult Intensive Care: those with a 'sovereign' mode of reasoning and those with an 'accommodating' mode of reasoning. 'Sovereign nurses' make their own judgements based on self-chosen and valued principles, regardless of group norms. 'Accommodating nurses' try to reconcile and conform their own view with the perceived group norms. Active and passive nurses were also identified.

Active nurses who participate actively in situations with ethical problems invest themselves in them, whereas passive nurses discount themselves and think about the risks of being committed to patients and tend to protect themselves.

Disillusionment

The result of nurses' inability to resolve moral problems can result in profound feelings of personal and professional disillusionment and erosion of personal integrity (Georges and Grypdonck, 2002). Passive attitudes can endanger a nurse's own moral integrity and result in a shift in moral orientation, which in turn can result in disengagement from patients and distancing of self from the nurse's own caring mission and values.

Moral issues are no longer seen as difficult, despite nurses' awareness of a violation (Raines, 2000; Van der Arend and Van den Hurk, 1995) and patients' rights are no longer seen as morally problematic. As a result, should nurses adopt a passive attitude, they are seen not only to accept the presence of moral problems but also to become less sensitive to them (Georges and Grypdonck, 2002).

Moral integrity

Nurses' attempts to maintain their own moral integrity is central to their moral experience. Sometimes, failure to achieve and maintain moral standards for patients can endanger nurses' own moral integrity and result in a shift in moral orientation. This can result in disengagement from patients, despite possible embarrassment, guilt and moral distancing of self from their own caring mission and values.

Nurses may feel that they require extra support and understanding from supervisors, friends and colleagues when suffering difficult ethical dilemmas or challenge. They must understand their right to this. Nurses must not be afraid to seek independent counselling to support them through difficult ethical issues. Discussing fears with someone else often puts events into perspective and provides courage for the nurse to proceed with the aim of fulfilling the duty of patient advocacy. This, in summary, means representing and educating patients of their rights, including to consent, working for their true benefit and never allowing their care to be compromised by elements of fear, lack of conviction or ignorance of the code of conduct. Accessing appropriate support can help in reducing resultant stress when encountering ethical dilemmas.

Cultural strategies for coping with stress

Two studies which focused on the ways of coping with stress by Chinese nurses have identified the different methods adopted by nurses to cope with stress in individual departments. One of the studies, by Li and Liang (2002), indicated that most nurses actively cope with occupational stress by:

- looking for support
- using body relaxation techniques
- engaging in self-analysis.

Managerial stress

Another study which explored the coping strategies among Chinese nurse managers (Xianyu and Lambert 2006), found that there was positive correlation in confrontive coping in relation to workload, conflict with physicians and inadequate preparation.

Problem-solving was positively correlated when in conflict with physicians. Avoiding a stressful event, instead of confronting it, did not help mental health quality. The researchers concluded that use of the strategy of escape-avoidance only prolongs the agony of dealing with an unpleasant situation and does little in the long-term resolution of a stressful event (Xianyu and Lambert, 2006).

Escape-avoidance strategies

A research study has shown a major coping strategy of nurses, from Japan and Thailand, to be self-control (Lambert et al., 2004a).

Another study of Japanese hospital nurses found a negative correlation between escape-avoidance strategies and effects on mental health, which simply reflected the inadequacy of using escape-avoidance strategies as a coping mechanism (Lambert et.al, 2004b).

The Royal College of Nursing support for members

The RCN is at the forefront in helping members recognise, accept and manage pressure and stress. Their guidance on 'coping with stress' is essential reading: *Healthy workplace, healthy you. Stress and you: a short guide to coping with pressure and stress* (RCN, 2015). Some helpful suggestions provided in the guide include:

- Aim for the healthy tension between being relaxed and energised.
- Regularly assess your stress response and the current stresses, as stress can creep up unawares.
- Plan for expected increases in stress.
- Find out what works best for you in terms of reducing and managing your stress.
- Try out new ideas that may work well for you. Remember, feeling stressed does not equate with not coping. It is OK to seek help when stressed.

- Remember that your employer carries a responsibility for your health and safety at work, which includes your emotional/mental health as well as your physical well-being.

Importance of leadership: work-related stress and how to tackle it

The Health and Safety Executive (HSE) reminds employers that they have a legal duty to protect employees from stress at work by doing a risk assessment and acting on it. There are six principal areas of work design which can affect stress levels. These are:

- demands
- control
- support
- relationships
- role
- change

The HSE advises employers to assess the risks in these areas to manage stress in the workplace (HSE, 2021). The GMC has issued guidance titled *How to transform UK healthcare environments to support doctors and medical students to care for patients* (West and Coia, 2019).

The importance of education to relieve stress

The importance of the numbers of health professionals in practice, is equal to the importance of ensuring optimum quality of their learning. 'Knowledge is power' is an important maxim.

One investment which can be cost-effective in terms of stress reduction for nurses is the process of clinical supervision as already discussed in Chapter 7. This has been a long-term recommendation for nurses and pays dividends for their well-being despite the need for accessing an external facilitator and cost for 'time out' for nurse attendance at the support sessions. Not all facilitators for such support, however, are required to be external to the organisation.

Management responsibility for safe staffing levels

There have been many debates on workforce shortages within health and care settings in recent years and yet there remain unanswered questions on the changes needed to remedy this crisis.

One of the factors in the problem of staff shortages is a vicious circle of increasing workloads deterring new recruits.

Nursing invisibility and attrition

A nursing study conducted twenty years ago by
Rodney and Varcoe revealed that:
Nursing services remain largely invisible to other providers,
to administrators and policymakers and to theorists in fields such
as bioethics and health economics. What remains invisible
is all too easy to dismiss and what does get measured does
not necessarily reflect the full worth of nursing services.

(Rodney and Varcoe, 2001)

Causes of nurse attrition

The current causes of attrition from nursing are complex and widespread. Falling morale, constant stress, falling real wages and the impact of Brexit has resulted in a general nursing shortage and is threatening the quality of care across the NHS. Emergency funding is in short supply and hiring agency staff is considered, rightly, to be an inefficient use of public money.

Staff shortages

Following the EU referendum in 2016, the number of nurses from the European Economic Area (EEA) registering to work in 2017 in Britain, fell by 32%. Some of the decrease was accounted for by applicants failing new and necessary language tests, but the fall was still significant. It has been compounded by a sharp increase in the number of EEA nurses opting to leave in the same period.

In absolute terms, an exodus of British nurses from the profession is even more troubling. In 2015, for the first time, more left the nursing and midwifery national register than joined it. In 2017, the net loss was nearly 5,000.

Healthy workplaces

RCN senior employment relations advisor, Kim Sunley, has urged employers to improve working conditions for nurses. She said that employers had a responsibility to create a healthy working environment and employees should seek advice from their union if necessary. Healthy, happy nurses deliver the best care. By creating a healthy workplace, including flexible working, well-designed shift patterns and a supportive culture, employers can reduce the risk of nurses becoming unwell due to stress (Dean, 2017). (See the RCN website for more information: rcni.com/resilience).

Nursing shortage factors

The literature suggests a multitude of factors contributing to the nursing shortage, including the ageing of current nurses. This shortage has repercussions for the next generation of nurses, contributes to the overall nursing workforce shortage and holds implications for the development of nursing research and continued practice development.

Most nurse academics come from a clinical background with little preparation for the complex role in education. Despite this, there is little exploration of their experiences transitioning to academia. The limited available evidence suggests that this new role may be accompanied by feelings of uncertainty, anxiety and isolation associated with changed responsibilities, an emphasis on scholarly activities and teaching and the unique culture of the academic environment (McDiarmid et al., 2012).

Nurse workloads affect patient outcomes

According to a Finnish study by Fagerström et al. (2014), overworked nurses may be linked to a 40% increase in risk of patient death. When nurses' workloads have exceeded 'optimum' levels, the chances of a patient safety incident increased by up to 30% and the chances of patient mortality spiked by around 40%.

The study, titled *Nursing workload, patient safety incidents and mortality: an observational study*, marks the first study to analyse daily the relationship between nurse workload and patient outcomes.

The RAFAELA workload system

The researchers from Abo Akademi University in Finland were able to obtain detailed information about nursing workload thanks to the RAFAELA patient classification. This method was pioneered in Finnish hospitals in the 1990s and aims to uphold staffing levels in accordance with patients' care needs. The system was developed to help with the systematic and daily measurement of nursing intensity (NI) and allocation of nursing staff. The article highlights the benefits of using a systematic measurement of NI. The system has now been rolled out across almost all hospitals in Finland and implementation has started elsewhere in Europe and Asia. The RAFAELA system aims to uphold staffing levels in accordance with patients' care needs and its structure consists of three parts as an alternative to classical time studies:

1. Oulu Patient Classification instrument
2. Registration of available nursing resources
3. Professional Assessment of Optimal Nursing Care Intensity Level method.

Relation between workload and patient welfare

Instead of using fixed nurse-to-patient ratios, the RAFAELA system uses daily data on patient's care needs and the workload per nurse to ensure an appropriate number of staff on the wards. When several factors that could skew the data were accounted for, including ward specifics, days of the week and the time of year, the research team found an association between daily workload and patient welfare.

The study's lead author, Fagerström, concluded that a reduced workload would mean that nurses have more time for caring and observing each patient, which may reduce the risk for adverse events and accordingly prevent the patient's health condition from deteriorating.

Evidence found that a staffing measure based on daily measurements of individual patient care needs and the recommended nursing workload is slightly better in predicting incidents and mortality rates, as compared to the standard patient-to-nurse ratio. The authors, however, emphasised how it remained unclear which method was able to best avoid patient safety incidents and deaths. To determine this, the authors said larger studies over a longer period are necessary (Fagerström et al., 2014).

Staffing for safe and effective care

The following predictions and demands for the future of the workforce were made in 2020 by the RCN at a debate titled *Nursing shortages in England*, following a petition delivered by RCN members to the Prime Minister in February. This petition, with over 200,000 signatories, is part of the RCN *Staffing for Safe and Effective Care* campaign which calls for action to remedy the staffing shortages as a priority.

Staffing shortages are the responsibility of multiple decision-makers across all levels of the health and care system. Ultimately, much of this is outside the control of frontline staff and Trusts. It requires political will and decisive action to ensure there are enough skilled healthcare staff to provide safe and effective care.

Nurses, however, have been embroiled in a row with the government over their pay for several months. The RCN said analysis by London Economics has shown that pay for nurses has declined at twice the rate of the private sector in the last decade. Nurses' real-terms earnings have fallen by 6% compared with 3.2% for private sector employees, it was found.

What are nurses demanding from the government?

The RCN has been campaigning for a pay rise above inflation, having argued that the post COVID crisis pay award followed years of squeezes on nurse's salaries.

According to the union, the government's offer left an experienced nurse more than £1,000 worse off in real terms (Itvnews, 2022).

Student nurses

For government to begin to fix the workforce crisis, there are two urgent matters that need to be addressed. Firstly, nursing students in higher education need investment and secondly a law must be secured to protect their ability to provide safe and effective care for the future.

All nursing students on courses from September 2020 will now receive a payment of at least £5,000 a year which they will not need to pay back. This is encouraging as it is expected to benefit more than 35,000 students every year.

Funding for nursing students is crucial for attracting more people to study nursing as debt can act as a disincentive, especially to prospective mature students who may already shoulder debt from a previous degree in another subject. Everything possible must be done to remove financial barriers for nursing students. This should be either full grants for tuition, or forgiveness of tuition loans for people who enter public service (RCN, 2020).

Students will receive at least £5,000 a year, with up to £3,000 further funding available for eligible students, including allowances for:

- specialist disciplines that struggle to recruit, including mental health
- an additional childcare allowance, on top of the £1,000 already on offer
- areas of the country which have seen a decrease in people accepted on some nursing, midwifery and allied health courses over the past year.

This means that some students could be eligible for up to £8,000 per year, with everyone getting at least £5,000. The funding will not have to be repaid by recipients. Students will also be able to continue to access funding for tuition and maintenance loans from the Student Loans Company. The announcement comes alongside the latest push in the biggest nursing recruitment drive in decades.

Prior to the tragedy of the COVID-19 pandemic, in 2019 former Prime Minister Boris Johnson said of the NHS,

I have heard loud and clear that the priority of the British people is to focus on the NHS – and to make sure this treasured institution has everything it needs to deliver world-class care. Nurses epitomise everything that makes the NHS so revered across the world – skill, compassion, energy and dedication. On the steps of Downing Street last week, I said we will deliver 50,000 more nurses and this new financial support package is a crucial part of delivering this. There can be no doubting our commitment to the NHS and over the coming months we will bring forward further proposals to transform this great country. As we enter the Year of the Nurse and Midwife, we are embarking on the biggest nursing recruitment drive in decades, backed by a new universal support package.

(Johnson, 2019)

Nursing a popular career choice?

The King's Fund is an English health charity that shapes health and social care policy and practice. Their vision is that the best possible health and care is available to all. It provides a range of consultancy and advisory services which bring together a deep understanding of the health and care system, policy expertise and experience of supporting and developing leaders and organisations.

A spokesperson for the King's Fund argues that nursing as a career is experiencing a surge in popularity, with an 8% rise reported by the Nursing Standard in the number of students starting courses in 2021. The increase has been attributed to the profession's high profile during the pandemic.

Student attrition and practice hours

An annual investigation of nursing student attrition by the Nursing Standard showed one in three students didn't complete their course in 2020 as planned. It was a highly unusual year due to the pandemic but the drop-out rate has hovered around 25% for years now, demonstrating the challenge faced by the profession.

The number of practice hours required of undergraduates by the NMC in the UK is almost three times higher than that stipulated for nursing students in Australia or the US. And, even with the best intentions, capacity to provide high-quality learning experience is much constrained.

A nursing undergraduate described how she was one of five students on a ward on one day and while the staff were wonderful it was impossible for them to keep track of so many students and ensure learning and patient safety. So, is it time to reduce the practice hours and focus on getting the best experiences for students on those placements? (Munn, 2021).

Staffing; the future

The RCN recognises the government's pledge for 50,000 more nurses in five years and hopes to see the plans for how this will be delivered. Any increase to the nursing workforce must be across all health and care settings, not just in hospitals. Underpinning the pledge with costed and funded solutions will help this target make a meaningful difference to nursing staff and the people in their care.

Stressful shift patterns: 12-hour shifts

People are living longer with ever more complex needs. Resources to meet these needs are limited. Emphasis on high technical care targets and tasks can limit focus on the individual. There can be a greater focus on those who can be cured.

Unquestioned taking on of doctors' roles takes qualified nurses away from fundamental care. The long 12-hour shifts can be stressful and exhausting over time for all nurses. Such shifts are a less costly alternative than the traditional staff overlap between early and late shifts.

The resourcing problems are historical within the NHS. Some of the so-called 'solutions' to the resource problems in healthcare can be argued to have had damaging consequences for nurses. An example of this was the apparent, unquestioned acceptance of the introduction of 12-hour shifts as long ago as the 1980s. Such long shifts can, or should, pose questions about care continuity and consistency for patients and staff welfare.

These shifts originated from the USA where mentally ill patients were thought to benefit from longer nursing shifts to help their need for therapeutic interaction. They were then introduced to the UK but to many more care areas where the physical demand was different from mental health nursing or Intensive care units where there are less patients allocated to one nurse and patient interaction is generally on a one- to -one basis.

It has been suggested that 12 -hour shifts were introduced to save money, by eliminating the 'costly' historical period of overlap of staff in the afternoon. This period, however, was perceived as a good means of providing further teaching opportunities for learners and for allowing continuity of patient care. Working either early or late shifts, nurses were on the wards in a more consistent manner. It is well known that many nurses follow these onerous 12- hour shifts (3 or 4 days a week) working further 12-hour bank shifts elsewhere on their days off. Such practice for those who need to work these hours is acknowledged as an understandable effort to maintain a decent standard of living. But how do nurses, whether older or young and fit, manage such consecutively long shifts which have become the norm?

The 'right staff'

One of the action areas in the NHS England's strategy, titled *Compassion in practice nursing, midwifery and care staff – our vision and strategy* (2012) is 'ensuring we have the right staff, with the right skills in the right place'. Dr Ruth May (Regional Chief Nurse, Midlands and East of England), as the senior responsible officer, led this work nationally. On her behalf, Pauline Milne (Head of Clinical Workforce Development and Planning, Health Education East of England) invited the National Nursing Research Unit (NNRU) of King's College, London and Southampton University to undertake research into 12-hour shifts, using existing data sets and published evidence to explore the prevalence, views and potential impact of these shifts.

Can 12-hour shifts reduce costs without any deleterious effects?

There are reports that some NHS Trusts have moved away from 12-hour shifts and reintroduced 8-hour shifts to enable nurses to spend more time with their patients (Sprinks, 2012). The study authors recommended that an evaluation of such a development is imperative and new nurses (who have only ever worked 12-hour shifts) may need re-educating into the purpose and value of the afternoon overlap for this time to be fully utilised. But many Trusts continue to have 12-hour shifts in operation, based on an untested assumption that it is a cost-effective system.

Wisdom of 12-hour shifts?

The study by Kings College, London and Southampton University in 2015, raised a significant challenge to the assumption that 12-hour shifts can reduce costs without any deleterious effects. The review and analysis of data presented, has suggested that there has been an increase in needle stick injuries and musculoskeletal disorders and that nurses who work 12 hours or longer were more likely to rate the quality of care as poor and gave a lower patient safety rating to the environment and few reported benefits.

A stronger evidence base was recommended with a fully controlled trial or natural experiment if possible and in-depth qualitative work to understand better, nurses' needs and preferences in this complex area.

Several gaps are identified in the evidence base

- Research that takes account of the other working pattern variables (e.g., choice, shift sequence, breaks, overtime, etc.) that are likely to influence the outcomes examined.
- Exploration of how 12-hour shifts may have different effects for different staff (e.g., by role/grade of staff, age, or domestic circumstances).
- Absence of specific information about healthcare support workers.
- Little UK-based research.
- Long-term understanding of potential deleterious effects.
- No economic analysis.

Study conclusion

At present, in the absence of a more complete picture of both the effects and the costs of 12-hour shifts, the study recommended that managers should proceed with caution (Ball et al., 2015).

Clarifying workforce accountability in law

There is a gap between the numbers of nursing staff we currently have and the number of people who need healthcare. In part, this is due to no person or organisation being legally accountable for growing and developing the nursing staff we need now, or in the future, to deliver patient care. In England, the RCN are calling for the forthcoming NHS Long-Term Plan Bill (2019) to be published with a framework which sets out explicit roles, responsibilities and accountabilities for workforce supply and planning, for government and throughout all levels of decision-making.

Legislation for safe staffing

The Welsh Nurse Staffing Levels Act (2016) aims to protect nurse staffing levels in acute care services and Scotland passed legislation on safe staffing in 2019.

The RCN is not alone in calling for accountability to be addressed. In September 2019, NHS England recommended that the government review whether the national responsibilities and duties in relation to workforce functions are sufficiently clear. Polling by YouGov found that 80% of respondents in England agreed that 'the Government should have a legal responsibility to ensure there are enough nursing staff to meet the country's needs' (YouGov/RCN, 2019).

This call is also supported by other Royal Colleges and health organisations. Achieving accountability in law will enable decision-makers to begin to fix the workforce crisis by clarifying decisions, action plans and funding required for workforce growth to meet population needs. This will prevent health and care services struggling to provide care without enough nurses in future.

Recruitment

The NHS campaign *We Are Nurses* targets teenagers who are about to choose their degrees as well as career switchers considering going into nursing. (See the link: https://www. healthcareers.nhs.uk/we-are-the-nhs/nursing-careers for more information).

The measures will be part of the upcoming NHS People Plan, (NHS 2020/2021) which will set out work to reduce vacancies across the NHS and secure the staff needed for the future.

Conclusion

The RCN is at the forefront in helping minimise effects of stress for their members, be it in helping nurses with stress management and staff support or how nurses themselves can highlight risks of staff shortages (see Chapter 6). Those in authority must lead and evaluate practice development initiatives to support continuous improvement in care and quality standards and use of evidence-based practice by all accountable as patient advocates.

Managers' responsibility

A lower recruitment and high turnover rate of RNs have resulted in a global shortage of nurses. In the UK, prior to the COVID-19 epidemic, nurses' intention to leave rates were between 30 and 50% suggesting an elevated level of job dissatisfaction.

Determinants of nurse job dissatisfaction – findings from a cross-sectional survey analysis in the UK

In a study of RNs (RCN, 2017), data from a cross-sectional mixed-methods survey was developed by the RCN and administered to the nursing workforce across all four UK nations. It aimed to explore the levels of dissatisfaction and demoralisation – one of the predictors of nurses' intention to leave.

Findings

A considerable proportion of nurses reported feeling dissatisfied and demoralised. RNs reported how staffing issues and failures in leadership, left them feeling disempowered and demoralised. To reduce the negative impact of dissatisfaction and improve retention, more research needs to investigate the relationship dynamics within healthcare teams and how the burden experienced by RNs when unsupported by managers impacts on their ability to provide safe, good-quality care (RCN, 2017).

These findings in 2017, pre-date the COVID-19 pandemic outbreak which may have had a further detrimental effect on job satisfaction in the UK and the nursing workforce of other nations.

A recent study of systematic reviews, explored interventions to reduce adult nursing turnover, and concluded that more high-quality primary research is needed to inform decision-making by human resource managers and organisations to improve retention strategies. Respondents criticised failures in leadership and organisational support which caused negative feelings due to a lack of support from hospital management.

This lack of support was experienced in a range of ways from simple disregard to being made to feel incompetent and even blamed for the poor state of patient care. The disregard encountered by the RNs was not only for themselves but also, they felt, extended to a disregard for patient's needs with one respondent saying, 'I feel our patients are behind us, but I do feel that upper management are disengaged with patients and staff's real concerns and issues' (Senek et al., 2020).

Management styles

Managers should not be assumed to possess the necessary leadership skills. Preparation and assessment of suitability for these roles is required. The management style and ability to lead others, can be a positive or toxic influence which can affect the organisation's culture and in turn the lives of staff and patients for years.

Educational programmes

If students are not taught their rights in addition to the rights of patients, neither group will fare well. Students warrant education about their human rights e.g., to conscientious objection, in line with the responsibilities of higher education institutes where nurses are educated. Sound education can be a support source in ethically difficult, thus stressful, clinical areas.

Factors influencing stress

Stress affects people differently – the things that cause one person stress may not affect another. Factors like skills and experience, age or disability and level of support may all affect whether an employee can cope with stress.

Employees feel stress when they can't cope with pressures and other issues. Employers should match demands to employees' skills and knowledge. For example, employees can get stressed if they feel they don't have the skills or time to meet tight deadlines. Workforce planning and providing training and clinical support (clinical supervision) can reduce pressure and bring stress levels down with the aim of retaining optimum numbers of satisfied, resilient and appreciated staff.

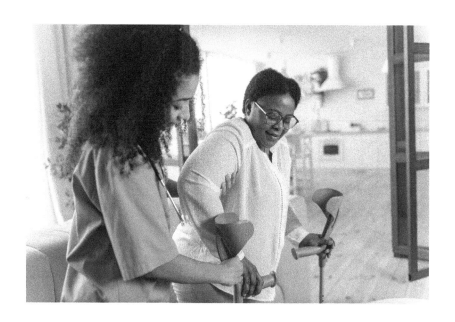

Chapter 18

Christianity and secularism

Whoever does not love, does not know God, for God is love.

(1, John 4:8)

Introduction

Christians now account for less than half of England and Wales' population for the first time in census history, at 46.2 per cent of the population in 2021 - 13.1 per cent down on the figure a decade earlier (Somerville, 2023).

Simon Calvert, deputy director at the Christian Institute, has said that "we have been warning for years that Christians are being pushed from the public square, yet the problem is getting worse. Christians and those with traditional views often find themselves silenced or bullied. It's particularly ironic when this happens at institutions that were originally founded on Christian principles and with endowments from Christian benefactors" (Calvert, 2023).

Christianity has suffered and continues to suffer great persecution. Nevertheless, Christianity will never die, according to its founder, Jesus Christ, who said: I am with you always, even to the end of the age (Matthew 28:20).

Christianity

This belief system, at its most basic, is the faith tradition that focuses on the figure of Jesus Christ who declared Himself to be 'the way, the truth and the life'. His parable of the Good Samaritan is so relevant to any health professional in any area of care, whether within or outside of the NHS, in hospital or community.

Faith and liberalism

A secular culture has dangers for those wishing to comply with the tenets of both faith, reason and conscience. Aggressive secularism can ignore the virtue of obedience and the gift of faith. Faith provides knowledge of something real and objective, not a feeling or an opinion and it compels obedience.

Liberalism

The concept of liberalism, which holds faith as an opinion and that all knowledge requires proof, endangers practitioners who wish to remain obedient to the tenets of their faith.

Aggressive secularism cannot and will not, trump the long-held belief system of those practitioners who believe in God and the sanctity of life, no matter how vulnerable or how it may be perceived as economically 'unproductive'. The concept of the ethical 'slippery slope' must be guarded against by those caring professionals who profess a faith and those who profess none.

Our purpose

The following words by St John Henry Newman can help all health care professionals to persevere through the good and bad times of their calling:
God has created me to do Him some definite service. He has committed some work to me which He has not committed to another. I have my mission. I may never know it in this life, but I shall be told it in the next. I am a link in a chain, a bond of connection between persons. Therefore, I will trust Him, whatever I am, I can never be thrown away. If I am in sickness, my sickness may serve Him, in perplexity, my perplexity may serve Him. If I am in sorrow, my sorrow may serve Him. He does nothing in vain. He knows what He is about. He may take away my friends. He may throw me among strangers. He may make me

feel desolate, make my spirits sink, hide my future
from me. Still, He knows what He is about.

(Newman, 1864)

Heart speaks to heart

Newman's relationship with Jesus Christ is always apparent in his writing as highlighted by his motto: *cor ad cor loquitor* (from the Latin, 'heart speaks to heart'). Newman's search for the Truth, which led to his reception into the Catholic Church in 1845, was slow and methodical. Newman's *Apologia Pro Vita Sua* (from the Latin, 'a defence of one's own life) is a genuine account of someone wanting to know God more fully. His defence of his religious opinions was published in 1864 in response to much criticism from some in the Church of England, after Newman left his position as the Anglican vicar of St Mary's, Oxford. His faith in God persisted amid his questions and doubts:

> *Of all points of faith, the being of a God is, to my own*
> *apprehension, encompassed with most difficulty and borne*
> *in upon our minds with most power.*

(Newman, 1864)

Healthcare is a charitable work

Healthcare is a primary work of charity and the health professions are privileged to be involved in such a calling, whether coming from a religious standpoint or not. Health concerns discussed within the chapters in this book may be seen to be implicated in 'a tyranny of secularism'. This was a phrase initiated by Pope St John Paul II who was a fierce defender of Christianity in the face of the forces of communism, capitalism and totalitarian atheism.

For Newman, love was the key and he advocated uncompromisingly the need to give human beings the deepest value. Many atheists and non-aggressive secularists who are pro-life, would concur with this view because of the immoral and the dangerous implications for the disabled and vulnerable threatened by, for example, the spectre of assisted suicide.

A disabled member of the House of Lords, Baroness Campbell of Surbiton has said about assisted suicide: 'Assisted dying is practised in Belgium, the Netherlands and elsewhere. Whatever the initial intentions were, decisions to end life in those places are now not taken only by the individual. It is not an autonomous act. The slippery slope is oiled by the vague euphemism of assisted dying (Campbell, 2015).

Truth is truth

There is much confusion in society and the secular world today has influenced medical practice in many ways. Today's young nurses and doctors and healthcare professionals ought to take much encouragement from Newman's resolve to choose the Truth above all else, simply because it is the Truth. Pope Leo XIII declared, 'truth cannot contradict truth' (Scriptorum, 2019).

It cannot be denied that health professionals with no religious affiliation can provide the best care to those in need, acting as Good Samaritans. The problem arises for all where there is a psychologically oppressive, anti-Christian, anti-life culture.

Conviction of conscience and awareness of God

It is well recognised by anthropologists that the most apparently, unsophisticated tribes have a belief in a greater power. It is argued that it is intrinsically human to have a constant awareness of God, stamped on our being as an operating system, installed, waiting to be launched. God remembers us before we remember God (Varden, 2018).

Coercion and ostracising of staff is not unknown when ethical dilemmas are apparent. Staff acting as the Good Samaritan, will fight for patients' welfare with conviction of conscience without concern for themselves. Staff of whatever religious denomination or none, who are pro-life, may consequently be considered as 'non team players' or even lacking in 'compassion' when disagreeing with a team consensus on some ethical issues.

Secularism

Secularism is defined in different contexts:

- Apropos religion, it can be defined as the indifference to, or rejection or exclusion of religion and religious considerations (Merriam-Webster dictionary, 2019).
- In political terms, secularism is the principle of the separation of government institutions and the people.
- As a philosophy, secularism seeks to interpret life on principles taken solely from the material world, without recourse to religion (Livingstone, 2006).

Such a philosophy has implications for committed Christians and others in healthcare and their freedom to conscientious objection. That freedom is now considered to be under threat by many Christians and non-Christians alike.

A tyranny of secularism

Secularism is not necessarily opposed to Christianity or other belief systems. Colin Hart, director of the Christian Institute, said of atheists: This tiny group of people lays great claims to have their beliefs at the front and centre of our national life. What the atheists lack in numbers, they certainly make up for in terms of their influence and boldness. They understand that their beliefs are a worldview which they are determined to impose on everyone else (Hart, 2014).

Free speech

Winston Churchill said in a debate in the House of Commons during the second World War:

"Indeed, Parliamentary democracy has flourished
under party government.
so long as there is full freedom of speech, free
elections and free institutions.
So, we must beware of a tyranny of opinion
which tries to make only one side of a question
the one which may be heard.
Everyone is in favour of free speech.
Hardly a day passes without its being extolled, but
some people's idea of it is that they are free to say
what they like, but if anyone says anything
back, that is an outrage

(Churchill, 1943)

Risks of militant secularism

The last census of 2011 found that less than 78,000 people (0.14% of the population) identified themselves as Secularist, Atheist, Humanist, Agnostic or as a free thinker. All of whom, of course, can be most caring individuals, alongside Christians in the workplace. The risk is that militant forms of secularism can become a tyrannical culture that leave no room for questioning or conscientious objection.

A Free Church minister in Scotland exhorts Christians to recognise that the 'new secularism' is trying to undermine and destroy their faith. Writing for the website *Christian Today*, David Robertson explained: 'The vast majority of the posts on secular message boards are anti-religious. The main purpose is to attack religion in general and Christianity in particular and in very particular, the Catholic Church and Evangelicals. This attitude quickly degenerates into personal abuse if the comments are challenged' (Robertson, 2014).

Christianity and secularism

Secularism has been described by one famous Catholic as follows:
We have to go to the heart of the tragedy being experienced by
modern man: the eclipse of the sense of God and man, typical of

a social and cultural climate dominated by secularism, which,
with its ubiquitous tentacles, succeeds at times in putting
Christian communities themselves to the test.

(Pope St John Paul II, 1995b)

Aggressive secularism

David Robertson, who is the director of the Solas Centre for Public Christianity, warned about the difference between secularists who are 'simply about the separation of church and state' and a 'new secularism which is much more militant and dangerous' (Robertson, 2014).

Certain healthcare scandals have revealed how overwhelming
the odds can be for health professionals who attempt to
act as the Good Samaritan where an aggressively secular
agenda can dictate the healthcare culture.
It is argued that aggressive secularism appears to come with
"values", such as being pro-abortion, pro-euthanasia and pro-
homosexuality. Dare any one in public life suggest, for
example, that marriage should be between a man and a
woman and they are automatically decried as homophobic.
Some secularists want the complete neuterisation
and privatisation of religion.
They want only their views and values to be taught and
allowed in public life. We need to recognise the new
secularism for what it is – an attempt to undermine and
destroy Christianity. We need to stand against its
fundamentalism and we need to stand up for the poor,
the young, the disabled and the marginalised, by proclaiming
the gospel of Christ against the elitism and intolerance of
our new fundamentalist atheists.

(Robertson, 2014)

Aggressive secularists, of course, reject any idea of God, but over and above that they claim that religion is repressive and responsible for most of the world's ills – which is why, they say, its influence needs to be removed.

Aims of the secular society

The mission statement of the national secular society states on its website:

> *In multi-cultural Britain, where the majority of the population actually have no faith, secularism is presented as the objective voice of reason working to establish successful democratic governance across the world. We campaign for a secular democracy with a separation of religion and state, where everyone's Human Rights are respected equally.*

(National Secular Society, 2022)

It has been argued, however, that their statement does not apply to those secularists who espouse aggressive secularism:

> *Aggressive secularists are not neutral, they are not tolerant and they are not fair. Secularism actually is a competing ideology or belief system – in effect it is a religion and it wants total dominance. Secularists may claim to defend tolerance and freedom of speech for all, but the reality is they will not allow any dissent.*

(Rose, 2018)

Christianity: the most persecuted religion

According to the widely respected Pew Research Centre report (2018), Christianity remains the world's most persecuted religion. All around the world, Christians are subject to real and sustained violence for the profession of their faith, the one that we proclaim most insistently today: that life is stronger than death, that love will ultimately triumph over hate (Fraser, 2019).

This persecution of Christianity, however, does not always arise from militantly secular positions. It can arise from fervent followers of a faith. To persecute others for their faith may indicate that the perpetrators have an insecure faith base from which they operate.

Of particular concern in this regard is Africa, where extremism threatens previously strong Christian communities. In Nigeria and other countries this violence clearly passes the threshold of genocide (Aid to the Church in Need, 2022).

A nineteenth century Pope, in his beautiful and insightful Encyclical on the wisdom of Christianity said that:

> *Nothing emboldens the wicked so greatly*
> *as the lack of courage on the part of the good.*
> *He reminds us that,*
> *Christians are born for combat,*
> *whereof the greater the vehemence,*
> *the more assured, God aiding, the triumph*

> (Pope Leo XIII, 1890)

Coronavirus

The following extract is from 'Return to Order', a special US campaign for the Defence of Tradition, Family and Property (TFP). It is one of several autonomous national TFP groups which claim to form the world's largest anti-communist and anti-socialist network of Catholic inspiration:

> *The coronavirus pandemic has the uncanny ability to*
> *turn our material paradises into hells. The cruise ship,*
> *the symbol of all earthly delights, became an infected*
> *prison for passengers who did everything possible*
> *to get out. Those who consider sport their god,*
> *now find empty stadiums and cancelled tournaments.*
> *Those who adore money now find decimated*
> *portfolios and quarantined workforces. The worshippers of*
> *education look at their empty schools and universities.*

The devotees of consumerism face bare supermarket shelves.
The world we worshipped is tumbling down. The things
for which we glory are now in ruins. Some might object that
taking a non-secular attitude toward the virus requires a
leap of faith. However, we must ask which is the greater leap
of faith – to confide in Holy Mother Church or the cold
hands of a State that had already shown itself incapable
of solving society's problems.

(Horvat, 2020b)

Humanism

The All-Party Parliamentary Humanist Group (APPHG) is pushing for the replacement of the daily prayers in the Houses of Parliament with a time of daily meditation. In their new report titled *A Time for Reflection* (APPHG, 2020), they also say that Church of England bishops should no longer sit in the House of Lords.

Prayer, however, is literally woven into the fabric of the Palace of Westminster. The floor tiles of Westminster Central Lobby are inscribed with these words in Latin:

'Nisi dominus edificaverit domum, in vanum
laboraverunt qui edificant eam' (unless the Lord builds
the House, they labour in vain that build it).

(Psalm 127)

Coronavirus impacts on faith

It has been argued that corona-phobia is rattling the globe. In this sense, the reaction to the coronavirus is extremely political and secular. It reflects a society that has turned its back on God. We face the crisis, trusting only in ourselves and our devices. Increasing secularism pushes for more 'control' over our lives, which can result in utilitarianism, absolute patient autonomy, which may be poorly understood (in terms of advance refusals and end of life wishes), eugenics, quality of life measurements and the 'greater good of society' (Horvat, 2020b). All these developments which can be ideologically prized by their adherents will encroach on the conscience of practitioners who wish to provide care which is not tainted and dominated by aggressive secularism.

Supernatural reality lost?

Horvat (2021) suggests,

Our metaphysical world is hollowed out and all that is left are ruins from times past. Thus, the sense of shame is deadened and suffocated by a postmodern wasteland without narratives or ideals. Shame occasionally returns in times of depression and boredom. However, it is quickly swept away by a loud and restless culture that bids us be merry amid our emptiness. It is not because we have lost certain habits or wear different clothes that we have no shame. We have lost the high standards and lofty principles that once governed our actions. We no longer live in a metaphysical world that supports a notion of shame. Only a rejection of our materialistic mindset and a return to God will restore our much-needed sense of shame.

(Horvat, 2021)

It is argued that not believing in anything, has nothing to offer as a foundation for many of our moral concerns. When the Christian worldview disappears from sight, secular culture will be walking on little but thin air. Without a meaningful moral story to underpin it, might will be right and power supreme (Fraser, 2022b).

Conclusion

New 'modern' or aggressively secular bioethicists who can influence government and the professions, must never trump the conscience of practitioners who wish to act as the Good Samaritan rather than agents of the state. Health professionals must be accountable, to their conscience, their patients, their professional registration body and their code of conduct and support each other. Being able to work in any field of care is the right of any health professional without fear of objection by their secular colleagues.

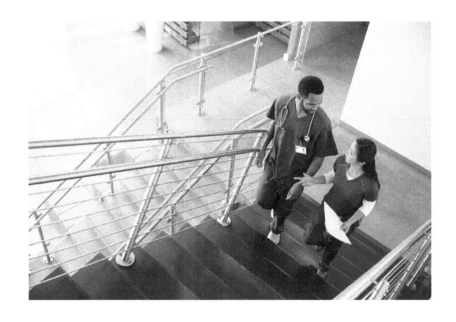

Chapter 19
The future: achieving the goal of the Good Samaritan in healthcare

---

The New Testament portrays God's love,
made visible in Jesus

as the source and substance of a new, compassionate
and selfless love
offered by Christians to all people.

Jesus adroitly describes this love through his
unforgettable story
of the Good Samaritan.

(Kavanaugh 2000)

Introduction

The parable of the Good Samaritan ends with Jesus giving a commandment to go out and do the same as the Samaritan had done. There are professional and personal aids to succeed in the role of the Good Samaritan (or the patient advocate), all of which can enhance the practitioner's courage, work satisfaction and ultimately, safety for patients.

Authentic human rights

Throughout this book, I argue that the role of the Good Samaritan in healthcare relates equally to politicians, health professionals and their often, non-clinical managers, whether Christian or not.

A journalist argues that genuine rights are not "sexual and reproductive" but include the freedom of religion, of conscience, of thought, speech and expression and of association (Caldwell, 2022).

The same astute journalist argues that the pro choice charities are in fact major abortion providers, organisations bloated on taxes channelled through the National Health Service, which pay their executives enormous salaries from the public purse, and which are growing increasingly bold in their attempts to dictate public policy. Their aims are to decriminalise, further liberalise and generally deregulate a legal framework which is already among the most permissive anywhere in the world. For the last five years the abortion industry and its friends in Parliament have been campaigning hard for these objectives. They dream of abortion on demand and up to birth enshrined as a human right.

British women, need to be truly heard in relation to this issue. They voice their views in favour of greater restrictions on abortion and just one per cent want abortion up to birth (https://righttolife. org.uk/polling).

The same journalist rightly argues that one doesn't have to be a Catholic,
or even a Christian, to reach the conclusion that
dismembering late-trimester
foetuses – fully formed unborn babies – limb by limb or
killing them by injecting them in the heart
with toxins
then delivering them as stillborn is
profoundly and regressively barbaric

(Caldwell, 2022)

He adds that proponents of abortion demonstrate a lack of respect accorded to authentic human rights rather than those which have evolved (i.e., made up to suit some destructive ideology or agenda).

Caldwell concludes that the attacks on these genuine rights are becoming the de facto equivalents of the Test Acts of the late 17th century when religious opinions were tested for conformity before a Catholic or nonconformist could either take any part in public life or avoid harsh financial and other penalties. They are concerned chiefly with sustained attacks on Christian morality and the value and sanctity of human life in particular, and like the Test Acts of old they mean that a person can be ruined for holding the "wrong" opinions. The proponents of assisted suicide and euthanasia, who have also detected a change in the tide in recent years, have been relentless in their campaign to legalise doctor-assisted death (Caldwell, 2022).

Such vicious intolerance is now endemic. Britain is in the grip of a grave social evil which threatens our way of life. Caldwell suggests that a new Prime Minister should look to remedy such a malevolent cultural revolution as an urgent issue whose importance is no less significant than the economic situation or Russia (Caldwell, 2022).

Protecting life, truth and freedom

John Deighan, the Chief Executive of the Society for the Protection of Unborn Children (SPUC), provides an excellent overview of the attacks on vulnerable, unborn life and on those attempting to defend it against a culture of death and disinformation.

"Recent coverage of issues around abortion have revealed an alarming willingness of journalists, politicians, and campaigners to make groundless emotional claims rather than assess objective reality. It has illustrated that we are in many ways now living in a post truth society. Declarations of feelings are to be accepted as reality irrespective of fact.

Of course, it works only one-way. Secularist (typically anti-Christian) pronouncements are given great weight, whereas their opponents' comments are not permitted even the air of publicity. In a recent meeting I had with a politician and civil servants, I asked about the measures to restrict the freedoms of pro-life people despite there being a complete absence of evidence of wrongdoing at pro-life gatherings. I was told that just because there is no evidence of harassment doesn't mean it isn't happening. How can justice prevail with such standards!?

Another ploy of the new anti-rationalists is that those who disagree with their views are not only 'wrong' but they are deemed to be 'dangerous'. On a series of moral issues, we now hear that those who uphold once common-sense viewpoints are claimed to be spreading "dangerous disinformation". I come across this expression a lot and have yet to see the substance of this supposed danger revealed. One journalist recently made such an allegation about a comment from SPUC, in which we merely noted the verifiable reality that the widespread provision of contraception didn't bring down abortion rates. It is of course a stratagem to shut up opponents and avoid debate or reflection. Government statistics can attest to the reality that abortion rates continue to climb despite society being awash with contraceptives.

SPUC's presence in schools to give talks on pro-life issues has also been deemed as dangerous by abortion crusaders. Vilification of pro-lifers is so widespread now that a perverse distortion of reality is being formed in the imaginations of our fellow citizens. It has paved the way for elderly, pro-life attendees at prayer vigils to be routinely intimidated and pro-life events to be invaded and cancelled.

Throughout history vilification has proven an effective means of radicalising the masses, so a response is needed. Reasoned voices in civic society need to displace the false narrative perpetrated by the current dominant minority which is suppressing alternative views. That puts special onus on good organisations to mobilise and educate their supporters. These need to become a new creative minority which can once more give society the values which encourage human flourishing. It is that vision that SPUC shares with the Association of Catholic Nurses. We are part of the solution that our wider society, whether it knows it or not, needs badly; before the secularist values which spread a culture of death lead our society to ruin" (Deighan, 2023).

The example of the Good Samaritan cannot be obliterated by new ideologies which reject authentic concern for the most vulnerable in society.

Nurses on the front line

Nurses can be described as the ultimate flexible workers. They have taken on some of the technical roles of doctors and still have their nurturing role with patients, while, understandably, not always achieving a perfect combination of these expressive and technical role expectations. Clinical supervision (support) can provide expert and effective clinical and educational support. Understanding the code of conduct (NMC, 2018) and the Equality Act (2010) and attending regular clinical support sessions, all can help to protect both the conscience of health professionals and their human right to conscientious objection. These rights, equate with the rights of their patients to evidence-based practice, holistic care, safety and comfort.

Role modelling

It is understood that role modelling can be the best form of teaching. Jesus completed the parable of the Good Samaritan by asking the lawyer which of the three protagonists seemed to be a good neighbour to the vulnerable victim, left half dead. The lawyer answered: 'He who showed mercy on him'. Then Jesus said to him, 'Go and do likewise'.

When the Samaritan saw the man, he took pity on him' (Luke 10:33)

The mercy shown by the Good Samaritan was not 'mercy killing', an offer of assisted suicide, a defeatist attitude in favour of 'futile' care beliefs, or the consideration of convenient sedation or an unethical and cheap 'end of life' care pathway.

The Good Samaritan health professional, learning from past and recent healthcare tragedies, will refuse to allow patient care to be compromised by unethical, economic and aggressively secular imperatives. The Divine Samaritan shows us the way: 'The Son of Man came not to be served but to serve' (Mark 10:45).

Service

'As for me and my house, I will serve the Lord' (Joshua 24:15).

> *The term 'service' has various meanings depending*
> *upon the context of the word. 'Service' is generally understood to*
> *be any duty or labour performed for another person.*
> *This definition relates to care in all its forms. In the opinion*
> *of the late Pope, St John Paul II, the parable that best articulated*
> *the heart of the healthcare mission and ministry of*
> *Jesus Christ was that of the Good Samaritan:*
> *Those involved professionally or voluntarily in the*
> *world of health are invited to fix their gaze on the divine*
> *Samaritan, so that their service can become a prefiguration of*
> *definitive salvation and a proclamation of new heavens*
> *and a new earth "in which righteousness dwells".*

(Pope St John Paul II, 2000, quoting St Peter, pt. 2, 3:13)

It is suggested that because true prophets dare to remind people of the need to respect human dignity, to be compassionate, to be particularly concerned for people who are poor, their lives are threatened. On the bandit-infested road, from Jerusalem to Jericho, the Good Samaritan not only risks his life for the victim but also, because of his actions, could suffer further marginalisation by both the Hebrew people and those of his own Samarian culture. Both cultures were greatly divided with distrust of each other and even hatred.

Christ, the storyteller, and the ultimate Good Samaritan, will, of course, give his life in the service of others (Arbuckle, 2007). The life of Jesus was a perfect example of loving concern and compassion, healing and saving lives.

Happy service providers

Nurses are generally responsible for coordination of the service provided, with a commitment to serve their patients' benefit. The key text to describe this is from St Peter 4:11, 'Whoever serves, [let it be] as one who serves by the strength that God supplies – in order that in everything God may be glorified through Jesus Christ'.

God is seen as glorious when all our serving is moment-by-moment receiving from God's supply. We receive this supply by faith. That is, we trust moment by moment that what we need, in serving Him, He will supply ('life, breath and everything'). This is the opposite of being anxious. Such serving is happy. And it makes God look no less authoritative, but infinitely more desirable. This is the glory He means to have. The giver gets the glory. Therefore, 'serve the Lord with gladness' (Psalm 100:2) (Piper, 2011).

All practitioners, however, must raise questions about the therapy that they are asked to give or omit. They must examine and respect their conscience as an honoured and sensitive guide, as to whether patient harm will result from decisions and subsequent orders which may be unequivocally unethical. Florence Nightingale said: 'No man, not even a doctor, ever gives any other definition of what a nurse should be than this – 'devoted and obedient'. This definition would do just as well for a porter. It might even do for a horse' (Nair, 2017).

The customer is king

In some non-healthcare settings, where service recipients are much less vulnerable than patients, customers or clients are so often considered as 'king' in the balance of power. The maxim that the 'customer is always right' is enshrined in service culture. This is a good mantra for health professionals to adopt, where people are utterly dependent on optimum service standards provided with true, not 'false compassion'.

Nursing and medicine are privileged professions with public expectations of responsibility and accountability for treatment and care. Despite the satisfaction derived from our vocation to care, to achieve the principles of our ethical code is not without difficulty when working within a culture of aggressive secularism, utilitarianism, 'the marketplace', 'modern bioethics and potential dismissal of the concept of conscientious objection.

Contemplating all the noted NHS healthcare scandals, we must evaluate how the calling to care is respected and cherished. Nurses traditionally are known for their virtues of tolerance, patience, empathy and compassion. They need to be mindful of the past and any potential care scandals on their watch. Several scandals have been examined in this book together with the systemic, managerial and organisational culture which can work against patient advocacy.

Is the past another country?

In 1861, a Jesuit priest, Jean Pierre de Caussade, authored a book which is becoming increasingly known today, titled: *Abandonment to Divine Providence*. It conveys what it means to walk in God's way and path without becoming an automaton. We know about the Sacraments of the church and de Caussade suggests considering the importance of another Sacrament, that of the *Present Moment*. This speaks to the intellect but also the heart and soul. The book describes the experience of total surrender of self to God and complete obedience to His will in every moment of living. It explores God's will and in particular the needs of those going through a time of pain and transition and trying to make sense of what God may be saying to them. God hides behind the simplest of daily activities; finding Him is a matter of total surrender to His will which is the message of this inspirational classic. Its encouragement to 'live in the moment,' accepting everyday obstacles with humility and love, has guided generations of seekers to spiritual peace.

Reflecting on past healthcare scandals should make all levels of healthcare staff redouble their efforts to prevent such tragedies in future. All health professionals should take pride in enacting their roles in which they continually weigh up potential harm, risk and benefit to patients, without considering the cost of acting as the patient advocate.

Medicine, like nursing, can be considered as a privilege. Both professions can be considered as an art, a science, and most importantly, a moral enterprise. Lessons, however, must be learned from past healthcare tragedies, backed by evil ideology, e.g., the Nazi regime.

Two British healthcare professionals were convicted for murdering their patients in the relatively recent past. Nurse Beverley Allitt, killed and injured children in her care in 1991 by drug overdoses. Her victims ranged from a seven-week-old baby to an 11-year-old child. Another paediatric nurse, Lucy Letby, in 2023, was sentenced to a whole life order for murdering babies in her care. An apparently 'good' nurse, who exemplified the fact that serial killers often have no recognisable profile. Dr Harold Shipman murdered a staggering number of his patients (estimated at 250 or more people). He has been described as the worst known serial killer. His killings were believed to have begun in the 1970s and were carried out for over 20 years. He personally gave lethal opioid overdoses to his mostly well, elderly patients in Yorkshire. No one appeared to question events, although those who had suspicions were afraid of being disbelieved, or those asking for investigation were not assisted. Such was the trust inspired in the community by this doctor. These practitioners who killed, needed help themselves with their problems.

However, the victims of these practitioners did not linger for days and weeks, suffering the effects of starvation and dehydration. This is the fate of those whose assisted feeding and hydration can be removed (in line with being considered by some as 'medical treatment'). Hope of recovery is not permitted and those deemed to be 'dying' on a flimsy basis, may be similarly treated with LCP-type practice being relentlessly pursued. This mindset must be vigilantly identified and stopped.

Betrayed trust, power addiction and corruption

The more recent multiple-level failures by NHS staff of trusting patients can act as a lesson for future managers and practitioners. Power and the need for admiration can become both pathological and addictive, not dissimilar to a heroin addict who will do anything to get their fix. It can be argued that medicine and nursing can attract or create murderous practitioners. Some are infamous, others never become known or see justice. Such people may inspire implicit trust in their patients and their relatives. They, too, can influence other practitioners, either through fear or indoctrination, which can result in corruption of conscience, but also the courageous act of whistleblowing which is described as patient advocacy (Jackson et al., 2010).

Them and us?

A bioethicist suggests that we ought to approach all persons with a kind of reverence, knowing that we are in the presence of something mysterious. The mystery is arguably greater in the case of people living with dementia, given their circumstances and the - at times - devastating impacts of cognitive decline. Yet perhaps their personhood and mode of being is deserving of greater reverence for this very reason (Symons, 2021).

> *The Catholic Church's perspective is invaluable in treating all people as sacred:*
> *... sick and disabled people are not some separate categories of humanity; in fact, sickness and disability are part of the human condition and affect every individual, even when there is no direct experience of it.*

(Congregation for the Doctrine of the Faith, 2008)

The soul of the person

Ludwig Wittgenstein described the unique ways in which human beings relate to each other as 'an attitude towards a soul'. This phrase provides a concise summary of the kind of attitude we ought to adopt towards people experiencing the effects of advanced dementia. It is argued that we need to 'look beyond the external markers of personhood that we usually rely on and instead focus on the inexhaustibly rich and unrepeatable character of the human soul' (Symons, 2021).

Non-monetary care costs

The feeling that satisfactory care for patients is not always an achievable aim is distressing for health professionals due to the work demands and the resource constraints. Developed nursing roles which are often technical in nature, may take nurses away from the fundamental requirement for meeting the expressive needs of patients. It was concluded by one study that the failure to play effectively, the expected role of the patient advocate, can result in nurses leaving their profession (Atashzadeh-Shoorideh et al., 2012).

Cost in the caring professions must not only be regarded in terms of financial outlay. Unresolved, constant stress and sickness needs attention as part of cost prevention in terms of staff sick leave. Such focus could mean a reduction in nursing attrition rates due to addressing the physical and mental health issues.

Patient safety

The aim of safe staffing for safer patient care requires a multifactorial approach. Factors to be considered include both government and managerial ultimate responsibility. The greater the authority within the health system for safe care and staff well-being, including sufficient staff resources, the grater the accountability. Stress is a huge factor among nurses as part of sickness rates, while the long 12-hour shifts can be stressful and exhausting over time. Such shifts are a cheaper alternative than staff overlap between the traditional early and late shifts which allowed for staff learning, increased care continuity and more rested nursing staff.

Dependence on overseas staff

Recruiting large numbers of nurses from overseas, may appear to be a welcome development to prop up the falling numbers of British nurses. Is this a fair development, however, for the patients in those countries who are now beginning to feel the effects of falling numbers of their own well-trained nurses such as in the Philippines? Such nurses can be considered as heroes and heroines for helping with their home economy by the historical and continuing practice of sending money back home to their relatives.

Morale

An element associated with staff attrition is the fact that some nurses feel not listened to, appreciated, or unable to achieve their role of patient advocate as revealed in surveys and the recent and past, healthcare scandals. Irrespective of cultural difference, assertiveness training is vital for all in nursing. Without this ability to defend patients' rights, feelings of inadequacy and failing patients can become intolerable and worse than the possible stress of having risen to the challenge.

Knowledge is power

Nurses need help in their pre- and post-registration training to develop skills in questioning, assertiveness and patient representation. This must involve knowledge of national and legal developments and questioning professional guidance. Accessing vital support in negotiating these developments and in exercising the right to conscientious objection as necessary is essential.

Obeying orders

Some of the NHS healthcare scandals involved orders given that required cooperation in carrying them out, which harmed and killed patients. Those expected to carry out unethical orders must question them with confidence and pride in their role as the patient advocate, in line with the code of conduct and a sensitive conscience, together with enlisting the appropriate support.

The 'unpopular' patient and patient 'labelling'

Felicity Stockwell published her seminal research, in 1972. This described nurses' relationships with patients who they perceived as 'difficult' and focused on negative stereotyping which then influenced preferential care to favoured patients. The widely held, contemporary view that nurses treated all patients in a non-judgemental fashion was challenged by this research.

Patients and families who are challenging to health professionals may find that the treatment and care may be less favourable. Such results can be seen in the labelling not only of patients as 'difficult' and regarded as 'unpopular', but also their prognosis deemed as 'poor' may have been coloured by a belief that they are better off dead. Patients can be labelled (inappropriately) as 'dying' and this results in their (unnecessary) death through lack of treatment and care.

The code of conduct in practice and the role of education

The role of patient advocate can be emotionally and physically demanding of the nurse and even more challenging when attempted within 'hostile' cultures, be they intimidating or militantly secular. Nurses, however, cannot disregard their responsibility for acting as the patient's advocate. Nurse-patient advocacy is an expectation of the code of conduct which is compiled by the NMC in collaboration with the public.

Educators need to be creative in retaining their workforce in a current era of numbers of retiring nurses and problems in staff recruitment and retention in economically challenging times. They must encourage their students to respect and internalise their nursing code of conduct to understand what it means to be a true professional. They must be educated in how defending and achieving the role of patient advocate can be helped by full knowledge and regular reference to the principles of the code. This is now incorporated into the process of revalidation for nursing reregistration which can give clear focus to its importance.

'Never again' nurse narratives

In 2006 Wolf and Zuzelo conducted a study into the experiences of nurses in 'never again' situations. Their study findings described the significant turning points in these 'never again' stories narrated by nurses. Those who had participated in previous, distressing situations of failed advocacy, vowed not to allow such situations to occur in future. Critical incidents revealed dilemmas in which nurses' autonomous, clinical practice was constrained by feelings of powerlessness.

Nurses submitted written accounts of critical 'never again' situations. Patient outcomes were fatal, close calls, dehumanising, or isolating. 'Never again' stories incorporated ethical dilemmas, deficits in nurses' knowledge, lack of confidence in clinical abilities and failure to act correctly. Patients' welfare was the centre of accounts. Circumstances threatened the trust of patients and family members in nurses and other providers. Patients' wishes were denied, because of haste, health providers' arrogance, or a desire not to be inconvenienced. Nurses' emotions mirrored a sense of failed responsibility for patients. Regret, however, was tempered by nurses' pledges to ensure better outcomes in the future (Wolf and Zuzelo, 2006). Such pledges can be facilitated by the support to nurses of structured and formalised, clinical supervision.

The importance of virtue
No matter to what depths a society may fall,
virtuous persons will always be beacons that light the
way back to moral sensitivity; virtuous physicians
are the beacons that show the way back to moral
credibility for the whole profession.

(Pellegrino, 1985)

Forgiveness

Where practitioners have experienced a personal sense of failure, it is vital to recall the words of Jesus who was all love, forgiveness and compassion. This was exemplified by another of His parables about the redeeming power of forgiveness, as shown by the father of the Prodigal Son. Jesus' compassion for His failed creatures was revealed in the forgiveness of Peter, who denied Him three times in a moment of weakness (Jn 21:9), the Samaritan woman at the well (Jn 4:4-26) and so many others, all felt His transforming power of forgiven sin. Even from the Cross, He asked His Father to forgive those who did not know what they were doing, in condemning Him to a cruel death.

Health culture, management responsibility

Researchers have concluded that ethical leaders create a context where people intuitively refrain from choosing unethical behaviour. Authors of a recent study on this subject have recommended that ethical leadership is a way to prevent corruption in organisations (Manara et al., 2020). Corruption causes serious harm not only for organisations but also for patients as microcosms of society in general.

Coronavirus effects on nurses

The COVID-19 pandemic appears to have highlighted the physical and mental vulnerability of nurses and doctors on the front line. The imperative for good care of staff applies not just at times of national crisis but as an ongoing challenge to ensure their physical and mental well-being to aid in their retention as truly educated and compassionate practitioners. This must include acceptance of their right to conscientious objection. This, in turn, can promote their acting as the Good Samaritan, for effective patient safety within holistic care approaches.

Nursing dedication

Against the grim statistic in the UK alone of reportedly tens of thousands of people who have died as a result of the COVID-19 pandemic, we know that each life is precious. Bereavement is harder when so many families were unable to be with their loved ones at the time of death. Yet against this time of suffering, sadness and grief, we have seen extraordinarily dedicated care by health professionals and carers. Their devotion and heroism have been celebrated by the public as a testimony to the intrinsic dignity of every human person and the respect owed to each human life, particularly in the last moments.

Professional education

Treatment and care benchmarks as pathways, if corruptible, are best discarded despite a prevailing view that without them practitioners are bereft of guidance. Perhaps a more realistic expectation for future, ethical practice will be improved education for undergraduate doctors and nurses. How do practitioners manage in other complex specialties where benchmark pathways are not always seen as essential as the LCP appeared to be?

'Those who are wise will shine like the brightness of the heavens and those who lead many to righteousness, like the stars for ever and ever' (Daniel 12:3).

Health professionals need more than a theoretical and practical base. Achieving a caring culture involves both managerial and educational involvement and reflection on clinical practice within an agreed philosophy of holistic care. Ethical role modelling is essential for future generations of healthcare practitioners and exploring, in safe environments, where things have gone wrong in the past. This should include discussion of the notorious NHS scandals which sadly, can appear to be ongoing. Root cause analysis is important for immediate incidents where harm may have inadvertently occurred but analysing a failed care culture in a wider context is also vital.

Precious life

Untimely deaths of millions around the world due to the pandemic have been recorded. While the large numbers of young men in the UK who kill themselves, comprise the highest cause of death of men under 45 years of age. Yet the gift of life in all its beauty, dignity and fragility, now faces a profound challenge in the UK through the latest attempt (of several) to legalise assisted suicide.

Assisted suicide and euthanasia

Repeated UK bills to allow assisted suicide are always framed as a compassionate response to those in the last stages of their life. However, such compassion must be denounced as 'false compassion' and its remedy is a 'true compassion'. This means accompanying, patiently, the vulnerable sick and dying, which is the required response to the needs of the valued dying person rather than allowing the common problem of fear of being a burden to be encouraged. Nurses should take comfort from the lessons of World War II where despite the excesses of the Nazi regime, it appears that nursing conscience was respected for those dissenting against euthanasia of the vulnerable.

Government's healthcare responsibility and accountability

One bereaved mother who suffered within a failing NHS trust midwifery service cautioned the new Minister for Health (as of June 2021) to finally listen to grieving relatives. She recounted the experience of attempts to be heard by successive Home Secretaries who promised change over repeated NHS maternity failings and coverups. The advice she gave was to 'focus on the fact that you represent people... and patient testimonies will guide you' (Hawkins, 2021).

Successive ministers for health had been approached for meetings, over nursing concerns about the LCP practices, which were not granted. This was attempted at the height of its use, before and following its independent review in 2013 and its recommended 'discarding', The same practices can be in use without the 'care pathway' label. Ministers cannot stubbornly ignore this fact.

Ministers with such responsibility must appreciate their own accountability for the LCP scandal which occurred under their long-held 'watch' and accountability must be owned by those ministers at the helm of health for any continuing similar LCP practice. Those at all levels who ignore bad practice reported to them are as culpable as the practitioners responsible for such practice. Listening to health professionals and the public must be considered as an important part of ministerial engagement. Ministers being content with a third party responding to valid concerns of those with 'frontline' experience and refusing to engage as was the case with the LCP has proved disastrous for timely intervention for saving lives. Health ministers must consider the parable of the Good Samaritan and its lessons, as applying to them, not just to health professionals. They must carefully listen when important discussion is requested about practitioners' concerns for patient safety.

Post-pandemic government issues

In the future, the government will have large debts, increasing areas of activity, a weakening currency and an increasing healthcare bill as the population ages. Legalise voluntary euthanasia – and what could possibly go wrong? In short, in a secular society that has abandoned moral principles for narratives, what is to stop the State from switching from spending money and saving lives to saving money and spending lives?

(Sutherland, 2021)

Our role as the Good Samaritan in healthcare is to minimise any damage suffered by individuals. It is certainly not to further any suffering by indifference or inaction which will cause them to lose hope or even be harmed.

Financial reward for unethical practice

The dangers of the financial incentives driven by the CQUIN process associated with LCP practice, should have been obvious to anyone with knowledge of people's human frailty and some awareness of those with obsessive, misguided economic considerations.

Secular bioethics

A bioethicist and theologian at Fordham University, Charles Camosy, argues that medicine, when detached from a transcendent dimension, is increasingly a threat to human dignity. In his new book; *Losing Our Dignity: How Secularised Medicine is Undermining Fundamental*

Human Equality; he predicts that the lives of millions of people with dementia will be at risk.

The central thesis of the book is that as medicine became secularised, it rejected the idea that fundamental human equality comes from sharing a common human nature which reflects the image and likeness of God – and replaced it with a vision of the person which insists on their being rational, self-aware, autonomous, productive and so on, to be morally and legally valuable.

But there is no principled reason why our secularised medical culture would stop with this population. After all, lots of disabled human beings are not rational, self-aware, autonomous and productive in the same way able-bodied human beings are. Why would we think that we will not eventually apply this horrific moral and legal vision to them? Camosy sounds the alarm and insists on our theological vision of the human person as one that is necessary to defend the fundamental equality of the most vulnerable human beings. A good proposition is that people with faith need to have equal seats at the table, refusing to be embarrassed by our theological beliefs. Camosy makes clear it is now absolutely necessary to proclaim our theological beliefs if we are going to preserve the concept of fundamental human equality (Cook, 2021).

Hope and healing

An African archbishop suggests that 'Hope is the theological virtue which receives the least attention. Yet it is the most needed to keep the flames of faith and love alive' (Job, 2019). No matter how dark it gets, when the material world fails us, there is a light called 'hope' when we have no solutions, when things are in the world's terms, hopeless.

A French philosopher has said: 'when you see the incredible resistance human beings can have to everything that has tried to destroy them, that is the incarnation of hope' (Levy, 2021).

Hope is a beacon against despair. It is a vital element in healing of the heart, the mind and soul, even though the possibility of a cure may be remote. Human beings need encouragement in practising this virtue as it is a positive orientation to life rather than despair. Hope is more than a light inside but a light for the way ahead.

Therapeutic relationships

The Spanish verb for hope is 'esperar' which also means 'to wait'. This definition seems appropriate, since hope can involve the process of waiting for clarification about what is to come. One of the healthcare provider's first duties to a client is to inspire hope through the development of a therapeutic relationship and the provision of appropriate and accurate health education and information (Miller, 1999).

Regardless of what scientific regime is required for the medical care of a person, health professionals should nurture faith and hope in themselves, their own potential and the one cared for. Hope is one of the three theological virtues, together with faith and charity. It can be argued that if we lose sight of the virtue of charity, we in turn can lose hope and then faith.

Faith and spirituality

Spirituality and the faith that it entails can provide people with a positive outlook on a life situation being experienced. The ageing person engaged in life struggles may, for example, hope for a resolution, hope for a closer relationship with a higher power, or hope for forgiveness. Spirituality and the intrapsychic strength of the ageing individual can provide a source of help when coping with stressful life events. This can take the form of intrinsic religiosity: prayer, a sense of meaning and purpose and transcendence (Fehring et al., 1997).

Having hope is also related to spiritual well-being (Burkhardt and Nagai-Jacobson, 2020). With God, all things are possible. St Jude Thaddeus is the patron saint of hopeless and difficult cases. It is suggested that in seeking God's will for our lives, we can let St Jude be our friend and companion (Job, 2019).

Research on the effects of hope and health in elderly people who are coping with cancer has found that hope is associated with spiritual well-being and results in:

- a greater number of goals being set by an individual
- more difficult goals chosen
- more personal happiness
- less distress
- better coping skills when dealing with difficult life situations
- faster recovery from physical illness and injury.

(Fehring et al., 1997)

Care vs cure

Patients need to know there is always something to offer whether it is purely relief of symptoms, physical, mental, emotional, or spiritual. Such holistic care can provide hope in patients at all stages of illness.

St Paul

Hope is beautifully described by Paul, the Apostle who, following his conversion by Jesus on the road to Damascus, never gave up his caring mission to bring the gospel to the people. He continued his mission despite his trials and repeated tribulations. He describes hope for us in his letter to the Romans:
We can boast about looking forward to God's glory. But that is not all we can boast about. We can boast about our sufferings. These sufferings bring patience, as we know, and patience brings perseverance, and perseverance brings hope, and this hope is not deceptive, because the love of God has been poured into our hearts by the Holy Spirit which has been given us.

(Romans 5:1–5)

Nurses as healers

Nurses may heal through their holistic approach to their patients as advocated by their code of conduct and their intrinsic orientation to care. The development of a therapeutic relationship can promote the possibility of patients' emotional healing, even where physical cure may not always be possible.

Healthcare professionals, while being expected to act as advocates for their patients, need to keep track of political and professional developments and how these may impact on the culture of their work setting and safety of their patients, together with the awareness of the vital virtue of compassion in healthcare practice.

Industrial action -preventable?

Strike action is a tragic decision which has untold consequences for patients, relatives, colleagues, and the nurses themselves who decide to strike. A public perception of betrayed trust may be the hardest consequence for the profession to overcome, hitherto viewed in general, as a body of Good Samaritans.

A member of the public suggests ways that:

*the Government could enhance the somewhat
parsimonious pay increase it is offering nurses.
First of all, it should put an end to the iniquitous practice of
charging staff for parking their cars on hospital premises.
These exorbitant costs could be picked up by the
private sector - parking - management companies that
could well afford this.
Secondly, full nursing bursaries should be
reintroduced for all trainees
so that on qualification they would not
have to repay large amounts of
student debts from their salaries.
This would also have the effect of encouraging
recruitment and reducing the number of
agency and foreign nurses being employed to
fill gaps, and again pay for itself*

(Shorter, 2023)

Conclusion

The culture of care

Legal, professional and government developments which can give rise to a culture at odds with ethical principles in practice, need to be monitored by all in healthcare. These developments can have inevitable implications on practice. Those involved in required monitoring include all tiers of management, educators and practitioners 'on the front line'. Those with an aggressive secularist vision, whether as members of ethical committees advising hospitals with their own modern bioethicist agenda of marketplace expediency, need challenge.

It is suggested that truly radical change to funding and delivery of healthcare will require a professionally executed grassroots campaign for change, followed by a referendum. The struggle must begin immediately and needs to be fronted by concerned doctors and nurses, including whistleblowers who have seen the destruction wreaked on vulnerable patients by an amoral bureaucracy (Heath, 2023). Any healthcare system, however, requires dedicated, professional oversight with a clear and agreed philosophy of care for those in real need, of timely treatment, recovery, rehabilitation and hope.

All in healthcare must understand and appreciate their strength in numbers as advocates to safeguard those most vulnerable at all stages of life. This safeguarding can include lobbying of MPs as part of one's civic duty to make efforts to ensure legislation is not passed which is a threat to the vulnerable, e.g., assisted suicide, as discussed in chapter 13.

When end - of - life care goes wrong

There seems, in many areas, to be rigid adherence to the LCP 'care' pathway which was heavily criticised a decade ago and officially recommended for discarding at the time (see chapter 10). Today, elderly and vulnerable people are still being put on an end-of-life 'death pathway'.

A report titled *When End of Life Care Goes Wrong* was commissioned by the Lords and Commons Family and Child Protection Group. It has exposed unacceptable practice according to its chair, DUP MP, Carla Lockhart.

The report concludes that the LCP is still being practised 'in all but name'. The report published in March 2023, details 16 cases where patients died after being given LCP-style treatment. The youngest was just 21. A retired neurologist comments: 'The contents of the report are tangible proof of the terrible loss of patient autonomy which has occurred in the NHS in the management of the elderly and disabled patients' (Pullicino, 2023).

The 16 cases showed doctors implementing a 'one-size fits all, tick-box approach'. In many of the case studies, patients were experiencing an end-of-life care pathway which was similar to the LCP in all but name.

One of the report's authors, retired palliative care consultant, Professor Sam Ahmedzai, said he was 'shocked' to hear how they had been treated 'at the hands of those who should have known better.' He noted that in 10 of the cases, relatives challenged doctors about whether the LCP was being applied but 'this was met with denial'. Some patients were subjected to 'indefensible end-of-life decisions' made 'unilaterally' by doctors.

Laura Jane Booth, 21, who had the genetic disorder Patau's syndrome, died in October 2016, after going into hospital for an eye operation. Her parents said: 'She had no nutrition for the entire three-and-a-half weeks she was in'. Even during three days in intensive care, 'still nobody did anything about Laura not feeding'. When she died, they still thought she was in hospital for routine surgery. 'Nobody ever told us that she was on an end-of-life care pathway' (Adams, 2023).

End-of-life pathways which use opioids, strong sedation and no hydration, are therefore facilitating 'best interest' decision-making and exclusion of the required judgement of the doctor and next of kin. The elderly should be able to rely on their doctor and close relative to decide for them if they do not have mental capacity (Pullicino, 2023).

'Best interests' decisions

An academic paper by Holm and Edgar (2008), has described 'best interest' as 'legal fiction,' as members of a best interest decision group are likely to put forward their own biases concerning acceptable quality of life or futility of treatment. They may be swayed by prevalent views in society or the convenience of the hospital and its staff. In many of the cases in the report, 'When End of Life Care Goes Wrong', the next of kin opposed a decision to start an end-of-life pathway but was overruled, and the patient died. Side-lining of close relatives in end-of-life decision making has been the source of great anguish and guilt in families. The exclusion of the doctor as the key decision-maker at this critical point reduces rational scientific input into management and makes an emotion-based conclusion more likely (Pullicino, 2023).

Care Quality Commission responsibility

Professor Pullicino who blew the whistle on LCP abuses more than a decade ago, believes that more must be done. He informed the journalist, Simon Caldwell of his misgivings about the responsible body, charged with patient care quality:

The report flags up shortcomings of the Care Quality Commission repeatedly, this is the body tasked with the safety of patients in the NHS. The CQC must bear full responsibility for the continued use of lethal pathways. They need to make dehydration a notifiable occurrence and sanction hospitals that dehydrate patients. The one body that could force a change and stop inappropriate deaths is doing nothing, despite repeated complaints made to it. The sick elderly necessarily take up a lot of hospital beds and therefore, consume a lot of resources. Despite the increase in the elderly population the number of hospital

beds in the UK has dramatically fallen.
It is impossible to avoid the connection
with the widespread use of end-of-life pathways.

(Caldwell, 2023)

A viewpoint from another Christian perspective, emphasises the need for compassion to be paramount at the end of a person's life and the danger of legalised assisted suicide:

No one should die by dehydration, and no
relative should suffer the distress of seeing
their loved one die in that way.
It is not difficult to provide hydration,
and it is unlawful to withhold it.
Sadly, legalising assisted dying would
only make things worse.
Once assisted dying is legalised,
the attitude and culture of the
medical profession changes.
When it is legal to help someone to die,
medics become used to the idea that
some lives are not worth preserving.

(Dieppe, 2023)

The LCP name may have changed, but the misapplication, misuse – and even abuse – persist.

Report proposals

Examining the many clinical failures, and what sometimes appears blatant abuse, the Report concludes with a series of proposed actions to address the problems:

1. A national inventory of local end of life care plans, policies and procedures currently being used in all healthcare settings

2. A national rapid response service to advise and support people who have a loved one currently experiencing poor quality end- of- life care
3. A fast-track advice helpline for recently bereaved families
4. A national register of cases where end -of- life care has fallen below standards or breaches guidelines
5. The urgent adoption of a uniform national system to capture patients' preferences for end- of- life care
6. Further high-quality research into social, medical and nursing aspects of end -of -life care

Doctors are called to save life, not kill, and it is urgent these problems be addressed by Parliament, and appropriate action taken to end such callous and inhumane treatment of those at the end of life (Rose, 2023).

The Good Samaritan, the future

My aim in authoring the book is to help all those practitioners with good will for their patients to be empowered to carry on providing compassionate, holistic care as good role models for those new to the profession. Whether in critical care or any other speciality, or working with patients in the community, in research or the voluntary sector, patients need someone who can be trusted to help them in their time of need.

Further to the well-documented care failings, causes of which may never be truly understood, patients must never be fearful of hospitalisation, or their health professionals. Learning must be derived for future practice to regain lost trust and enhance trust in healthcare by the public.

Respect for patient expectations of care

I acknowledge that some of the content of this book is much less positive than any health professional would wish for or would have imagined to be the case as a reflection of the revered NHS. My aim was to give a fair and balanced account of issues seldom discussed concerning the NHS. The negative aspects recounted do not negate the work of the numerous 'Good Samaritans' within the UK health and social care services, who, day by day, achieve constant, positive, and compassionate care outcomes for their patients and residents, having entered their chosen profession to do good.

Despite the unedifying and distressing NHS care scandals narrated in this book, many health professionals can be considered as heroes and heroines, on so many occasions and in multiple settings. This particularly applies during the challenge of caring for people in the coronavirus pandemic. Despite being a cause of such personal and professional stress, it has revealed great and unstinting courage and selflessness.

Nevertheless, the tragedies explored in this book, which involve the beginning, middle and end of life for so many people over so many years, reveal that the wish to act as the patient advocate can be opposed by growing philosophical arguments and ideologies. These can and have acted against a true vocation to care and can result in an apparent systemic lack of care. The concept of and the right to conscientious objection is increasingly under threat by aggressive secularists whose ideology of 'health care' mitigates against this right which is clearly relevant to ethical healthcare.

Ethical principles

Health professionals must not be forced into denial or embarrassment of accepted ethical principles and their conscience, which dictates holistic, hopeful, compassionate care. This aim, however, needs required support to enable confident, ethical practice. This can be accessed via legal, professional, educational, managerial, spiritual and finally, peer support.

The Nightingale School Fellowship prayer is an inspiration for our vocations, whether in nursing, medicine or the other professions, including government ministers and top managers in healthcare:

*'May we have the blessings of Grace that we
may never be false to the obligations of our calling'*

(Miller, 2020)

The following words of Jesus help us to reflect on the privilege of being a health professional who will offer compassionate care to every patient in keeping with conscience, professional codes and ethical principle: *For whatsoever you do to the least of your brothers and sisters, you do unto me* (Matthew 25:31–46).

An aggressive, secular culture will never negate the best example of what a caring health professional, can, and should be, at each level of an organisation, a Good Samaritan patient advocate. The parable helps us to believe we can do so much more than we realise despite possible difficulties, for patients in need.

Good Samaritans in healthcare do not pass by on the other side. They do not hold prejudice on account of patients' age, race, gender, religion, health, economic or social status. They give of themselves for the benefit of vulnerable, often lonely and broken people who so often have no one to communicate their needs, defend their rights and even their lives.

*In the evening of life, we shall be
judged on our love alone*

(St. John of the Cross)

Sources of support

For further information, or support, on any of the issues covered in this book, please visit the websites below:

Advisory, Conciliation and Arbitration Service (Acas), https://www.acas.org.uk/

Acas gives employees and employers free, impartial advice on workplace rights, rules and best practice and also offers training and help to resolve disputes.

Alliance defending freedom (ADF UK): https://adflegal.org/

A faith-based legal advocacy organisation defending fundamental freedoms and human dignity for people of all faiths.

Alliance of Prolife Students www.allianceofprolifestudents.org.uk

Anscombe Bioethics Centre www.bioethics.org.uk

Association of Catholic Nurses of England and Wales: http://www.catholicnurses. org.uk/

Bereavement support: Sue Ryder organisation: https://www.sueryder.org/how-we-can-help/online-bereavement-support

Care Not Killing https://www.carenotkilling.org.uk/

Christian Concern: Legal help for Christians: https://christianconcern.com/

Their Legal Defence Fund helps protect Christian religious freedom and restrain those who are unlawfully harassing and discriminating against Christian believers.

Citizens' Advice https://www.citizensadvice.org.uk/

Citizens' Advice is an independent organisation specialising in confidential information and advice to assist people with legal and other issues.

CRUSE Bereavement support: cis.cruse.org.uk

Dehydration lifeline: https://dehydrationlifeline.org/

Help for relatives of loved ones who are being denied fluids

Eden Care: www.edencareuk.com

Service for quality care of the dying, befriending and tackling social isolation. Set up originally for Muslim/Asian people but now available to all.

Medical Ethics Alliance: https://medethicsalliance.org.uk/contact/

The Alliance affirms the unique value of all human life, its inherent dignity and consequent right to protection in law.

Pro Life Nurses. Nurses against assisted suicide and euthanasia. A UK nursing network for support and information. https://www.prolifenurses.com/

Protect Charity: https://protect-advice.org.uk/

Protect works with organisations on improving their speak up arrangements and campaigns for better legal protection of whistle blowers to make whistleblowing work for individuals, organisations and society.

Society for the Protection of Unborn Children. https://www.spuc.org.uk/

The Good Counsel Network: info@goodcounselnetwork.com

Informs women about the risks to their physical and psychological health and presents them with realistic alternatives to abortion. Tel. 0207 723 1740

UK Catholic Medical Association: https://catholicmedicalassociation.org.uk/

Volunteering in palliative care: www.hospiceuk.org

References

Abortion Act (1967) Legislation.gov.uk. The National Archives. Available at: https://www.legislation.gov.uk/ukpga/1967/87/contents (Last accessed 2 May 2022).

ACAS (The Advisory, Conciliation and Arbitration Service) (2022) Definition Bullying. Available at: https://www.acas.org.uk/discrimination-bullying-and-harassment (Last accessed 26 April 2022).

ACP (2017) American College of Physicians Reaffirms Opposition to Legalization of Physician-Assisted Suicide: ACP also calls for improved hospice and palliative care. Available at: https://www.acponline.org/acp-newsroom/opposition-to-legalization-of-physician-assisted-suicide (Last accessed 9 April 2022).

Adams, S. (2023) Elderly and vulnerable people are still being put on an end-of-life 'death pathway', hard-hitting report reveals – even though it was officially abolished almost a decade ago. *Mail online*, 5 March. Available at: https://www.dailymail.co.uk/news/article-11821863/Elderly-vulnerable-people-end-life-death-pathway-report-reveals.html. (Last accessed 15 March 2023).

Adams, J. (2018) Ashya King has been cleared of cancer, three years after his parents were jailed for abducting him from an NHS hospital to seek treatment abroad. Available at: https://www.telegraph.co.uk/news/2018/03/03/ashya-king-cleared-cancer-three-years-parents-abducted-hospital/ (Last accessed 8 April 2022).

Adams, R. (2006) A Theory of Virtue: Excellence in Being for the Good. Oxford University Press. In: Gallagher, A., (2010) Moral Distress and Moral Courage in Everyday Nursing Practice. American Nurses Association (ANA) OJIN: The Online Journal of Issues in Nursing Vol. 16 No. 2. Available at: https://ojin.nursingworld.org/MainMenuCategories/EthicsStandards/Resources/Courage-and-Distress/Moral-Distress-and-Courage-in-Everyday-Practice.html#Adams (Last accessed 2 May 2022).

Aid to the Church in Need (2022) Persecuted and Forgotten? A report on Christians Oppressed for their Faith 2020–2022. Executive Summary. P. 10. Aid to the Church in Need. UK.

Airedale NHS Trust v Bland (1993) AC 789. Available at: https://www.e-lawresources.co.uk/Airedale-N-H-S--Trust-v-Bland.php (Last accessed 2 May 2022).

Alexander, L. (1947) The Nuremberg Code. International Law Commission, Geneva, United Nations. Available at: https://legal.un.org/ilc/texts/instruments/english/draft_articles/7_1_1950.pdf (Last accessed 29 April 2022).

Alexander, L. (1949) Medical science under dictatorship. New England Journal of Medicine 241 (2), pp. 39–47.

Altahayneh, Z., Khasawneh, A. and Abedalhafiz, A. (2014) Relationship between organisational justice and job satisfaction as perceived by Jordanian physical education teachers. Asian Social Science 10 (4), pp. 131–138.

Alton, D. (2020) Catholics call for a national inquiry into UK nursing home deaths. Catholic News Agency. Available at: https://www.catholicnewsagency.com/news/44616/catholics-call-for-public-inquiry-into-uk-nursing-home-deaths (Last accessed 9 April 2022).

Alton, D. (2021) Lord Alton highlights double standards of the Animal Welfare Bill failing to afford the same rights to unborn humans. Available at: https://righttolife.org.uk/news/lord-alton-highlights-double-standards-of-the-animal-welfare-bill-failing-to-afford-the-same-rights-to-unborn-humans (Last accessed 1 May 2022).

AMA (2020) Physician Assisted Suicide. Ethics. AMA. Available at: https://www.ama-assn.org/delivering-care/ethics/physician-assisted-suicide (Last accessed 29 April 2022).

American Academy of Neurology (1995) Report of The Quality Standards Subcommittee of the American Academy of Neurology. Practice parameters for determining brain death in adults [summary statement]. *Neurology. Special article*, 1995; 45:1012–1014. 1 May. Available at: https://n.neurology.org/content/neurology/45/5/1012.full.pdf7 (Last accessed 24 November 2022).

Angelucci, P. (2006) Grasping the concept of medical futility. *Nurs Manage.* 37(2): pp. 12–14.

An NHS trust and others (Respondents) v Y (by his litigation friend, the Official Solicitor) and another (Appellants) (2018) Available at: https://www.google.com/search?q=An+NHS+Trust+and+others+(Respondents)+v+Y+(by+his+litigation+friend%2C+the+Official+Solicitor)+and+another+(Appellants)+(2018)&rlz=1C1CHBF_en-GBGB900GB900&oq=An+NHS+Trust+and+others+(Respondents)+v+Y+(by+his+litigation+friend%2C+the+Official+Solicitor)+and+another+(Appellants)+(2018)&aqs=chrome..69i57.3814j0j9&sourceid=chrome&ie=UTF-8 (Last accessed 2 May 2022).

Animals (Scientific Procedures) Act (1986) Amendment Regulations 2012. Available at: https://www.legislation.gov.uk/ukdsi/2012/9780111530313 (Last accessed 2 May 2022).

Anscombe, G.E.M. (1958) Modern Moral Philosophy. *Philosophy* 33 (124) pp. 1–19. Available at: https://www.jstor.org/stable/3749051 (Last accessed 26 July 2022).

Ansseau, M., Dierick, M., Buntinkx, F., Cnockaert, P., De Smedt, J., Van Den Haute, M. and Vander Mijnsbrugge, D. (2004) High prevalence of mental disorders in primary care. *J Affect Disord* 78 (1), pp. 49–55. Available at:

https://pubmed.ncbi.nlm.nih.gov/14672796/ (Last accessed 29 April 2022).

APPHG (2020) Report: Time for reflection: a report of the all-party parliamentary humanist group on religion or belief in the UK parliament Available at: https://humanists.uk/wp-content/uploads/APPG-report_religion-in-parliament_Jan2020_print.pdf (Last accessed 29 April 2022).

Arbuckle, G. (2007) Retelling the Good Samaritan. Jesus' Parable is the Founding Story of Catholic Health Care. Health Progress. *Journal of the Catholic Health Association of the United States.* Available at: www.chausa.org (Last accessed 1 May 2022).

Archbishop of Canterbury, Welby, J. (2021) Assisted Dying Bill [HL] (Meacher Bill.) (Vol 815) Hansard. Debated on 22 October 2021.

Ashton, J. (2020) *Blinded by Corona.* Gibson Square Books Ltd. London, UK.

Ashworth, P. (2000) Editorial. Nurse-doctor relationships; conflict, competition, or collaboration. *Intensive and Critical Care Nursing* 16, pp. 127–128.

Assisted Dying (No 2) Bill [HL]. (2015). (Marris Bill) (Vol 599).

Astrup J., Symon L., Branston, N.M. and Lassen, N.A. (1977) Cortical evoked potential and extracellular K+ and H+ at critical levels of brain ischemia. *Stroke.* 8:51–7. In: Davis, S.M. and Donnan, G.A. (2021) Ischemic Penumbra: A Personal View. *Cerebrovascular Diseases: 30th Anniversary Review.* Cerebrovasc Dis 2021; 50:656–665. DOI: 10.1159/000519730. Received: August 9. Accepted: September 16, 2021. Published online: November 4, 2021. Departments of Medicine and Neurology, Melbourne Brain Centre at the Royal Melbourne Hospital, University of Melbourne, Victoria, VIC, Australia. Available at: https://www.karger.com/Article/Pdf/519730#page8 (Last accessed 25 November 2022).

Atashzadeh-Shoorideh, F., Ashktorab, T. and Yaghmaei, F. (2012) Iranian intensive care unit nurses' moral distress: a content analysis. *Nurs Ethics* 19 (4), pp. 464–478.

Atherton, D. and Peyton, M. (2013) Faith and Martyrdom, the Holy Hand of St Edmund Arrowsmith. Available at: http://saintsandrelics.co.uk/ p 10. (Last accessed 5 April 2022).

Aylin, P., Best, P., Bottle, A. and Marshall, C. (2003) Following Shipman: a pilot system for monitoring mortality rates in primary care. *Lancet* 362, pp. 485–491.

Bakeer, H.M., Nassar, R.A. and Sweelam, R.K.M. (2021) Investigating organisational justice and job satisfaction as perceived by nurses, and its relationship to organizational citizenship behaviour. Available at: https://journals.rcni.com/nursing-management/evidence-and-practice/investigating-organisational-justice-and-job-satisfaction-as-perceived-by-nurses-and-its-relationship-to-organizational-citizenship-behaviour-nm.2021.e1973/full. (Last accessed 7 July 2021).

Baker, R. (1997) The History of Medical Ethics. In: Bynum, W.F. and Porter, R. (1997) *Companion Encyclopaedia of the History of Medicine.* Routledge, Oxford, UK. Chapter 37, Vol. 2, pp. 852–887.

Baldwin, M.A. (2003) Patient advocacy, a concept analysis. *Nursing Standard* 17 (21), pp. 33–39.

Baldwin, S. (2006) Organisational justice. Brighton Institute for Employment Studies. Available at: http://employment-studies.co.uk/system/files/resources/files/mp73.pdf (Last accessed 4 April 2022).

Ball, J., Maben, J., Murrells, T. and Day, T. (2015) National Nursing Research Unit, King's College London. Griffiths, P. University of Southampton & NIHR Collaboration for Applied Health Research & Care. 12-hour shifts: prevalence, views and impact. Report to Dr Ruth May, National Lead 'Compassion in Practice: Action Area'.

Barnard, G.W. (2011) The Dissolution of the Monasteries. Available at: https://onlinelibrary.wiley.com/doi/abs/10.1111/j.1468-229X.2011.00526.x (Last accessed 29 April 2022).

Barnhart, K., Bartels, D., Brunnquell, D., Cranford R., Moldow, G, and Sandler V. (2004) Model Guidelines for Addressing Medical Futility in End-of-life Care. Resource Center, University of Minnesota Center for Bioethics.

Bass, B.M. (1990) From Transactional to Transformational Leadership: Learning to Share the Vision. *Organizational Dynamics*, pp. 18, 19–31. https://doi.org/10.1016/0090-2616(90)90061-S

Bass, B.M. (1999) Two decades of research and development in transformational leadership. *European Journal of Work and Organizational Psychology*, 8(1), 9–32. American Psychological Association. https://doi.org/10.1080/135943299398410 Available at https://psycnet.apa.org/record/2010-19281-002 (Last accessed 21 March 2023).

BBC NEWS (2019) Vincent Lambert: Frenchman at centre of end of life debate dies 11 July. Available at: https://www.bbc.co.uk/news/world-europe-48911187 (Last accessed 1 May 2022).

Bear, T., Philipp, M., Hill, S. and Mündel, T. (2016) A preliminary study on how hypohydration affects pain perception. *Psychophysiology* 53 (5) 605–610.

Beauchamp, T.L. and Childress, J.F. (1994) *Principles of Biomedical Ethics*. 5th ed. Oxford University Press: New York.

Bellieni, C.V. and Buonocore, G. (2013) Abortion and subsequent mental health: review of the literature. *Psychiatry and clinical neurosciences* 67 (5), pp. 301–310.

Benedict, S. and Shields, L. (eds.) (2014) *Nurses and Midwives in Nazi Germany. The 'Euthanasia Programs'*. Charles Sturt University. Aust. Routledge. Books. google.com Available at: https://researchoutput.csu.edu.au/en/publications/nurses-and-midwives-in-nazi-germany-the-euthanasia-programs (Last accessed 4 May 2022).

Bible Gateway (1993) The Good Samaritan. Adapted from the New Revised Standard Version. Catholic Edition. Available at: https://www.biblegateway.com/passage/?search=Luke%2010%3A25-37&version=NRSV (Last accessed 1 May 2022).

Bilger, M. (2019) Vincent Lambert's father slams hospital starving his son to death. Life News.com 9 July. Available at: https://www.lifenews.com/2019/07/09/vincent-lamberts-father-slams-hospital-starving-his-son-to-death-its-murder-in-disguise/ (Last accessed 28 April 2022).

Blackwell, T. (2014) Should doctors tell people they're dying? Why soft-pedalling the grim reality could help patients live longer. *National Post*. Available at: https://nationalpost.com/news/canada/should-doctors-tell-people-theyre-dying-why-soft-pedaling-the-grim-reality-could-help-patients-live-longer (Last accessed 11 July 2022).

Bland, L. and Hall, L.A. (2010) Eugenics in Britain: The View from the Metropole. In: Bashford, A. and Levine, P. (eds.), (2012) The Oxford Handbook of the History of Eugenics. Oxford University Press: Oxford. pp. 213–227.

Blau, E. (1995) *Krishnamurti: 100 Years*. New York: Stewart, Tabori and Chang.

Bliss, J., Cowley, S. and While, A. (2000) Inter professional working in palliative care in the community: a review of the literature. *J Interprof Care* 14 (3), pp. 281–290

Bloomfield, J. and Pegram, A. (2013) Care, compassion and communication. *Nursing Standard ART & SCIENCE, Essential skills clusters 1*. **doi:** 10.7748/ns.29. 25. e7653. 25 March. pp. 45-50. (Last accessed 4 July 2022).

BMA (2018/2021) Clinically-assisted nutrition and hydration (CANH) New guidance to support doctors making decisions about CANH for adults who lack capacity in England and Wales. 22 October. Last reviewed 16 July 2021. Available at: https://www.bma.org.uk/advice-and-support/ethics/adults-who-lack-capacity/clinically-assisted-nutrition-and-hydration (Last accessed 28 April 2022).

BMA (2020) The BMA's policy position on physician-assisted dying and how it has been reached. Available at: https://www.bma.org.uk/advice-and-support/ethics/end of life/physician-assisted-dying (Last accessed 28 April 2022).

BMA (2020, updated 2021 & 2022). COVID-19. Guidance for doctors on the impact of coronavirus on your work, training, education and well-being as a medical professional. BMA. Available at: https://www.bma.org.uk/advice-and-support/covid-19#.

Boi, S. (2000) Nurses' experiences in caring for patients from different cultural backgrounds. *Journal of Research in Nursing*. 5 (5), pp. 382–389.

Booth, T. (1985) Home Truths – Old People's Homes and the Outcome of Care. Aldershot: Gower.

Bostridge, M. (2011) *Florence Nightingale: the Lady with the Lamp*. Available at: http://www.bbc.co.uk/history/british/victorians/nightingale_01.shtml (Last accessed 9 May 2022).

Bradshaw, A. (2016) An analysis of England's nursing policy on compassion and the 6Cs: the hidden presence of M. Simone Roach's model of caring. *Nursing*. (1) pp. 78–85. Available at: https://pubmed.ncbi.nlm.nih.gov/26059388/ (Last accessed 28 April 2022).

Brazier, J. and Tsuchiya, A. (2015) Improving cross-sector comparisons: going beyond the health-related QALY. *Applied Health Economics and Health Policy* 13 (6), pp. 557–565.

Brockhaus, H. (2023) Pope Francis laments new euthanasia law in Portugal on feast of Our Lady of Fatima. *Catholic News Agency*. 13 May. Available at: Pope Francis laments new euthanasia law in Portugal on feast of Our Lady of Fatima | Catholic News Agency (Last accessed 14 May 2023).

Brown, J., Kitson, A. and McKnight, T. (1992) *Challenges in Caring: Explorations in nursing and ethics.* Chapman and Hall, London.

Brown, P.J., Rutherford, B.R., Yaffe, K., Tandler, J.M., Ray, J.L., Pott, E., Chung, S. and Roose, S.P. (2016) The depressed frail phenotype: the clinical manifestation of increased biological aging. *Am J Geriatr Psychiatry* 24 (11), pp. 1084–1094. Available at: https://pubmed.ncbi.nlm.nih.gov/2761 8646/ (Last accessed 28 April 2022).

Bubna-Kasteliz, B. (2017) Correspondence: Maintaining fluid at the end of life. *Catholic Medical Quarterly* 67(4).

Bubna-Kasteliz, B. and Bodagh, I. (1993) Subcutaneous route for fluid replacement. *Care of the Elderly Journal.*

Buckle-Henning, P. (2011). Disequilibrium, development and resilience through adult life. September 2011. *Systems Research and Behavioral Science* 28(5). Abstract available at: https://www.researchgate.net/publication/264760476_ Disequilibrium_Development_and_Resilience_Through_Adult_Life (Last accessed 3 May 2022).

Bucknell, T. and Thomas, S. (1997) Nurses' reflections on problems associated with decision-making in critical care settings. *Journal of Advanced Nursing* 25, pp. 229–237.

Burkhardt, M.A and Nagai-Jacobson, M.G. (2020) Spirituality and health. In: *Dossey, B.M., Keegan, L. (eds.), (2020) Holistic Nursing, A Handbook for Practice. 6th ed. Burlington, MA USA: Jones & Bartlett Learning, pp. 135–162.*

Burns J. M. and Login, I. S. (2002) Confounding factors in diagnosing brain death: a case Report. BMC, *BMC Neurol* 2, 5., Accepted 26 June 2002, Published 26 June. DOI https://doi.org/10.1186/1471-2377-2-5. Available at: https://bmcneurol.biomedcentral.com/articles/10.1186/1471-2377-2-5#article-info (Last accessed 17 November 2022).

Caldwell, S. (2021a) Bishops urge Catholics to act to stop Meacher Bill. *Catholic Herald* 25 August.

Caldwell, S. (2021b) Canadian mum requests euthanasia for disabled four-year-old. *Catholic Herald* 16 August.

Caldwell, S. (2021c) An indelible mark on the soul. *Catholic Herald* 26 August.

Caldwell, S. (2022) Thérèse Coffey is being smeared because she values human life. *Catholic Herald*. 8 September 2022.

Caldwell, S. (2023) When end-of-life 'care' is a death sentence. *TCW Defending Freedom (formerly The Conservative Woman)*. 5 March 2023. Available at:

https://www.conservativewoman.co.uk/when-end-of-life-care-is-a-death-sentence/ (Last accessed 15 March 2023).

CALM (2020) The ONS figures on suicide rates for 2020. Available at: https://www.thecalmzone.net/2021/09/the-ons-figures-on-suicide-rates-for-2020-a-message-from-simon-our-ceo/ (Last accessed 3 May 2022).

Calvert. S. (2023) In: *Somerville, E. (2023) University cancels Lent because 'it's too Christian'. The Daily Telegraph, 30 January. P. 9.*

Campbell, J. (2014) Assisted Dying Debate. Hansard, UK Parliament 18 July. Available at: https://hansard.parliament.uk/Lords/2014-07-18/debates/14071854000545/AssistedDyingBill (Last accessed 12 May 2022).

Campbell, J. (2015) Assisted Dying Bill [HL] Debate between Baroness Campbell of Surbiton and Lord Ashton of Hyde. 16 January. Available at: https://www.parallelparliament.co.uk/lord/baroness-campbell-of-surbiton/vs/lord-ashton-of-hyde (Last accessed 26 January 2023).

Capsim Management Solutions Inc. (2020) Five ways to shape ethical decisions: virtue approach. Available at: https://www.capsim.com/blog/five-ways-shape-ethical-decisions-virtue-approach (Last accessed 3 May 2022).

Care not Killing (2012) Euthanasia is out of control in Belgium – new ten-year review. Report on the first decade of legalised euthanasia exposes 'the absence of any effective control'. Available at: https://www.carenotkilling.org.uk/articles/belgian-euthanasia-out-of-control/ (Last accessed 3 May 2022).

Carr, C. (2018) UN committee wants to make abortion and assisted suicide a 'universal human right'. Available at: https://www.dailysignal.com/2018/11/15/un-committee-wants-to-make-abortion-and-assisted-suicide-a-universal-human-right/ (Last accessed 3 May 2022).

Catholic Bishops' Conference of England and Wales, (2020) Organ Donation: A brief guide for Catholics. *Spring*. pp. 1–3.

Catholic Herald (2021) No duty to die. 1 July. HC 343. London., p 77.

Cavanaugh, T.A. (2017) Hippocrates' Oath and Asclepius' Snake: The Birth of the Medical Profession. Oxford University Press: Oxford.

Centre for Policy on Ageing – Rapid Review (2014) The effectiveness of care pathways in health and social care. Available at: http://www.cpa.org.uk/information/reviews/CPA-Rapid-Review-Effectiveness-of-care-pathways.pdf (Last accessed 9 April 2022).

Cerit, B. and Dinc, L. (2013) Ethical decision-making and professional behaviour among nurses. A correlational study. *Nurs Ethics*. March 20 (2), pp. 200–212.

Charter of the United Nations (2016) Article 55c Chapter IX – International Economic and Social Cooperation. 23 August. Codification Division Publications. Available at: https://legal.un.org/repertory/art55.shtml (Last accessed 4 May 2022).

Cherny, N., Ripamonti, C., Pereira, J., Davis, C., Fallon, M., McQuay, H., Mercadante, S., Pasternak, G. and Ventafridda, V. (2001) Expert Working Group of the European Association of Palliative Care Network. Strategies to manage the adverse effects of oral morphine: an evidence-based report. *J Clin Oncol* 19, pp. 2542–2554.

Chitty, C. (2007) *Eugenics, Race and Intelligence in Education.* P.2. Continuum International Publishing Group, London.

Chochinov, H. (2007) Dignity and the essence of medicine: the A, B, C and D of dignity conserving care. *BMJ* 335, p 184.

Chowdhury, S. (2022) NHS staff told to take 'extra caution' extracting organs after 'brain-dead' baby starts breathing. *Sky News*, 29 September. Available at: https://news.sky.com/story/amp/nhs-staff-told-to-take-extra-caution-extracting-organs-after-brain-dead-baby-starts-breathing-12707621 (Last accessed 2 October 2022).

Churchill, W. (1943) October 13, United Kingdom Parliament, Commons, Coalmining Situation, Speaking: The Prime Minister (Winston Churchill), *Hansard, HC* Deb, volume 392, cc920-1012. Available at: https://api.parliament.uk/historic-hansard/commons/1943/oct/13/coalmining-situation (Last accessed 21 November 2022).

Clery, E., McLean, S. and Phillips, M. (2007) Quickening death: the euthanasia debate. In: Park, A., Curtice, J., Thomson, K., Phillips, M. and Johnson, M. (eds.), British Social *Attitudes: The 23rd Report. 2006/2007th edition.* Available at: https://methods.sagepub.com/book/british-social-attitudes-the-23rd-report (Last accessed 4 May 2022).

Cole, A. (2015) Response to the NICE draft guidelines on end of life care for adults. In: *Barrie, J. The Catholic Union: 12 September.* Available at: https://catholicunion.org.uk/2015/09/nice-guidelines-on-end of life-care/ (Last accessed 29 April 2022).

Cole, A. (2019) Reports: Futile treatments? Futile Lives? Joint meeting of the medical ethics alliance and the midlands branch of the CMA in Birmingham 20th Oct. *Catholic Medical Quarterly.* Volume 69 (1) Available at: www.cmq.org.uk (Last accessed 27 April 2022).

Cole, A. (2022) The use and misuse of the ReSPECT form. Correspondence, Catholic Medical Quarterly, Volume 72 (4) November. Available at: http://www.cmq.org.uk/CMQ/2022/Nov/use_and_misuse_of_the_respect_fo.html (Last accessed 23 March 2023).

Cole, A. and Duddington, J. (2021a) Good Samaritans or Angels of Death? *Catholic Herald* 14 March.

Cole, A. and Duddington, J. (2021b) The seven false pillars of the case for euthanasia. *Catholic Herald* 20 May.

Compendium of the Catechism of the Catholic Church (2005) The Virtues. Section 377-378. https://www.vatican.va/archive/compendium_ccc/documents/archive_2005_compendium-ccc_en.html (Last accessed 2 August 2022).

Congregation for the Doctrine of the Faith (1997) (Renamed the Dicastery for the Doctrine of the Faith, 5 June 2022). *Catechism of the Catholic Church.* No. 2276–2279. Part Three, Life in Christ. Section Two, The Ten Commandments, Chapter Two: 'You shall love your neighbour as yourself'. Article 5, The Fifth

Commandment: You shall not kill. Available at: http:// www.scborromeo.org/ ccc/p3s2c2a5.htm (Last accessed 8 April 2022).

Congregation for the Doctrine of the Faith (2008) (Renamed the Dicastery for the Doctrine of the Faith, 5 June 2022). Instruction Dignitas Personae: On Certain Bioethical Questions. No 22. Available at: https://www.google. com/search?q= Congregation+for+the+Doctrine+of+the+Faith+(2008)+Instruction+Dignitas+P ersonae%3A+On+Certain+Bioethical+Questions.+No+2 2.&rlz=1C1CHBF_ en-GBGB900GB900&oq=Congregation+for+the+ Doctrine+of+the+Faith+(20 08)+Instruction+Dignitas+Personae%3A+On+ Certain+Bioethical+Questions.+ No+22.&aqs=chrome...69i57.5882j0j4&s ourceid=chrome&ie=UTF-8 (Last accessed 8 April 2022).

Congregation for the Doctrine of the Faith (2020a). (Renamed the Dicastery for the Doctrine of the Faith, 5 June 2022). Note on the morality of using some anti-Covid-19 vaccines 21 December. Available at: https://www.vatican.va/ roman_curia/congregations/cfaith/documents/rc_con_cfaith_doc_20201221_ nota-vaccini-anticovid_en.html (Last accessed 8 April 2022)

Congregation for the Doctrine of the Faith (2020b). (Renamed the Dicastery for the Doctrine of the Faith, 5 June 2022). Letter: 'Samaritanus bonus, on the care of persons in the critical and terminal phases of life'. 14 July. Available at: https://www.vatican.va/roman_curia/congregations/cfaith/ documents/rc_ con_cfaith_doc_20200714_samaritanus-bonus_en.html (Last accessed 8 April 2022).

Conscientious Objection (Medical Activities) Bill [HL] (2018) Last updated 19 September 2019. *Chapter 6.* Available at: https://bills.parliament.uk/ bills/2003#timeline (Last accessed June 2021).

Constantini, M., Pellegrini, F., Di Leo, S., Beccaro, M., Rossi, C., Flego,G., Romoli, V., Giannotti, M., Morone, P., Ivaldi, G.P., Cavallo, L., Fusco, F., Higginson, I.J. (2014) The Liverpool Care Pathway for cancer patients dying in hospital medical wards: A before-after cluster phase II trial of outcomes reported by family members. *Palliat Med.* 2014;28(1):10–7. 10.1177/0269216313487569 [PubMed] [CrossRef] [Google Scholar] In: *Seymour, J. and Clark, D. (2018) The Liverpool Care Pathway for the Dying Patient: a critical analysis of its rise, demise and legacy in England. Wellcome Open Res. Available at: https:// pubmed.ncbi.nlm.nih.gov/29881785/ (Last accessed 30 July 2022).*

Convention on the Rights of the Child (1989) In: European Issues Human Rights in International Law. Strasbourg: Council of Europe, Publishing and Documentation Service, (1992), pp. 118–144.

Cook, M. (2018) Wow! How many people are Flemish doctors REALLY euthanising? Available at: https://mercatornet.com/wow-how-many-people-are-flemish-doctors-really-euthanasing/23127/ (Last accessed 9 April 2022).

Cook, M. (2019) Back to the source, the Hippocratic Oath examined. *Bio Edge: Bioethics news from around the world.* Available at: https://bioedge.org/

bioethics-d75/back-to-the-source-the-hippocratic-oath-re-examined/ (Last accessed 9 April 2022)

Cook, M. (2020) Does assisted suicide make economic sense? Coronavirus special. *Bio Edge: Bioethics news from around the world*, Available at: https://bioedge. org/endoflife-issues/assisted-suicide-makes-good-economic-sense-argue-scottish-academics/14 March. (Last accessed 9 April 2022).

Cook, M. (2021) Secular bioethics threatens human dignity, says US bioethicist. *Bio Edge: Bioethics news from around the world* 17 July. Available at: https:// bioedge.org/uncategorized/secular-bioethics-threatens-human-dignity-says-us-bioethicist/ (Last accessed 17 July 2021).

Cooper, B. (FRCP) (2021) Better NHS managers. *Letters to the Editor. The Daily Telegraph* 10 October.

Copp, L.A. (1986) The nurse as advocate for vulnerable persons. *J Adv Nurs* 11 (3), pp. 255–263.

Corner, J. (2003) The multidisciplinary team – fact or fiction? *European Journal of Palliative Care* 10 (2), *Supplement*, pp. 10–12.

Cornwell, J. (2011) Care and compassion in the NHS. Patient experience. Organisational culture. *The King's Fund.* Available at: https://www.kingsfund. org.uk/blog/2011/02/care-and-compassion-nhs-patient-experience (Last accessed 30 April 2022).

Cornwell, J. and Goodrich, J. (2009) Exploring how to enable compassionate care in hospital to improve patient experience. *Nursing Times*, Apr 21 105 (15), pp. 14–16.

Coronavirus Act (2020) *Legislation.gov.uk. Delivered by National Archives.* Available at: https://www.legislation.gov.uk/ukpga/2020/7/enacted (Last accessed 30 April 2022).

CQC (2020) Review of Do Not Attempt Cardiopulmonary Resuscitation decisions during the COVID-19 pandemic Interim report. https://www.cqc.org.uk/ news/stories/cqc-review-use-dnacpr-during-pandemic November (Last accessed 6 July 2022).

Craig, G. (2002) Terminal Sedation. *Catholic Medical Quarterly* 52(1): pp. 14–17.

Craig, G. (2004) Challenging Medical Ethics 1. No Water – No Life. Hydration in the Dying. p 130. Enterprise House, Northampton, UK.

Craycroft, K. (2022) Why 'Common Good' is Elusive. Available at: https:// catholicherald.co.uk/ch/why-common-good-is-elusive/ (Last accessed 4 May 2022).

Culhane, A. (2020) COVID-19 cuts prostate cancer referrals in half. Available at: https://www.urologynews.uk.com/features/features/post/covid-19-cuts-prostate-cancer-referrals-in-half (Last accessed 5 May 2022).

Dalal, S. and Bruera, E. (2004) Dehydration in cancer patients: to treat or not to treat. *The Journal of Supportive Oncology. Review.* 2(6): 467–79, 483.

Data Protection Act (1998/2018) HMSO. Available at: https://www.gov.uk/data-protection#:~:text=The%20Data%20Protection%20Act%202018%20

is%20the%20UK's%20implementation%20of,used%20fairly%2C%20 lawfully%20and%20transparently (Last accessed 4 May 2022).

Davies, M. (2021a) Legalising assisted suicide would cross a 'moral line' says English bishop. *Catholic Herald* 24 May.

Davies, M. (2021b) Don't let 'false compassion' legalise assisted suicide, say bishops of England and Wales. *Catholic News Agency*. Available at: https:// www.catholicnewsagency.com/news/247835/dont-let-false-compassion-legalise-assisted-suicide-say-bishops-of-england-and-wales (Last accessed 9 April 2020).

Davis, S.M. and Donnan, G.A. (2021). Ischemic Penumbra: A Personal View. *Cerebrovascular Diseases: 30th Anniversary Review*. Cerebrovasc Dis 2021; 50:656–665. DOI: 10.1159/000519730. Received: August 9. Accepted: September 16, 2021. Published online: November 4, 2021. Departments of Medicine and Neurology, Melbourne Brain Centre at the Royal Melbourne Hospital, University of Melbourne, Victoria, VIC, Australia. Available at: https://www.karger.com/Article/Pdf/519730#page8 (Last accessed 25 November 2022).

Davoodvand, S., Abbaszadeh, A. and Ahmadi, F. (2016) Patient advocacy from the clinical nurses' viewpoint: a qualitative study. Available at: https://www. ncbi.nlm.nih.gov/pmc/articles/PMC4958925/ (Last accessed 30 April 2020.

Dawson, T. (2017) Blog. The death with dignity myth. the abundant life (*CareNet website*) Available at: https://www.care-net.org/abundant-life-blog/debunking-the-death-with-dignity-myth (Last accessed 30 April 2022).

Dean, E. (2017) Stress at work: the reality of the front line. *Nursingstandard.com*. Available at: https://pubmed.ncbi.nlm.nih.gov/28327011/ (Last accessed 30 April 2022).

de Bellaigue, C. (2019) Death on demand: has euthanasia gone too far? *The Guardian* 18 January.

de Caussade, J.P. (2008) Abandonment to Divine Providence. LSC communications. Dover books on Western philosophy. Dover publications Inc. New York. London UK.

DEFRA (2021) Animal Welfare (Sentience) Bill. (2021) [HL]. Session 2021/22. Available at: https://bills.parliament.uk/bills/2867 (Last accessed 30 April 2022).

Deighan J. (2023) Protecting life, truth and freedom. Catholic Nurse Journal. Easter. www.catholicnurses.org.uk

Del Rio, M.I., Shand, B., Bonati, P. and Palma, P. (2011) Hydration and nutrition at the end of life: A systematic review of emotional impact, perceptions and decision-making among patients, family and health care staff. *Psycho-Oncology* 21 (9), pp. 913–921.

DH (1983) The Mental Health Act. Code of Practice. London Stationary Office. Available at: https://assets.publishing.service.gov.uk/government/uploads/ system/uploads/attachment_data/file/435512/MHA_Code_of_Practice.PDF (Last accessed 30 April 2022).

DH (2000a) NHS Plan. Available at: https://www.google.com/search?q=DH+(Department+of+Health)+(2000)+NHS+Plan.+HMSO.&rlz=1C1CHBF_en-GBGB900GB900&oq=DH+(Department+of+Health)+(2000)+NHS+Plan.+HMSO.&aqs=chrome..69i57j0i546l4.9398j0j4&sourceid=chrome&ie=UTF-8 (Last accessed 30 April 2022).

DH (2000b) The NHS cancer plan: a plan for investment, a plan for reform. London: Crown Copyright Reference Source [Google Scholar] [Ref list]

DH (2007) The Mental Health Act. (Amended, most recently from Mental Health Act 1983) Available at: https://www.google.com/search?q=DH+(Department+of+Health)+(2007)+The+Mental+Health+Act.+(Amended%2C+most+recently+from+Mental+Health+Act+1983)&rlz=1C1CHBF_en-GBGB900GB900&oq=DH+(Department+of+Health)+(2007)+The+Mental+Health+Act.+(Amended%2C+most+recently+from+Mental+Health+Act+1983)&aqs=chrome..69i57.5715j0j4&sourceid=chrome&ie=UTF-8 (Last accessed 30 April 2022).

DH (2008) Department of Health in collaboration with Comic Relief investigate elder abuse,

Hospital, HealthCare, Europe. https://hospitalhealthcare.com/news/dh-and-comic-reliefinvestigate-elder-abuse/ (Last accessed 7 July 2022).

DH (2009) Safeguarding Adults. Report on the Consultation of the review on 'No Secrets: Guidance on developing and implementing multi agency policies and procedures to protect vulnerable adults from abuse'. Available at: https://assets.publishing.service.gov.uk/government/uploads/system/uploads/attachment_data/file/194272/No_secrets__guidance_on_developing_and_implementing_multi-agency_policies_and_procedures_to_protect_vulnerable_adults_rom_abuse.pdf (Last accessed 30 April 2022).

DH (2008–2010) Valuing People Now: Government 3-year big plan. *Summary Report*, March 2009 to September 2010. Including findings from *Learning Disability Partnership Board Self Assessments 2009–2010*. Available at: https://assets.publishing.service.gov.uk/government/uploads/system/uploads/attachment_data/file/215891/dh_122387.pdf (Last accessed 30 April 2022).

DH (2012) Compassion in practice. Nursing Midwifery and Care staff. Our Vision and Strategy. Available at: https://www.england.nhs.uk/wp-content/uploads/2012/12/compassion-in-practice.pdf (Last accessed 30 April 2022).

DH (2013) *More care, less pathway: a review of the Liverpool Care Pathway.* Available at: https://assets.publishing.service.gov.uk/government/uploads/system/uploads/attachment_data/file/212450/Liverpool_Care_Pathway.pdf (Last accessed 30 April 2022).

Department for Business Innovation and Skills (2015) Whistleblowing: guidance for employers and code of practice. Available at: https://www.gov.uk/government/publications/whistleblowing-guidance-and-code-of-practice-for-employers (Last accessed 30 April 2022).

Department for Constitutional Affairs UK (2005) The Mental Capacity Act (MCA) HMSO. Available at: https://www.gov.uk/government/publications/mental-capacity-act-code-of-practice (Last accessed 30 April 2022).

Department for Constitutional Affairs (2007) The Mental Capacity Act – Code of Practice, pp 203–206. TSO. Available at: https://www.gov.uk/government/publications/mental-capacity-act-code-of-practice (Last accessed 30 April 2022).

Department for Health and Social Care (2008) End of Life Care Strategy: promoting high quality care for adults at the end of their life. July. Available at: https://www.gov.uk/government/publications/endoflife-care-strategy-promoting-high-quality-care-for-adults-at-the-end-of-their-life (Last accessed 30 April 2022).

Department for Health and Social Care (2020) Organ Donation (Deemed Consent) Act. Available at: https://www.legislation.gov.uk/uksi/2020/520/made (Last accessed 30 April 2022).

Department for Health and Social Care (2021) NHS Constitution for England, Guidance. Available at: https://www.gov.uk/government/publications/the-nhs-constitution-for-england/the-nhs-constitution-for-england (Last accessed 9 July 2022).

Department for Health and Social Care (2022) Summary of changes to COVID-19 guidance for adult social care providers (updated 3 May) Available at: https://www.gov.uk/government/publications/infection-prevention-and-control-in-adult-social-care-covid-19-supplement/summary-of-changes-to-covid-19-guidance-for-adult-social-care-providers (Last accessed 17 May 2022).

Dieppe, T. (2023) When End of Life Care Goes Wrong. *Christian Concern.* 13 March. Available at: https://christianconcern.com/comment/when-end-of-life-care-goes-wrong/ (Last accessed 17 March 2023).

Derbyshire, S.W.G. and Bockmann, J.C. (2019) Reconsidering foetal pain. Available at: https://jme.bmj.com/content/46/1/3 (Last accessed 30 April 2022).

de Stoutz, N., Bruera, E. and Suarez-Almazor, M. (1995) Opioid rotation for toxicity reduction in terminal cancer patients. *Journal of Pain and Symptom Management* 10 (5) July. Available at: https://pubmed.ncbi.nlm.nih.gov/7673770/ (Last accessed 3 July 2022).

Doogan, M. and Wood, C. v Greater Glasgow and Clyde Health Board (2014) CSIH 36. Available at: https://www.supremecourt.uk/cases/uksc-2013-0124.html (Last accessed 30 April 2022).

Dorries, N. (2015) Assisted Dying (Marris) Bill, Debate. 11 September. Hansard, UK Parliament Available at: https://hansard.parliament.uk/commons/2015-09-11/debates/15091126000003/AssistedDying(No2)Bill (Last accessed 11 May 2022).

Doshi, J.A., Sonet, E.M., Puckett, J.T and Glick, H. (2018) The need for a new patient-centered decision tool for value-based treatment choices. In *oncology [blog]. Center for Health Incentives and Behavioral Economics at the Leonard Davis Institute.* Available at: https://www.hmpgloballearningnetwork.com/

site/jcp/article/advocating-new-patient-centered-tools-value-based-treatment-choices-oncology (Last accessed 3 May 2022).

Dossey, B.M. (1999) Florence Nightingale: Mystic, Visionary, Healer. October. Springhouse Publishing Co, U.S.

Doughty, S. (2007) We'll fight 'backdoor euthanasia' and risk jail say doctors. *Daily Mail.* 30 March. Available at: https://www.dailymail.co.uk/health/article-445585/Well-fight-backdoor-euthanasia-risk-jail-say-doctors.html (Last accessed 12 July 2022).

Downie, R. and Macnaughton, J. (2007) *Bioethics and the humanities: attitudes and perceptions.* Routledge-Cavendish: Abingdon. pp. 36–41.

Drakeford, M. (2021) Appointment of Rt Hon Baroness Heather Hallett to lead UK-wide COVID-19 inquiry. *Press release.* Appointment of Rt Hon Baroness Heather Hallett to lead UK-wide Covid-19 inquiry | GOV.WALES (Last accessed 4 May 2022).

Drinka, T.J.K., Miller, T.F. and Goodman, B.M. (1996) Characterising motivational styles of professionals who work on interdisciplinary healthcare teams. *Journal of Interprofessional Care* 10, pp. 51–61.

Drought, T. (2007) Parrhesia as a conceptual metaphor for nursing advocacy. *Editorial comment.* Available at: https://www.academia.edu/48810427/Parrhesia_as_a_conceptual_metaphor_for_nursing_advocacy (Last accessed 10 May 2022).

Dunlop, M.J. (1986) Is a science of caring possible? J *Adv Nurs.* 11 (6), pp. 661–670.

Dunne, K and Docherty, P. (2011) Donation after circulatory death. *Continuing Education. In Anaesthesia Critical Care & Pain* 11 (3), pp. 82-86. BJA Education, Oxford Education. Available at: https://reader.elsevier.com/reader/sd/pii/S1743181617302548?token=FE8D7FE014884457D7AFCE9116943B6C0A9AC187623111CB8D5FE7107DB3D85BC698DA6C773F6CED10BAB78A6FC05393 (Last accessed 4 May 2022).

Dyer, C. (2017) Law, ethics and emotion: the Charlie Gard case. *BMJ* 358. Available at: https://www.bmj.com/content/358/bmj.j3152/rapid-responses (Last accessed 30 April 2022).

ECHR (2009) European Convention for the Protection of Human Rights and Fundamental Freedoms.

Elan Jones, S. (2015) Assisted Dying (No 2) Bill [HL]. (*Marris Bill*) (Vol 599) Debated on 11 September. Hansard UK Parliament. Available at: https://www.google.com/search?q=Elan+Jones%2C+S.+(2015)+Assisted+Dying+(No+2)+Bill+%5BHL%5D.+(Marris+Bill)+(Vol+599)+Debated+on+11+September.+Hansard+UK+Parliament.&rlz=1C1CHBF_en-GBGB900GB900&oq=Elan+Jones%

Eliot, T.S. (1941) The Four Quartets. (*No 2 of four quartets. East Coker*) Available at: http://www.davidgorman.com/4quartets/2-coker.htm (Last accessed 1 May 2022).

Ende, J. (2017) American College of Physicians Reaffirms Opposition to Legalisation of Physician-Assisted Suicide: ACP also calls for improved hospice and palliative care. Available at: https://www.acponline.org/

acp-newsroom/opposition-to-legalization-of-physician-assisted-suicide (Last accessed 30 April 2022).

End of Life Law in Australia (2021) Voluntary assisted dying. *University for the real world, Aust.* 5 October. Available at: https://end of life.qut.edu.au/assisteddying (Last accessed 1 May 2022).

Equality Act (2010) HMSO. Available at: https://www.legislation.gov.uk/ukpga/2010/15/contents (Last accessed 3 May 2022).

Equality and Human Rights Commission (1998) *Human Rights Act.* HMSO. Available at: https://www.equalityhumanrights.com/en/human-rights/human-rights-act (Last accessed 3 May 2022).

Esterhuizen, P. (1996) Is the professional code still the cornerstone of clinical nursing practice? *Journal of Advanced Nursing* 23 (1) Available at: https://onlinelibrary.wiley.com/doi/10.1111/j.1365-2648.1996.tb03131.x (Last accessed 3 May 2022).

Euronews (2022) MPs in Italy back a new law that would legalise a form of euthanasia. 11 March. https://www.euronews.com/amp/2022/03/11/mps-in-italy-back-a-new-law-that-would-legalise-a-form-of-euthanasia (Last accessed 25 July 2022)

Fagerström, L., Lemming, K. and Anderson, M.H. (2014) The RAFAELA system: a work-force planning tool for nurse staffing and human resource management. *Nursing Management, Art & Science* 29 April 21 (2), pp. 1–8. Available at: https://www.scribd.com/document/242082815/the-rafaela-system-a-workforce-planning-tool-for-nurse-staffing-pdf (Last accessed 10 May 2022).

Falconer, C. (2006) Doctors face prison for denying right to die. *Evening Standard, London Lite; thisislondon.co.uk.*

Falconer, C. (2014) Assisted Dying Bill (HL Bill 6) Available at: https://www.carenotkilling.org.uk/public/pdf/falconer-bill---overview,-arguments,-problems.pdf (Last accessed 3 May 2022).

Farmakidis, A. (2005) Excerpt: From The death of Ivan Ilyich by Leo Tolstoy, (1886) In: *Academic Medicine: Medicine and the Arts.* Vol. 80, No. 9. p 856.

Farmer, A. (2020) Nazi echoes in the clinics of death. *TCW Defending freedom. (Formerly The Conservative Woman)* Available at: https://www.conservativewoman.co.uk/nazi-echoes-in-the-clinics-of-death/ (Last accessed 15 April 2022).

Fergusson, D.M., Horwood, L.J. and Ridder, E.M. (2006) Abortion in young women and subsequent mental health. *Journal of Child Psychology and Psychiatry* 47 (1), pp. 16–24.

Fehring, R.J., Miller, J. and Shaw, C. (1997) Spiritual well-being, religiosity, hope, depression and other mood states in elderly people coping with cancer. *Oncol Nurs Forum.* May; 24 (4), pp. 663–671

Finlay, I. (2008) NHS. Hospital Feeding. Hansard, Volume No. 701 Part No. 93. Available at: https://publications.parliament.uk/pa/ld200708/ldhansrd/index/080515.html#contents. (Last accessed 4 July 2022).

Finlay, I. (2020) Access to Palliative Care and Treatment of Children Bill [Hl]. Available at: https://bills.parliament.uk/bills/2536 (Last accessed 3 May 2022).

Finlay, I. (2021a) Assisted Suicide Bill. Assisted dying risks being seen and used as a cheap solution for human suffering. 7 January.*The House Magazine* Available at: https://www.politicshome.com/thehouse/article/assisted-dying-will-only-worsen-the-current-provision-of-care-for-the-terminally-ill (Last accessed 3 May 2022).

Finlay, I. (2021b) Assisted Dying Bill, 2nd reading, *Hansard,* 22 October. Available at: https://www.parallelparliament.co.uk/lord/baroness-finlay-of-llandaff/debate/2021--22/lords/lords-chamber/assisted-dying-bill-hl (Last accessed 31 July 2022).

Fleming, D. (2019) The compassionate state? Voluntary Assisted Dying, neoliberalism and the problem of virtue without an anchor. Available at: https://www.abc.net.au/religion/compassionate-state-voluntary-assisted-dying-neoliberalism-and/10937504 (Last accessed 3 May 2022).

Fletcher, M. (2000) Doctors are more caring than nurses. *British Medical Journal* 320, p.1083.

Fohr, S A. (1998) The Double Effect of Pain Medication: Separating Myth from Reality. *Journal of Palliative Medicine* 1: 315–328. In: Doctrine of Double Effect. First published Wed Jul 28 ,2004 substantive revision Mon Dec 24, 2018. Stanford Encyclopaedia of Philosophy, Copyright © 2018 by Alison McIntyre <amcintyre@wellesley.edu> Available at: https://plato.stanford.edu/entries/double-effect/#:~:text=According%20to%20the%20principle%20of,about%20the%20same%20good%20end (Last accessed 5 May 2022).

Francis, R. (2013) Final report of the independent inquiry into care provided by Mid Staffordshire NHS Foundation Trust. Available at: https://assets.publishing.service.gov.uk/government/uploads/system/uploads/attachment_data/file/279124/0947.pdf (Last accessed 3 May 2022).

Fraser, G. (2019) As the Sri Lanka attacks show, Christians worldwide face serious persecution. *The Guardian* 21 April.

Fraser, G. (2022a) Christianity is not just for Christmas. *The Daily Telegraph, Features & Art*. 24 December.

Fraser, G. (2022b) Secularisation is leading Britain astray. The Church must stop trying to be cool. *Unherd.com. The Post*. 1 December. Available at: https://unherd.com/2022/12/secularisation-is-leading-britain-astray/ (Last accessed 9 January 2023).

Frigerio, B. (2018) How Alfie died, all the facts. La Nuovo Busso La Quotidiano. 1 May. The original article by Benedetta Frigerio in Italian is: Ecco come hanno fatto morire Alfie (Translation by Patricia Gooding Williams) Available at: https://lanuovabq.it/it/how-alfie-died-all-the-facts (Last accessed 3 May 2022).

Fullbrook, S. (2007) Autonomy and care: acting in a person's best interest. *Br J Nurs*. 16 (4), pp. 236–237.

Fulp, M. (2007) Working Toward a Definition of Futile Care in the United States Health Care System. *Theses and Dissertations*. 3187. Available at: https://commons.und.edu/theses/3187 (Last accessed 11 July 2022).

Gadow, S. (1984) Touch and technology: two paradigms of patient care. *Journal of Religion and Health* 23, pp. 63–69.

Galloway, D. (2021) Assisted suicide discussion. *Nana Akua Show*. GB News.

Gartside, B. (2019) The obsession with free speech at universities is a betrayal of ordinary students. *The Times*.

Gelling, L. (1999) Ethical principles in healthcare research. *Nursing Standard* 13 (36), pp. 39–42.

Georges, J. and Grypdonck, M. (2002) Moral problems experienced by nurses when caring for terminally ill people: a literature review. *Nursing Ethics* 9 (2), March, Arnold, pp. 155–178.

Giacino, J. T., Katz, D. I., Nicholas, M.D., Schiff, D., Whyte, J., E.J., Ashwal, S., Barbano, R., Hammond, F.M., Laureys, S., Ling, G. S.F., Nakase-Richardson, R., Seel, R., Yablon, S., Thomas, S. D., Getchius, S.D., Gronseth, G.S. and Armstrong, M.J. (2018) Practice guideline update recommendations summary: Disorders of consciousness: Report of the Guideline Development, Dissemination and Implementation Subcommittee of the American Academy of Neurology; the American Congress of Rehabilitation Medicine; and the National Institute on Disability, Independent Living and Rehabilitation Research. *Neurology*, August. Available at: https://www.ncbi.nlm.nih.gov/pmc/articles/PMC6139814/ (Last accessed 4 May 2022).

Gilbert, P and Procter, S. (2006) Compassionate mind training for people with high shame and self-criticism: Overview and pilot study of a group therapy approach. *Clinical Psychology and Psychotherapy* 13, pp. 353–379.

Gillon, R. (1985) Confidentiality. *British Medical Journal* 291, pp. 1634–1636.

Gillon, R. (1994) Medical ethics: four principles plus attention to scope. *British Medical Journal* 309, pp. 184–188.

Gillon R. (2003) Ethics needs principles – four can encompass the rest – and respect for autonomy should be 'first among equals'. *J Med Ethics* 2003; 29:307–12. Available at: https://jme.bmj.com/content/29/5/307 (Last accessed 13 May 2022).

Glick, S.M. (2004) Letter: Terminal sedation in the Netherlands. *Annals of Internal Medicine* 966. Available at: https://www.acpjournals.org/doi/abs/10.7326/0003-4819-141-12-200412210-00016 (Last accessed 3 May 2022).

GMC (2014) National training survey: bullying and undermining. Working with doctors working for patients. Available at: https://www.gmc-uk.org/about/what-we-do-and-why/data-and-research/-/media/documents/national-training-survey-2016-key-findings-68462938.pdf (Last accessed 30 April 2022).

GMC (2022a) Good Medical Practice. Available at: https://www.gmc-uk.org/ethical-guidance/ethical-guidance-for-doctors/good-medical-practice#: ~:text=It%20says%20that%20as%20a,patient%20safety%20is%20 being%20compromising%20%20%20GMC%20(2022b)%20 (Last accessed 30 April 2022).

GMC (2022b) Meeting patients' nutrition and hydration needs. Treatment and care towards the end of life: good practice in decision making. Good Medical Practice. London: *GMC*. Available at: https://www.gmc-uk.org/ ethical-guidance/ethical-guidance-for-doctors/treatment-and-care-towards-the-end of life (Last accessed 4 May 2022).

Godlee, F. (2018) Editor's choice: Lessons from Gosport. *BMJ*, July 2018 362: k29237. Available at: https://www.bmj.com/content/362/bmj.k2923 (Last accessed 3 May 2022).

Goldbeck-Wood, S. (2016) Lack of qualified workforce in abortion care. *The Today Programme. BBC News*. Available at: https://www.bbc.co.uk/news/ av/health-38414436 (Last accessed 3 May 2022).

Goldberg, A. (2019) Is death by organ donation around the corner? Available at: https://www.mercatornet.com/careful/view/is-death-by-organ-donation-around-the-corner/22482 (Last accessed 3 May 2022).

Goldring, M. (2012) Death by indifference: 74 deaths and counting. *Mencap report finds NHS still unsafe for people with a learning disability*. Available at: https://www.mencap.org.uk/press-release/mencap-report-finds-nhs-still-unsafe-people-learning-disability (Last accessed 3 May 2022).

Gooch, N. (2018) End of life. Belgium's shame. *Catholic Herald 2* August.

Govier, I. (2000) Spiritual care in nursing: a systematic approach. Art & Science, literature review. *Nursing Standard* 14 (17), pp. 32–36.

Grace, P.J. and McLaughlin, M. (2005) When consent isn't informed enough. *American Journal of Nursing* 105 (4), p 82.

Grimley-Evans, J. (1997) Rationing healthcare by age: the case against. *British Medical Journal* 314, p 822.

Grimstad, J. (2007) The living will boondoggle. Available at: https://ilofs.org/ newsletters/SFONews_200707.pdf (Last accessed 3 May 2022).

Grogan, C. (2017) Holy See tells UN a 'right to abortion' defies moral, legal standards. Available at: https://www.catholicnewsagency.com/news/40986/ holy-see-tells-un-a-right-to-abortion-defies-moral-legal-standards (Last accessed 3 May 2022).

Guys and St Thomas NHS Trust (2015) Managing your breathlessness using a handheld fan. *Leaflet number 4182/VER 1*.

Hackett, K. (2020) DNACPR notices: review finds 'unacceptable and inappropriate' use early in pandemic. Care Quality Commission says older and vulnerable people most at risk. *Nursing Standard* 4 December. Available at: https://rcni.com/nursing-standard/newsroom/news/dnacpr-notices-review-finds-unacceptable-and-inappropriate-use-early-pandemic-169711Last (Last accessed 3 May 2022).

Hain, R. (2005) A time to die. Rapid response, editor's choice. Available at: https://www.bmj.com/rapid-response/2011/10/31/assisted-dying-terminally-ill-bill-0-g (Last accessed 3 May 2022).

Hale, B. (2014) Supreme Court judgement appeal case. *Greater Glasgow and Clyde Health Board v Doogan, M. and Wood, C.* Available at: https://www.supremecourt.uk/cases/uksc-2013-0124.html (Last accessed 3 May 2022).

Halliday, J. (2022) NHS mental health hospital staff filmed 'mocking and slapping' patients. NHS. The Guardian. 28 September. Available at: https://amp.theguardian.com/society/2022/sep/28/nhs-mental-health-hospital-staff-filmed-mocking-and-slapping-patients (Last accessed 29 September 2022).

Hamilton, M. and Essat, Z. (2008) Minority ethnic users' experiences and expectations of nursing care. Available at: https://journals.sagepub.com/doi/10.1177/1744987108088638 (Last accessed 3 May 2022).

Hammer, J. (2020) The Defiance of Florence Nightingale. *Smithsonian Magazine.* Available at: https://www.smithsonianmag.com/history/the-worlds-most-famous-nurse-florence-nightingale-180974155/ (Last accessed 3 May 2022).

Hanks, R.G. (2008) The lived experience of nursing advocacy. *Nursing Ethics* 15 (4), pp. 468–477.

Hansford, P. and Meehan, H. (2007) Gold Standards Framework: improving community care clinical practice development. *End of Life Care* 1 (3) pp. 56-61.

Harding-Clark, M. (2006) *The Lourdes Hospital inquiry – An inquiry into postpartum hysterectomy at Our Lady of Lourdes Hospital, Drogheda.* p 316. The Stationary Office, Dublin. Retrieved 15 January 2011 from www.dohc.ie/publications/lourdes.html. In: *Gallagher, A., (2010) Moral Distress and Moral Courage in Everyday Nursing Practice 21 March. OJIN: The Online Journal of Issues in Nursing* Vol. 16 No. 2. (Last accessed 2 May 2022).

Hardy, L.K. (1982) Nursing models and research – a restricting view. *Journal of Advanced Nursing* 7, pp. 447–451.

Harris, N.M. (2001) The euthanasia debate. *J R Army Med Corps.* 147 (3), pp. 367–370.

Hart, C. (2014) Christians warned over 'dangerous' new secularism. *The Christian Institute* 26 May. Available at: https://www.christian.org.uk/news/christians-warned-over-dangerous-new-secularism-2/ (Last accessed 1 May 2022).

Hawkins, S. (2021) Revealed: Over 30 deaths in Nottingham University Hospitals scandal. *Channel 4 News* 30 June. Available at: https://www.youtube.com/watch?v=pan_Y_87Qrw (Last accessed 3 May 2022).

Hayman, S. (2021) Assisted Dying Bill [HL] (Meacher Bill.) (Vol 815) *Hansard.* Debated on 22 October

Health and Care Act (2022) Legislation.gov.uk. Available at: https://www.legislation.gov.uk/ukpga/2022/31/contents/enacted (Last accessed 28 January 2023)

Heath, A. (2023) The NHS is dead -and it's dragging the rest of the country down with it. *The Daily Telegraph, Comment*, 12 January.

Heffernan, M. (2012) Dare to disagree. *Technology, Entertainment and Design (TED) talks Online. Ideas worth spreading.* Available at:https://m.youtube.com/watch?v=PY_kd46RfVE&feature=emb_rel_end (Last accessed 24 November 2022).

Hemsley, B., Balandin, S., Worrall, L. (2012) Nursing the patient with complex communication needs: time as a barrier and a facilitator to successful communication in hospital. J Adv Nurs; Jan. 68(1): pp. 116-26. doi: 10.1111/j.1365-2648.2011.05722. x. Epub 2011 Aug 10.

Herdman, E.A. (2004) Nursing in a post emotional society. *Nursing Philosophy 5*, pp. 95–103.

Hewlett, S. (1996) Consent to clinical research: adequately voluntary or substantially influenced. *Journal of Medical Ethics* 22, pp. 232–237.

Higginson, I. and Hall, S. (2007) Rediscovering dignity at the bedside. *Editorials, BMJ 335*, p 168.

Hodgson, R. (1992) A nursing muse. *British Journal of Nursing* 1 (7), pp. 330–333.

Hogan, R. and Kaiser, R.B. (2005) What We Know about Leadership. *Review of General Psychology*, pp. 9, 169–180. https://doi.org/10.1037/1089-2680.9.2.169 (Last accessed 21 March 2023).

Hollins, S.C (2021) Amendment to the Motion, Part of Assisted Dying Bill. [HL]22 October 2021. My Lords, I speak with 40...: 22 Oct 2021: House of Lords debates - TheyWorkForYou (Last accessed 31 July 2022).

Holm, S., Edgar, A. B. (2008) Best Interest: A Philosophical Critique [Book Review]. *Health Care Analysis* 16 (3):197–207.

Holy See Press Office (2017) Presentation of the 25th World Day of the Sick and the New Charter for Healthcare Workers, 06.02.2017. Summary of Bulletin, Holy See Press Office. Available at: https://press.vatican.va/content/salastampa/en/bollettino/pubblico/2017/02/06/170206b.html# (Last accessed 1 December 2022).

Horvat II, J. (2020a) The Coronavirus Is a Call to Return to God. *Return to Order. A special campaign for Tradition, Family, Property.* Available at: https://tfpuk.org.uk/archives/2271 (Last accessed 3 May 2022).

Horvat II, J. (2020b) The stunning triumph of Hobbes in the covid crisis. *The imaginative Conservative.* Available at: https://theimaginativeconservative.org/2020/08/stunning-triumph-thomas-hobbes-covid-crisis-john-horvat.html (Last accessed 3 May 2022).

Horvat II, J. (2021) What has happened to our sense of shame? The Imaginative Conservative Available at: https://theimaginativeconservative.org/2021/02/what-has-happened-our-sense-shame-john-horvat.html (Last accessed 3 May 2022).

Houllebecq, M. (2021) Weekend Essay: How France lost her dignity. A civilisation that legalises euthanasia loses all respect. *UnHerd* 24 April. This essay appeared in *Le Figaro* on 5 April 2021. Translated for UnHerd by Dr Louis Betty. Available at: https://unherd.com/2021/04/how-france-lost-her-dignity/ (Last accessed 3 May 2022).

House of Commons Health Committee (2009) Patient Safety, *Sixth report of session 2008–2009*. HC 151 – 1. London. The Stationary Office, pp. 86–87. Available at: https://publications.parliament.uk/pa/cm200809/cmselect/cmhealth/151/151i.pdf (Last accessed 3 May 2022).

House of Commons House of Lords Joint Committee on Human Rights (2020). The Government's response to COVID-19: human rights implications. https://committees.parliament.uk/publications/2649/documents/26914/default/ (Last accessed 7 July 2022).

Howard, P. (2018) Decriminalisation of Abortion. *Catholic Medical Quarterly* 68 (1) Available at: http://www.cmq.org.uk/CMQ/2018/Feb/decriminalisation_of_abortion.html (Last accessed 3 May 2022).

HSE (2021) Work related stress. *HSE.* Available at: https://www.hse.gov.uk/statistics/causdis/stress.pdf (Last accessed 3 May 2022).

Hudson, P.L., Schofield, P., Kelly, B., Hudson, R., O'Connor, M., Kristjanson, L.J., Ashby, M. and Aranda, S. (2006) Responding to desire to die statements from patients with advanced disease: recommendations for health professionals. *Palliative Medicine, Review,* Oct 20 (7): pp. 703-10. Available at: https://pubmed.ncbi.nlm.nih.gov/17060269/ (Last accessed 4 May 2022).

Human Fertilisation and Embryology Act (1990) *Legislation.gov.uk. The National Archives.* Available at: https://www.legislation.gov.uk/ukpga/1990/37/contents (Last accessed 3 May 2022).

Human Rights Act (1998) Legislation.gov.uk. *The National Archives.* Available at: https://www.legislation.gov.uk/ukpga/1998/42#:~:text=1998%20CHAPTER%2042,Rights%3B%20and%20for%20connected%20purposes. (Last accessed 3 May 2022).

Human Rights Watch (2006) So Long as They Die, Lethal Injections in the United States. Available at: https://www.hrw.org/reports/2006/us0406/4.htm (Last accessed 3 May 2022).

Hunt, P. (2021) Why I remain firmly against assisted dying. *The Daily Telegraph* 3 October. Available at: https://www.telegraph.co.uk/news/2021/10/03/assisted-dying-will-always-open-bullying-exploitation/ (Last accessed 3 May 2022).

Hurwitz, B. (2013) Healthcare Serial Killings: was the Case of Harold Shipman Unthinkable? *Bioethics, Medicine and the Criminal Law. Medicine, Crime and Society.* (eds.). Griffiths, D. and Sanders, A. Vol 2. Cambridge University Press: UK. pp. 13-42.

Hurwitz, B. (2015) Medical humanities and medical alterity in fiction and in life. Available at: https://www.ncbi.nlm.nih.gov/pmc/articles/PMC5146638/ (Last accessed 13 May 2022).

Hutchison, M. (1997) Healing the whole person: the spiritual dimension. Holism and spiritual care in nursing practice. *Christian nursing page. Marg Hutchison*, Sydney, Australia. marghut@bigpond.net (Last accessed 3 May 2022).

Ibegbu, J. (2000) Rights of the Unborn Child in International Law. Towards a convention. Vol. I. New York: Edwin Mellen Press. Available at: http://groups. csail.mit.edu/mac/users/rauch/nvp/misc/ibegbu.html (Last accessed 3 May 2022).

ITVnews (2022) Explainer. What happens if nurses vote for strike action - and how many will take part? Sunday 6 November 2022. Available at: https://www.itv. com/news/2022-11-06/what-happens-if-nurses-vote-for-strike-action-and-how-many-will-take-part (Last accessed, 6 November, 2022).

Inghelbrecht, E., Bilsen, J., Mortier, F. and Deliens, L. (2011) Continuous deep sedation until death in Belgium: a survey among nurses. *J Pain Symptom Management* 41 (5), pp. 870–879.

Jackson, D., Peters, K., Andrew, S., Edenborough, M., Halcomb, E., Luck, l., Salamonson, Y. and Wilkes, L. (2010) Understanding whistleblowing: qualitative insights from nurse whistleblowers. J American Nursing. Leading Global Nursing Research. 66 (10) 2194–2201.

Jameton, A. (1993) Dilemmas of moral distress: moral responsibility and nursing practice. *AWHONN's Clinical Issues in Perinatal and Women's Health* 4 (4), pp. 542–551.

Jameton, A. (1994) Nursing Practice: The Ethical Issues. Englewood Cliffs NJ: Prentice Hall. In: Konishi, E. Davis, A. and Aiba, T. (2002) The ethics of withdrawing artificial food and fluid from terminally ill patients: an end of life dilemma for Japanese nurses and families. Nursing Ethics 9 (1).

Jenkins, R. (2011) Moral Imperialism. *Encyclopedia of Global Justice*. Springer, London. p 432.

Job, F.A. (2019) Emeritus Archbishop. Imprimatur. In: *Igwebuike Ani, M. (2019) Prayer in Hopelessness*. Newbourne Nig Ltd: Nigeria.

Joffe, J. (2006) In: *Keown, J. (2012) The Law and Ethics of Medicine: Essays on the Inviolability of Human Life. Oxford*. Available at: https://oxford. universitypressscholarship.com/view/10.1093/acprof:oso/9780199589555. 001.0001/acprof-9780199589555 (Last accessed 3 May 2022).

Joffe, A.R., Anton, N.R., Duff, J.P. (2010). The APNEA test: Rationale, Confounders, and riticism. *Journal of Child Neurology*. Available at: https:// journals.sagepub.com/doi/abs/10.1177/0883073810369380 (Last accessed 13 June 2022).

Johnson, B. (2019) Nursing students to receive £5000 payment a year. Department of Health and Social Care (2019) Gov.uk 18 December. Available at: https:// www.gov.uk/government/news/nursing-students-to-receive-5-000-payment-a-year (Last accessed 3 May 2022).

Johnstone, M.J. (2011) Nursing and justice as a basic human need. *Nurs Philos* 2011 12 (1), pp. 34–44.

Johnstone, P., Ratan, A. and Hickey, N. (2015) Prevention of dehydration in hospital inpatient. *Br J Nurs.*, June 11–24 24 (11), pp. 568–570, 572–573.

Jones, H. (2015) Assisted Dying (No 2) Bill [HL]. (Marris Bill) (Vol 599) Debated on 11 September. Hansard. Available at: https://hansard.parliament.uk/commons/2015-09-11/debates/15091126000003/AssistedDying(No2)Bill (Last accessed 11 May 2022).

Jones, R. K., Nash, E., Cross, L., Philbin, J. and Kirstein, M, (2022). Medication Abortion Now Accounts for More Than Half of All US Abortions. Policy Analysis *Guttmacher Institute*. Available at: https://www.guttmacher.org/article/2022/02/medication-abortion-now-accounts-more-half-all-us-abortions (Last accessed 4 May 2022).

Julian of Norwich. In: *Kirvan, J. J. (Editor) (2008) All will be well. (30 Days with a Great Spiritual Teacher series). P. 34.* 1 April. Ave Maria Press. University of Notre Dame. Indiana. USA.

Juthani, M. (2021) In: *Katella, K. (2021) 8 Lessons we can learn from the COVID-19 pandemic. 14 May. Yale Medicine,* Available at: https://www.yalemedicine.org/news/8-lessons-covid-19-pandemic (Last accessed 3 May 2022).

Kavanaugh, K. (2000) St Teresa of Avila. The Way of Perfection. Study Edition. ICS Publications. Institute of Carmelite Studies. Washington DC.

Kearney, D. (2013) Critics of Liverpool Care Pathway deserve our thanks. Letters, *Catholic Herald* 24 May.

Kearney, D. (2019) Offering a second chance: abortion pill reversal. *Catholic Medical Quarterly* 69 (2) Available at: www.cmq.org.uk PAPERS 12. (Last accessed 3 May 2022).

Kearney, D. (2021) Abortion pill rescue update. In Haec Tempora: news from our CMA (UK) president, sent to all CMA (UK) members. 27 October 2020. *Catholic Medical Quarterly* 2021 71 (1). Kelly, B. (1993) The real world of hospital nursing practice as perceived by nursing undergraduates. *J. Prof Nurs* ; 9, 1: pp. 27 – 33.

Kelly, C. (1998) Investing or discounting self: are moral decisions shaped by conditions in the workplace? *Adv Prac Nurs Q*. 4 (20), pp. 8–13.

Ketafian, S. (1989) Moral reasoning and ethical practice in nursing. Measurement issues. *Nurs Clin North Am* 24, pp. 509–521.

King, N., Thomas, K., Martin, N., Bell, D. and Farrell, S. (2005) 'Now nobody falls through the net': practitioners' perspectives on the Gold Standards Framework for community palliative care. *Palliative Medicine* 19 (8), pp. 619–627.

Kinley, J. and Hockley, J. (2010) A baseline review of medication provided to older people in nursing care homes in the last month of life. *International Journal of Palliative Nursing*: Research. Vol. 16, No. 5.

Kirby, J. (2022) We're all the prisoners of an unreformed NHS. *The Daily Telegraph, Comment*, 18 November.

Kline, R. (2013) Bullying: the silent epidemic in the NHS. *Public World*: Democracy at Work. 15 May 2013. Available at: http://publicworld.org.gridhosted.co.uk/blog/bullying_the_silent_epidemic_in_the_nhs (Last accessed 4 May 2022).

Knight, J. (2003) The Patients' Protection Bill. Available at: https://www.theyworkforyou.com/lords/?id=2003-03-12a.1402.0&s=section%3Adebates+section%3Awhall+section%3Alordsdebates+section%3Ani+speaker%3A13103 (Last accessed 3 May 2022).

Knight, I. (2020a) This fairy tale row is strictly for toddlers. *The Sunday Times* 22 November.

Knight, D. (2020b) Epicenter Nurse: Fraud, Greed, Negligence Fueled COVID Deaths. Round Table Report. Available at: https://roundtablereport.com/?p=6542. (Last accessed 7 July 2022).

Kohnke, M. F. (1982). Advocacy, risk and reality. St. Louis, MO: The C. V. Mosby Co: USA

Kuokkanen, L., Leino-Kilpi, H., Katajisto, J., Heponiemi, T., Sinervo, T. and Marko, E. (2014) Does organisational justice predict empowerment? Nurses assess their work environment. *Journal of Nursing Scholarship* 46 (5), pp. 349–356.

Lambert, V., Lambert, C., Itano, J., Inouye, J., Kim, S., Kuniviktikul., W., Sitthimongkol, Y., Pongthavornkamol, K., Gasemgitvattana, S. and Ito, M. (2004a) Cross-cultural comparison of workplace stressors, ways of coping and demographic characteristics as predictors of physical and mental health among hospital nurses in Japan, Thailand, South Korea and the USA (Hawaii) *Int. J. Nurs. Stud.* 41, pp. 85–87.

Lambert, V., Lambert, C. and Ito, M. (2004b) Workplace stressors, ways of coping and demographic characteristics as predictors of physical and mental health of Japanese hospital nurses. *Int. J. Nurs. Stud.* 41, pp. 85–97.

Lampl, Y., Gillad, R., Eschel, Y., Boaz, M., Rapoport, A., and Sadeh, M. (2002) Diagnosing Brain Death Using the Transcranial Doppler with a Transorbital Approach. *Arch Neurol*; 59(1):58–60. doi:10.1001/archneur.59.1.58 Accepted for publication September 4, 2001. Available at: https://jamanetwork.com/journals/jamaneurology/fullarticle/781174#27024342 (Last accessed 17 November 2022).

Lancet (2020) Redefining vulnerability in the era of COVID-19. Available at: https://www.thelancet.com/journals/lancet/article/PIIS0140-6736(20)30757-1/fulltext (Last accessed 11 May 2022).

Lawlor, P.G. (2002) Delirium and dehydration: some fluid for thought? *Support. Care Cancer.* 2002; 10: pp. 445–454.

Lawson, D. (2020) The inconvenient truth: we practise eugenics. *The Sunday Times* 22 November.

Learning Disabilities Mortality Review (LeDeR) Programme: Fact Sheet 24 (2019) Available at: https://www.bristol.ac.uk/media-library/sites/sps/leder/2099_DNACPR_PDF.pdf (Last accessed 24 March 2023).

Le Fanu, J. (2012) Bad days for Big Pharma. Features: *Catholic Herald* 3 August.

Le Fanu, J. (2021) The right to die could become a burden. The Surgery, Doctor's Diary. *The Daily Telegraph* 20 September.

Leininger, M. (1978) The Phenomenon of Caring, Part V, Caring: The Essence and Central Focus of Nursing. *American nurses Foundation Nursing Research Report*. Vol 12 (1).

Levin Y. (2008) Imagining the Future: Science and American Democracy. New Atlantis Books. Encounter Books. New York, London.

Levy, B.H. (2021) Cancel culture is churning out imbeciles. In: *The Daily Telegraph, Walden, C. Features and Arts 16 October.*

Lewis, I. (2006) Dignity in care campaign launch. Available at: https://www.hsj. co.uk/dignity-in-care-campaign-launched/1715.article (Last accessed 11 May 2022).

Li, L. and Liang, S. (2002) Investigation on the nurses' response to tension in the new era and counter measures. *J. Nurs. Sci.* 17, pp. 16–18.

Life Site News (2021) Covid nurse explains becoming a whistleblower: I recorded them murdering patients. Available at: https://www.lifesitenews. com/news/nyc-covid-nurse-turned-whistleblower-people-were-just-dying-from-gross-negligence-medical-malpractice/ (Last accessed 3 May 2022).

Livingstone, E.A. (2006) Secularism. *The Concise Oxford Dictionary of the Christian Church.* 2nd ed. Oxford University Press: Oxford, UK.

Loeb Classical Library (1923) Hippocrates of Cos: The Oath 147, pp. 298–299.

Longczak, H. (2019) 20 Reasons why Compassion is so important in Psychology. *Positivepsychology.com.* Compassion. Available at: https://positive psychology.com/why-is-compassion-important/ (Last accessed 7 July 2022).

Lords and Commons Family and Child Protection Group (2023) Report: When End of Life Care Goes Wrong, Available at: https://vfjuk.org/product/when-end-of-life-care-goes-wrong-report/ (Last accessed 17 March 2023).

Lutzen, K., Nordstrom, G. and Evertzon, M. (1995) Moral sensitivity in nursing practice. *Scand J Caring Sci* 9, pp. 131–138.

MacDonald, G. (2020) 'Assisted suicide an NHS moneysaver', 'disturbing report says. *The Christian Institute.* 18 March. Available at: https://www. christian.org.uk/news/assisted-suicide-an-nhs-moneysaver-disturbing-report-says/ (Last accessed 31 July 2022).

MacDonald, G. (2022a) Urgent: Assisted Suicide Bill Moves a Step Closer. Autumn Appeal. Our Duty of Care. 27 September.

MacDonald, G. (2022b) Alert: Petition launched to include mental health conditions in the McArthur Bill. Autumn Appeal. Our Duty of Care. 29 September.

MacIntyre, A. (1981) After Virtue. Indiana: University of Notre Dame. In: Fleming (2019) The compassionate state? Voluntary Assisted Dying, neoliberalism and the problem of virtue without an anchor ABC religion and Ethics. Available at: https://www.abc.net.au/religion/compassionate-state-voluntary-assisted-dying-neoliberalism-and/10937504 (Last accessed 11 May 2022).

Mackintosh, D. (2015) Demise of the LCP: villain or scapegoat? *J Med Ethics.* August; 41(8): pp. 650–1. 10.1136/medethics-2014-102424 [Pubmed] [CrossRef] [Google Scholar]. In: *Seymour, J. and Clark, D. (2018) The Liverpool Care Pathway for the Dying Patient: a critical analysis of its rise, demise and legacy in England. Wellcome Open Res. Available at: https:// pubmed.ncbi.nlm.nih.gov/29881785/ (Last accessed 30 July 2022).*

Macmillan Cancer Charity (2021) A holistic needs assessment (HNA) Macmillan, London. Available at: https://www.macmillan.org.uk/healthcare-professionals/innovation-in-cancer-care/holistic-needs-assessment (Last accessed 11 May 2022).

Magnussen, J. and Mulder, J. (2001) Opioid Neurotoxicity. *Communication.* May/June. Available at: https://www.pharmacistsmb.ca/files/2001/May-June/Opioid_Induced_Neurotoxicity.pdf (Last accessed 15 April 2022).

Malone, B. (2005) RCN Magazine Spring edition. *RCN,* London: 48. In: Finlay, N., James, C., Irwin, J. (2006). Nursing education changes and reduced standards of quality care. Br J Nurs; 15, 13. pp. 700 – 702.

Manara, M.U., van Gils, S., Nübold, A. and Zijlstra, F.R.H. (2020) Corruption, fast or slow? Ethical leadership interacts with Machiavellianism to influence intuitive thinking and corruption. Frontiers in Psychology. December. Available at: https://www.frontiersin.org/articles/10.3389/fpsyg.2020.578419/full (Last accessed 6 April 2022).

Mandlestam, M. (2011) *How We Treat the Sick. Neglect and Abuse in Our Health Services.* Jessica Kingsley Publishers, London. p 187.

Mannix, K. (2022) 'Being a listener'. Conference: Why end of life companionship matters. *The Centre for the Art of Dying Well, St Mary's University, Twickenham,* London, 22 September.

Marcuse, H.N. (1964/1991) One Dimensional Man. Beacon Press, Boston MA.

Marris, R. (2015) Assisted Dying (No 2) Bill [HL]. (Marris Bill) (Vol 599) Debated on 11 September. Hansard. Available at: https://hansard.parliament.uk/ commons/2015-09-11/debates/15091126000003/AssistedDying(No2)Bill (Last accessed 11 May 2022).

Martin, F. (2012) Caring for the elderly is hospitals' core business. In: *National Health Executive (NHE) Integrated care and social care.* Sept/Oct 2012 1 October. Available at: https://www.nationalhealthexecutive.com/Interviews/ caring-for-the-elderly-is-hospitals-core-business (Last accessed 11 May 2022).

Maryland, M. and Gonzalez, R.I. (2012) Patient advocacy in the community and legislative arena. American Nurses Association, Online Journal of Issues in Nursing, No. 1. January. Available at: https://ojin.nursingworld.org/ MainMenuCategories/ANAMarketplace/ANAPeriodicals/OJIN/Tableof Contents/Vol-17-2012/No1-Jan-2012/Advocacy-in-Community-and-Legislative-Arena.html (Last accessed 11 May 2022).

Maslach, C. and Jackson, S. (1981) The measurement of experienced burnout. *Journal of Occupational Behavior.* 2: pp. 90–113. In: Wilkinson,

H., Whittington, R., Perry, L. and Eames, C. (2017) Examining the relationship between burnout and empathy in healthcare professionals: a systematic review. Burnout Research. 6 Sep.: 18–29. MCID: PMC5534210. PMID: 28868237. Available at: https://pubmed.ncbi.nlm.nih.gov/28868237/ (Last accessed 11 May 2022).

Matthews, J.J., Hausner, D., Avery J., Hannon, B., Zimmerman, C. and al Awamer, A. (2020) Impact of medical assistance in dying on palliative care: a qualitative study. *Palliative Medicine*. Available at: https://pubmed.ncbi.nlm.nih.gov/33126842/ (Last accessed 11 May 2022).

McCullagh, P. (1996) Thirst in relation to withdrawal of hydration. *Catholic Medical Quarterly*. XLVI 3 (269) 5–12. 76. Available at: http://www.cmq.org.uk/CMQ/1996/Thirst-and-PVS.html (Last accessed 28 April 2022).

McCullough, L.B. (1998) Introduction. In: John Gregory's Writings on Medical Ethics and Philosophy of Medicine. Philosophy and Medicine, vol 57. Springer, Dordrecht. Available at: https://link.springer.com/book/10.1007/978-0-585-32315-2 (Last accessed 4 May 2022).

McDiarmid, F., Peters, K., Jackson, D. and Daly J. (2012) Factors contributing to the shortage of nurse faculty: a review of the literature. *Nurse Education Today* 32 (5), July 2012, pp. 565–569.

McDonald, L. (2013) What would Florence Nightingale say? *British Journal of Nursing* 22 (9) p 542. Available at: https://nightingalesociety.com/what-would-florence-nightingale-say/ (Last accessed 11 May 2022).

McDonald, V. and Lintern, S. (2021) Revealed over 30 deaths in Nottingham maternity units' scandal. *Channel 4 News* 30 June 2021. Available at: https://www.channel4.com/news/revealed-over-30-deaths-in-nottingham-maternity-units-scandal (Last accessed 11 May 2022).

McFarland, G. K. and McFarlane, E.A. (1997) Nursing Diagnosis & Intervention: Planning for Patient Care. 3rd ed. Missouri, St Louis: Mosby.

McLeod, A. (2014) Nurses' views of the causes of ethical dilemmas during treatment cessation in the ICU: a qualitative study. Available at: https://doi.org/10.12968/bjnn.2014.10.3.131 (Last accessed 4 May 2022).

MCPIL (2011) National Care of the Dying Audit – *Hospital Generic Report Round* 3. Available at: https://www.whatdotheyknow.com/request/169193/response/419788/attach/5/Audit%202011.pdf?cookie_passthrough=1 (Last accessed 4 May 2022).

Meacher Bill (2021) (Assisted Dying Bill) [HL]. A Bill to enable adults who are terminally ill to be provided at their request with specified assistance to end their own life and for connected purposes. Private Members' Bill. Originated in the House of Lords, Session 2021–22. Last updated: 26 January 2022 at 19:28. Available at: https://bills.parliament.uk/bills/2875 (Last accessed 4 May 2022).

Meilaender, G. (2017) Pathos, bathos and euthanasia. Celebrating the 'gift' of death? Available at: https://www.commonwealmagazine.org/

pathos-bathos-and-euthanasia (Last accessed 4 May 2022) Mellish, J.M. and Wannenburg, I. (1992) *Unit Teaching and Administration for Nurses.* 3rd edn. Butterworths, Durban.

Mencap (2007) Report: Death by Indifference. Available at: https://www.mencap.org.uk/sites/default/files/2016-06/DBIreport.pdf (Last accessed 4 May 2022).

Mencap (2010) Getting it right charter. Available at: https://www.mencap.org.uk/sites/default/files/2016-07/Getting%20it%20Right%20charter.pdf (Last accessed 4 May 2022).

Mencap (2012) Death by Indifference: 74 deaths and counting. A progress report 5 years on. Available at: https://www.mencap.org.uk/sites/default/files/2016-08/Death%20by%20Indifference%20-%2074%20deaths%20and%20counting.pdf (Last accessed 4 May 2022).

Menzies, I. (1960) A case-study in the functioning of social systems as a defence against anxiety. A report on a study of the nursing service of a general hospital. Available at: https://doi.org/10.1177/001872676001300201 (Last accessed 20 April 2022).

Merriam-Webster Dictionary (2019) Secularism. Merriam-Webster Incorporated. Available at: https://www.merriam-webster.com/dictionary/secularism (Last accessed 30 April 2022).

Meštrović, S. (1997) Post emotional Society. London: Sage, pp. 9-10. In: *Herdman, E. A. (2004) Nursing in a post emotional society. Nursing Philosophy 5, pp. 95–103.* Available at: https://pubmed.ncbi.nlm.nih.gov/15189550/ (Last accessed 4 May 2022).

Michael, J. (2008) Healthcare for all. The report of the independent inquiry into access to healthcare for people with learning disabilities. Available at: https://easy-read-online.co.uk/media/1231/healthcare%20for%20all%20easy%20read.pdf (Last accessed 4 May 2022).

Military tribunal no. 1. (1950) *United States v. Karl Brandt et al.,* the medical trial. In: *Trials of War Criminals Before the Nuremberg Military Tribunals Under Control Council Law 10.* Washington, DC: Superintendent of Documents, US Government Printing Office.

Miller, W.R. (1999) Integrating Spirituality into Treatment: Resources for Practitioners. *American Psychological Association.* Available at: https://psycnet.apa.org/record/1999-02703-000 (Last accessed 4 May 2022).

Miller, J. (2021) What is your must? 25 January. *One Spirit Interfaith Foundation.* (Last accessed 30 July 2022). First published on www.sundarispirit.co.uk https://www.interfaithfoundation.org/news/2021/1/25/what-is-your-must. (Last accessed 29 July 2022).

Miller, C. (2022) Legalisation of abortion and maternal mortality in Ethiopia. Ethiopian Medical Journal 2022; 60.

Mohamed, I. A. H. and Otman, N.M.N. (2021) Exploring the Link between Organizational Learning and Transformational Leadership: A Review.

Scientific Research Open Access Library Journal, 8, 1–19. doi: 10.4236/oalib. 1107242. Available at: https://www.scirp.org/journal/paperinformation. aspx?paperid=109383#ref1 (Last accessed 21 March 2023).

Mohammed, M., Cheng, M., Rouse, A. and Marshall, T. (2001) Bristol, Shipman and clinical governance: Shewhart's forgotten lessons. *Lancet;* 357, pp. 463–467.

Molassiotis, A., Xian-Liang, L. and Kwok, S.W. (2020) Impact of advanced nursing practice through nurse-led clinics in the care of cancer patients: A scoping review. *Eur J Cancer Care* (Engl) Available at: https://pubmed.ncbi. nlm.nih.gov/33169476/ (Last accessed 11 May 2022).

Morgan, B. (2012) Organ donation: *Church in Wales debate on presumed consent.* Available at: https://www.bbc.co.uk/news/uk-wales-16659597 (Last accessed 11 May 2022).

Moth, R., Mason, P. and Sherrington, J. (2020) Coronavirus and Access to Treatment, *Roman Catholic Diocese of Westminster* (RCDOW) ONLINE. Available at: https://www.cbcew.org.uk/coronavirus-and-access-to-treatment/

Munby, J. (2010) Legal implications of neglect and abuse. In: *Mandlestam, M. (2011) How We Treat the Sick. Neglect and Abuse in Our Health Services,* p 296. Jessica Kingsley Publishers: London.

Munn, F. (2021) Could curtailing practice hours improve students' experience of clinical placements? *Nursing Standard online, Editorial* 30 August. Available at: https://rcni.com/nursing-standard/opinion/editorial/could-curtailing-practice-hours-improve-students-experience-of-clinical-placements-177561 (Last accessed 11 May 2022).

Murphy, S. (2004) Establishment Bioethics. *Catholic Education Resource Centre.* Available at: https://www.catholiceducation.org/en/science/ethical-issues/establishment-bioethics.html (Last accessed 11 May 2022).

Murray, D. (2022) There's no cause for optimism in broken Britain. *The Daily Telegraph, Comment,* 24 December.

Nair, S. (2017) Twenty quotes on nursing and life from the 'Lady with the Lamp', Florence Nightingale. Available at: https://yourstory.com/2017/05/20-quotes-nursing-life-lady-lamp-florence-nightingale. (Last accessed 5 May 2022).

National Secular Society (2022). Secularism: Mission statement/Key aims. Available at: https://www.secularism.org.uk/ (Last accessed 28 April 2022).

Negarandeh, R., Oskouie, F., Hmadi, F. and Nikravesh, M. (2008) The meaning of patient advocacy for Iranian nurses. *Nurs Ethics* 15 (4), pp. 457–467.

Newman, J.H. (1864) Apologia Pro Vita Sua. London, Longman, Green, Longman, Roberts & Green.

NHS (2016a) National Health Service Staff Survey. Available at: https://www. england.nhs.uk/statistics/2017/03/07/the-2016-nhs-staff-survey-in-england/ (Last accessed 28 April 2022).

NHS (2016b) National framework for improvement and leadership. Available at: https://www.england.nhs.uk/2016/12/new-nhs-leadership-framework/ (Last accessed 28 April 2022).

NHS (2020) End of life care. (Updated version) Available at: https://www.nhs.uk/conditions/end of life-care/ (Last accessed 28 April 2022).

NHS (2022) Diagnosis, Brain death. NHS Guidelines. 8 September. Available at: https://www.nhs.uk/conditions/brain-death/https://www.nhs.uk/conditions/brain-death/diagnosis/ (Last accessed 24 November 2022).

NHS Blood and Transplant (2020) Donation after circulatory death. Available at: https://www.odt.nhs.uk/deceased-donation/best-practice-guidance/donation-after-circulatory-death/ (Last accessed 28 April 2022).

NHS Digital (2020) Sickness absence due to mental Health by staff group 2015 to 2020. Available at: https://digital.nhs.uk/search?query=nhs+staff+sicknes s+mental+health+2020 (Last accessed 10 May 2022).

NHS England (2012) Compassion in practice nursing, midwifery and care staff – our vision and strategy. Available at: https://www.england.nhs.uk/wp-content/uploads/2012/12/compassion-in-practice.pd (Last accessed 27 January 2023).

NHS England (2014) The Six Cs. Available at: https://www.ombudsman.org.uk/sites/default/files/2016-10/Care%20and%20Compassion.pdf (Last accessed 28 April 2022).

NHS England (2019) The NHS's recommendations to Government and Parliament for an NHS Integrated Care Bill. September. Available at: https://www.england.nhs.uk/wp-content/uploads/2019/09/BM1917-NHS-recommendations-Government-Parliament-for-an-NHS-Bill.pdf

NHS England and NHS Improvement (2020) Leading the acceleration of evidence into practice: a guide for executive nurses. Available at: https://www.england.nhs.uk/publication/leading-the-acceleration-of-evidence-into-practice-a-guide-for-executive-nurses/ (Last accessed 28 April 2022).

NHS Inform (2020) Spirituality. Available at: https://www.nhsinform.scot/care-support-and-rights/palliative-care/practical-help/spiritual-care. (Last accessed 11 July 2022).

NHS People Plan (2020/21) We are the NHS: People Plan - action for us all. Availableat: https://www.england.nhs.uk/wp-content/uploads/2020/07/We-Are-The-NHS-Action-For-All-Of-Us-FINAL-March-21.pdf (Last accessed 27 January 2023).

NICE (2004) Improving Supportive and Palliative Care for Adults with Cancer. Available at: https://www.nice.org.uk/guidance/csg4 (Last accessed 28 April 2022).

NICE (2015) Care of dying adults in the last days of life. NICE guideline NG31. Available at: https://www.nice.org.uk/guidance/ng31/ (Last accessed 28 April 2022).

NICE (2020) COVID-19 rapid guideline: critical care in adults. [NG159]. Published 20 March. Last updated 3 September 2020. Available at: https://www.nice.org.uk/guidance/ng159 (Last accessed 10 May 2022).

Nichols, V. (2014) Cardinal Vincent Nichols addresses Catholic healthcare students. *Independent Catholic News*. (ICN) Available at: https://www.indcatholicnews.com/news/25952 (Last accessed 12 May 2022).

NMC (2010) Standards for preregistration nursing education. Available at: https://www.nmc.org.uk/globalassets/sitedocuments/standards/nmc-standards-for-pre-registration-nursing-education.pdf. (Last accessed 28 April 2022).

NMC (2013) Raising Concerns. Available at: https://www.nmc.org.uk/standards/guidance/raising-concerns-guidance-for-nurses-and-midwives/ (Last accessed 28 April 2022).

NMC (2018) The Code of Professional Conduct: standards of practice and behaviour for nurses, midwives and nurse associates. 10 October. NMC: London. Available at: https://www.nmc.org.uk/standards/code/ (Last accessed 8 February 2022).

Norberg, A., Hirschfield, M., Davidson, B., Davis, A., Lairi, S., Lin, J.Y., Phillips, L. and Pittman, E. (1994) Ethical reasoning concerning the feeding of severely demented patients: an international perspective. *Nursing Ethics* 1 (1), pp. 3–13.

NSPCC (2020) Gillick competency and Fraser guidelines. NSPCC Learning. Last updated: 10 Jun 2020. Available at: https://learning.nspcc.org.uk/child-protection-system/gillick-competence-fraser-guidelines (Last accessed 28 April 2022).

Nsiah, C., Siakwa, M. and Ninnoni, J.P.K. (2019) Research article Registered Nurses' description of patient advocacy in the clinical setting. Available at: https://onlinelibrary.wiley.com/doi/epdf/10.1002/nop2.307 (Last accessed 12 July 2022).

Nurse Staffing Levels Act (Wales) (2016) *Legislation.gov.uk*. The National Archives. Available at: https://www.legislation.gov.uk/anaw/2016/5/section/1/enacted (Last accessed 28 April 2022).

Nys, T. (2016) Autonom, Trust and Respect. *J Med Philos*. Feb; 41(1): pp. 10–24. Available at: https://www.ncbi.nlm.nih.gov/pmc/articles/PMC4882631/ (Last accessed 2 May 2022).

Ockenden, D. (2021) *Interim Maternity Review, Shrewsbury and Telford Health Authority*. Available at: https://www.donnaockenden.com/downloads/news/2020/12/ockenden-report.pdf (Last accessed 1 May 2022).

Ockenden, D. (2022) Ockenden review: summary of findings, conclusions and essential actions. *Maternity Review, Shrewsbury and Telford Health Authority*. Available at: https://www.gov.uk/government/publications/final-report-of-the-ockenden-review (Last accessed 28 April 2022).

Oliver, M. (2012) Donating in good faith or getting into trouble: religion and organ donation revisited. *World Journal of transplantation* 2 (5), p 69. Available at: https://www.ncbi.nlm.nih.gov/pmc/articles/PMC3782236/ doi: 10.5500/wjt.v2.i5.69. (Last accessed 2 May 2022).

Oliver, M., Woywodt, A., Ahmed, A. and Saif, I. (2011) Organ donation, transplantation and religion. Editorial, *Nephrol Dial Transplant*. 26 Feb; (2):437-44. Available at: https://academic.oup.com/ndt/article/26/2/437/1894177 (Last accessed 2 May 2022).

Omery, A. (1985/1986) The moral reasoning of nurses who work in an adult intensive care setting. [Abstract]. *Diss Astr*; 46: 3007 B.

Onwuteaka-Philipsen, B.D., Brinkman-Stoppelenburg, A., Penning, C., de Jong-Krul, G.J.F., van Delden, J.J.M. and van der Heide, A. (2012) Trends in end of life practices before and after the enactment of the euthanasia law in the Netherlands from 1990 to 2010: a repeated cross-sectional survey. Available at: https://euthanasiadebate.org.nz/wp-content/uploads/2012/10/netherlands_euthanasia.pdf (Last accessed 9 April 2022).

Ostwal, S.P., Sallins, N. and Deodhar, J. (2017) Reversal of opioid-induced toxicity. *Indian J Palliat Care*, Oct–Dec. 23 (4), pp. 484–486.

Palliative Care Clinical Studies Collaborative (2014) In: Hosie et al. (2016) Measuring delirium point-prevalence in two Australian palliative care inpatient units. Article in: International Journal of Palliative Nursing 2016 22 (1), pp. 13–21.

Parkinson, M. (2010) My year as National Dignity Ambassador. London: Department of Health, p. 28. Available at: https://www.dignityincare.org.uk/_assets/Resources/Dignity/My_year_as_National_Dignity_Ambassador.pdf (Last accessed 11 May 2022).

Parris, M. (2020) It's shameful how we have treated our elderly. Available at: https://www.spectator.co.uk/article/Its-shameful-how-we-have-locked-down-our-elderly (Last accessed 11 May 2022).

Pearson, A. (2020) We need our NHS to resume normal service. *The Daily Telegraph*.

Pearson, A. Vaughan, B. and FitzGerald, M. (1996) *Nursing Models for Practice*. Butterworth-Heinemann: Oxford.

Pellegrino, E.D. (1985) The virtuous physician and the ethics of medicine. In: *Virtue and Medicine (1985) Dordrecht: Springer, pp. 237–255.* Available at: https://link.springer.com/chapter/10.1007/978-94-009-5229-4_1 (Last accessed 11 May 2022).

Pemberton, M. (2020) The final insult. *Daily Mail* 12 September.

Percival T. (1803) Strand, London, Manchester: S. Russell for J. Johnson, St. Paul's Church Yard and R. Bickerstaff; Medical Ethics; or, a Code of Institutes and Precepts, Adapted to the Professional Conduct of Physicians and Surgeons; In Hospital Practice. In private, or general Practice. III. In relation to Apothecaries. In Cases which may require a knowledge of Law. To which is added an Appendix; containing a discourse on Hospital duties; also notes and illustrations. [Google Scholar]. In: *Patuzzo, Sa Goracci, G· and Cilibert. R (2018) Thomas Percival. Discussing the foundation of Medical Ethics. Acta Biomed.* 2018; 89(3): 343–348. Available at: https://www.ncbi.nlm.nih.gov/pmc/articles/PMC6502118/ doi: 10.23750/abm. v89i3.7050 PMCID: PMC6502118PMID: 30333457 *(Last accessed 5 May 2018).*

Pereira, J. (2011) Legalising euthanasia or assisted suicide: the illusion of safeguards and controls. *Curr. oncology* 18 (2), pp.38–45.

Perl, J.M. (2007) A "Dictatorship of Relativism"? Symposium in Response to Cardinal Ratzinger's Last Homily An issue of: *Common Knowledge*. Duke

University Press Duke University Press - A "Dictatorship of Relativism"? (dukeupress.edu) (Last accessed 7 August 2022).

Petre, J. (2016) Veteran condemned to die by the NHS: Doctors at leading hospital put great-grandfather with a chest infection on notorious 'death pathway' after wrongly deciding he could not be saved. *Mail online* 24 July. Available at: https://www.pressreader.com/uk/the-scottish-mail-on-sunday/20160724/282291024591374 (Last accessed 9 April 2022).

Pew Research Centre (2018) Report: Global Uptick in Government Restrictions on Religion in 2016. Nationalist parties and organisations played an increasing role in harassment of religious minorities, especially in Europe. 21 June. Available at: https://www.pewresearch.org/religion/2018/06/21/global-uptick-in-government-restrictions-on-religion-in-2016/ (Last accessed 5 May 2022).

PHSO (2011) Report: Care and Compassion. Available at: https://www.ombudsman.org.uk/sites/default/files/2016-10/Care%20and%20Compassion.pdf (Last accessed 28 April 2022).

PHSO (2016) Report: Mr Joseph Boberek. 27 June.

PHSO (2021) What we can and can't help with. Available at: https://www.ombudsman.org.uk/making-complaint/what-we-can-and-cant-help (Last accessed 10 May 2022).

Pike, A.W. (1991) Moral outrage and moral discourse in nurse-physician collaboration. *J Prof Nurse* 7, pp. 351–363.

Piper, J. (2011) What does it mean to serve God? Available at: https://www.desiringgod.org/articles/what-does-it-mean-to-serve-god (Last accessed 5 May 2022).

Ponnu, C. and Chuah, C. (2010) Organisational commitment, organisational justice and employee turnover in Malaysia. *African Journal of Business Management* 4 (13), pp. 2676–2692.

Pontifical Council for Pastoral Assistance to Health Care Workers (2017) The New Charter for Health Care Workers. Preface. *The National Catholic Bioethics Centre: Upholding the Dignity of the Human Person in Health Care and Biomedical Research for Fifty Years, 1972–2022.* 600 Reed Road, Suite 102, Broomhall, PA, 19008, USA. ISBN 978-0-935372-69-4.

Pope Benedict XVI (2005a) *Deus Caritas Est*, para. 31a. Available at: https://www.vatican.va/content/benedict-xvi/en/encyclicals/documents/hf_ben-xvi_enc_20051225_deus-caritas-est.html (Last accessed 5 May 2022).

Pope Benedict XVI (2005b) *Deus Caritas Est*, para. 31b. Available at: https://www.vatican.va/content/benedict-xvi/en/encyclicals/documents/hf_ben-xvi_enc_20051225_deus-caritas-est.html (Last accessed 5 May 2022).

Pope Francis (2016) Post-synodal apostolic exhortation of the Holy Father Francis, on love in the family: 'Amoris Lætitia'. (The Joy of Love). Available at: https://www.vatican.va/content/dam/francesco/pdf/apost_exhortations/documents/papa-francesco_esortazione-ap_20160319_amoris-laetitia_en.pdf (Last accessed 5 May 2022).

Pope Leo XIII (1890) Sapientiae Christianae, Encyclical on Christians as Citizens. 10 January. Available at: https://www.vatican.va/content/leo-xiii/en/encyclicals/documents/hf_l-xiii_enc_10011890_sapientiae-christianae.html (Last accessed 21 November 2022).

Pope St John Paul II (1995a) The Gospel of Life: On the Value and Inviolability of Human Life. Chapter 1 – The voice of your brother's blood cries to me from the ground, excerpt from the Papal Encyclical, Evangelium Vitae Encyclical 25 March. Available at: https://www.vatican.va/content/john-paul-ii/en/encyclicals/documents/hf_jp-ii_enc_25031995_evangelium-vitae.html (Last accessed 5 May 2022).

Pope St John Paul II (1995b) The Gospel of Life: On the Value and Inviolability of Human Life. Loss of the sense of God. *Papal Encyclical, Evangelium Vitae.*

Pope St John Paul II (1999) Message for the celebration of XXXIII World Day of Peace, w2.vatican.va. 8 December. Available at: https://www.vatican.va/content/john-paul-ii/en/messages/peace/documents/hf_jp-ii_mes_08121999_xxxiii-world-day-for-peace.html (Last accessed 5 May 2022).

Pope St John Paul II (2000) Contemplate the face of Christ in the sick (message for the VIII World Day of the Sick), *Libreria Editrice Vaticana.* Available at: https://www.vatican.va/content/john-paul-ii/en/messages/sick/documents/hf_jp-ii_mes_19990806_world-day-of-the-sick-2000.html (Last accessed 5 May 2022).

Pope St John Paul II (2004a) Address to the participants in the international congress on 'life-sustaining treatments and vegetative state: scientific advances and ethical dilemmas. Saturday 20 March. Available at: https://www.vatican.va/content/john-paul-ii/en/speeches/2004/march/documents/hf_jp-ii_spe_20040320_congress-fiamc.html (Last accessed 5 May 2022).

Pope St John Paul II (2004b) Address of the participants in the 19th international conference of the Pontifical Council for Health Pastoral Care. 12 November. Available at: https://www.vatican.va/content/john-paul-ii/en/speeches/2004/november/documents/hf_jp-ii_spe_20041112_pc-hlthwork.html (Last accessed 5 May 2022).

Proffitt, A. (2019) Assisted dying: why the RCP should be opposed. *Royal College of Physicians.* Available at: https://www.rcplondon.ac.uk/news/assisted-dying-why-rcp-should-be-opposed (Last accessed 5 May 2022).

Protection from Harassment Act (1997) Legislation.gov.uk Available at: https://www.legislation.gov.uk/ukpga/1997/40/contents (Last accessed 5 May 2022).

Public Health England (2018) Tailoring Immunisation Programmes Report and Recommendations. Available at: https://assets.publishing.service.gov.uk/government/uploads/system/uploads/attachment_data/file/705096/Tailoring_Immunisatio_report_including_Protocols_and_research_appendix.pdf (Last accessed 5 May 2022).

Public Health England (2020) Deaths of people identified as having learning disabilities with COVID-19 in England in the spring of 2020. Available at: https://assets.publishing.service.gov.uk/government/uploads/system/uploads/

attachment_data/file/933612/COVID-19__learning_disabilities_mortality_ report.pdf (Last accessed 26 July 2022).

Public Interest Disclosure Act (1998). GOV.UK. Available at: https://www.gov.uk/ government/publications/whistleblowing-and-the-public-interest-disclosure-act-1998-c23/whistleblowing-and-the-public-interest-disclosure-act-1998-c23-accessible-version#:~:text=The%20Public%20Interest%20Disclosure%20 Act%201998%20(%20PIDA%20)%20protects%20whistleblowers%20 from,making%20a%20public%20interest%20disclosure (Last accessed 18 April 2023).

Public Interest Disclosure Act (2014) updated by the Protected Disclosures (Amendment) Act (2022) *Charity Commission for England and Wales. Gov. UK.* Available at: https://www.gov.uk/government/publications/guidance-for-auditors-and-independent-examiners-of-charities/the-public-interest-disclosure-act--2#:~:text=1.-,What%20does%20the%20Act%20do%3F,blow%20 the%20whistle%20on%20wrongdoing (Last accessed 10 April 2023).

Pugh, J. (2015) Assisted Dying (No 2) Bill [HL]. (Marris Bill) (Vol 599) Debated on 11 September. Hansard UK Parliament. Available at: https://hansard. parliament.uk/commons/2015-09-11/debates/15091126000003/Assisted Dying(No2)Bill (Last accessed 11 May 2022).

Pullicino, P. (2015) The new end of life guideline is lethal: the troubling Liverpool Care Pathway needs replacing but not with NICE's dangerous and distorted plan. *The Daily Telegraph.*

Pullicino, P. (2012) The dangers of abandonment of evidence-based medicine in the use of the Liverpool Care Pathway. *Catholic Medical Quarterly* 62 (4), November. Available at: http://www.cmq.org.uk/CMQ/2012/Nov/LCP-Pullicino.html (Last accessed 5 May 2022).

Pullicino, P. (2016) Comment: Old should never be denied treatment. *Mail online* 30 November.

Pullicino, P. (2020) Catholics call for a national inquiry into UK nursing home deaths. *Catholic News Agency* 23 May. Available at: https://www. catholicnewsagency.com/news/44616/catholics-call-for-public-inquiry-into-uk-nursing-home-deaths (Last accessed 5 May 2022).

Pullicino, P. (2023) Relatives must be empowered in end-of-life care decisions. *TCW Defending Freedom (formerly The Conservative Woman).* 7 March. Available at: https://www.conservativewoman.co.uk/relatives-must-have-priority-in-end-of-life-care-decisions/ (Last accessed 15 March 2023).

Purba, A.K. (2020) How should the role of the nurse change in response to Covid-19? Coronavirus. Discussion. Available at: https://www.nursingtimes.net/ clinical-archive/public-health-clinical-archive/how-should-the-role-of-the-nurse-change-in-response-to-covid-19-26-05-2020/ (Last accessed 5 May 2022).

Quest, T., Herr, S., Lamba, S. and Weissman, D. (2013) IPAL-EM Advisory Board. Demonstrations of clinical initiatives to improve palliative care in the emergency department: a report from the IPAL-EM Initiative. *Ann. Emerg Med* 61, pp. 661–667.

Raglan, F.J. (1969) Voluntary Euthanasia Bill [H.L.] HL Debate 25 March. Vol. 300 cc1143–1254. Available at: https://api.parliament.uk/historic-hansard/lords/1969/mar/25/voluntary-euthanasia-bill-hl (Last accessed 11 May 2022).

Raines, M.L. (2000) Ethical decision-making in nurses. Relationships among moral reasoning, coping style and ethics stress. *JONAS Health Law Ethics Regul* 2 (1), pp. 29–41.

Ramsey, P. (1968) The morality of abortion. In: Labby, D.H. (1968) (ed.) *Life or Death: Ethics and Options*. University of Washington Press, Seattle and London, pp. 60–93.

Randall, D. (2021) Neutrality is a retreat from this important debate on assisted dying. Letters. *BMJ* 6 October.

RCN (2009) RCN neutral on assisted suicide. July. Available at: http://news.bbc.co.uk/1/hi/health/8167454.stm (Last accessed 29 April 2022).

RCN (2010) Spirituality Survey – Report on members' views on spirituality and spiritual care in nursing practice 24 June 2011. Available at: https://silo.tips/download/rcn-spirituality-survey-a-report-by-the-royal-college-of-nursing-on-members-view (Last accessed 11 May 2022).

RCN (2015) Stress and you: a short guide to coping with pressure and stress. London RCN. Available at: https://www.rcn.org.uk/professional-development/publications/pub-004966 (Last accessed 11 May 2022).

RCN (2017) The UK nursing labour market review, *R Coll Nurs. RCN*, London. Available at: https://www.rcn.org.uk/professional-development/publications/pub-006625 (Last accessed 11 May 2022).

RCN (2018) When someone asks for your assistance to die. RCN guidance on responding to a request to hasten death. *RCN*. 2nd edition. December. Available at: https://www.rcn.org.uk/professional-development/publications/pub-005822 (Last accessed 11 May 2022).

RCN (2019) YouGov/Royal College of Nursing commissioned survey results. *Nursing Workforce*. September. Available at: https://www.rcn.org.uk/professional-development/publications/pub-007927 (Last accessed 11 May 2022).

RCN (2020/2021) SenseMaker: the lived experience of nursing in Northern Ireland during a pandemic. Available at: https://www.rcn.org.uk/professional-development/publications/sensemaker-nursing-in-northern-ireland-during-a-pandemic-2020-2021-uk-pub-009-870 (Last accessed 11 May 2022).

RCN (2020) Beyond the Bursary: Workforce Supply, *RCN*, London. Available at: https://www.rcn.org.uk/professional-development/publications/rcn-beyond-the-bursary-workforce-supply-uk-pub-009319 (Last accessed 11 May 2022).

RCN (2021a) Advice: what to do when staffing levels become a safety risk. *RCN bulletin* 391, Spring. Available at: https://www.rcn.org.uk/get-help/rcn-advice/covid-19-and-staffing-levels (Last accessed 11 May 2022).

RCN (2021b) Staff safety at risk unless nursing shortages are addressed) Available at: https://www.rcn.org.uk/news-and-events/news/uk-staff-safety-at-risk-unless-nursing-shortages-are-addressed-170920 (Last accessed 13 May 2022).

RCOG (2010) Termination of pregnancy for fetal abnormality in England, Scotland and Wales. Available at: https://www-temp.rcog.org.uk/guidance/browse-all-guidance/other-guidelines-and-reports/termination-of-pregnancy-for-fetal-abnormality-in-england-scotland-and-wales/ (Last accessed 29 April 2022).

RCOG (2019) Better for Women report: Improving the health and well-being of girls and women. Available at: https://www.rcog.org.uk/better-for-women#:~:text=Improving%20the%20health%20and%20wellbeing%20of%20girls%20and%20women&text=This%20report%20identifies%20simple%20and,the%20cornerstone%20of%20healthy%20societies (Last accessed 26 July 2022).

RCP (2019) The RCP clarifies its position on assisted dying. Available at: https://www.rcplondon.ac.uk/news/rcp-clarifies-its-position-assisted-dying (Last accessed 29 April 2022).

RCUK (2016) The Respect Process. Available at: https://www.resus.org.uk/respect (Last accessed 28 April 2022).

RCUK (2020) Resuscitation Council UK introduces version 3 of ReSPECT form. Available at: https://www.resus.org.uk/about-us/news-and-events/resuscitation-council-uk-introduces-version-3-respect-form (Last accessed 5 July 2022).

RCUK (2022) CPR Decisions, DNACPR and ReSPECT. Available at: https://www.resus.org.uk/public-resource/cpr-decisions-and-dnacpr (Last accessed 5 July 2022).

Reisman, D. (1997) Foreword. In: Meštrović, S. (ed.) Post emotional Society. London: Sage, pp. 9-10. In: Herdman, A. (2004) Nursing in a post emotional society. *Nursing Philosophy* 5, pp. 95–103.

Rest, J. (1982) A psychologist looks at the teaching of ethics. Hastings Centre Report 12 (1), pp. 29–36.

Right to Life News (2021) Matt Hancock confirms Government 'not recommending' introduction of assisted suicide. Available at: https://righttolife.org.uk/news/matt-hancock-confirms-government-not-recommending-introduction-of-assisted-suicide (Last accessed 5 May 2022).

Ritzer, G. (1993) The McDonaldisation thesis: is expansion inevitable? *International Sociology* 11, pp. 291–309.

Roach, M.S. (1992) The Human Act of Caring: A Blueprint for the Health Professions, Ottawa: Revised Ed. *Canadian Hospital Association.*

Roberts, D. (2008) Learning in clinical practice: the importance of peers. *Nursing Standard* 23, pp. 35–41.

Robertson, D. (2014) Christians warned over 'dangerous' new secularism. *The Christian Institute.* 26 May.

Robinson, C. (2020) Marie Stopes International hoping to recruit more students into abortion care'. *Right to Life.*

Robinson, P. (2022) Deafening Silences: propaganda through censorship, smearing and coercion. Coronavirus, UK Column, 20 September. Available at: https://www.ukcolumn.org/article/deafening-silences-propaganda-through-censorship-smearing-and-coercion (Last accessed 28 September 2022).

Rodney, P. and Varcoe, C. (2001) Towards ethical enquiry in the economic evaluation of nursing practice. *Can J Nurs Res* 33, pp. 35–57.

Rollins, M.D. and Rosen, M.A. (2014) Anaesthesia for fetal surgery and other intrauterine procedures. Available at: https://pubmed.ncbi.nlm.nih.gov/11754150/ (Last accessed 11 May 2022). In: *Chestnut, D.H. (ed.), Chestnut's Obstetric Anaesthesia Principles and Practice. 5th ed. Philadelphia PA: Elsevier Saunders, pp. 128–147.*

Roman Catholic Diocese of Westminster (2020) Catholic Church issues guidelines for Catholics on organ donation following change in the law. Available at: https://rcdow.org.uk/news/catholic-church-issues-guidelines-for-catholics-on-organ-donation-following-change-in-the-law/ (Last accessed 26 July 2022).

Rose, D. (2010) 'Watchdog closes care homes over fears for "the very basics of life"'. *The Times,* 29 September.

Rose, L. (2018) The myth of secular neutrality. The Christian Coalition for Education Conference in Oxford, Saturday 24 November. In: *Anglican Mainstream, an information resource for Orthodox Anglicans (2018) 26 November.* Available at: https://anglicanmainstream.org/the-myth-of-secular-neutrality/ (Last accessed 11 May 2022).

Rose, L. (2023) Description Executive Summary. When 'End of Life Care' Goes Wrong – Lords and Commons Printed Report. *Voice for Justice UK.* Available at: https://vfjuk.org/product/when-end-of-life-care-goes-wrong-report/ Last accessed 17 March 2023).

Rosenstein, D. (2011) Depression and end of life care for patients with cancer. Available at: https://www.ncbi.nlm.nih.gov/pmc/articles/PMC3181973/ (Last accessed 11 May 2022).

Roush, K. (2011) Speaking out on social justice. *Am. J. Nurs.* 111 (8), p 11.

Rudge, C. (2017) Ex-transplant chief: my doubts about new donor plans. In: Templeton, K., Health Editor. *The Sunday Times* 8 October. Available at: https://www.dailymail.co.uk/news/article-4960272/Ex-transplant-chief-says-WON-T-donate-plans-ahead.html (Last accessed 11 May 2022).

Rudman, A. and Gustavsson, J.P. (2011) Early-career burnout among new graduate nurses: a prospective observational study of intra-individual change trajectories. *Int J Nurs Stud.* (2011), Mar 48 (3), pp. 292–306. Available at: https://pubmed.ncbi.nlm.nih.gov/20696427/ (Last accessed 29 April 2022).

Saad, L. (2013) U.S. Support for Euthanasia Hinges on How It's Described. Support is at low ebb on the basis of wording that mentions "suicide". Available at: https://news.gallup.com/poll/162815/support-euthanasia-hinges-described.aspx (Last accessed 29 April 2022).

Saarto, T. and Wiffen, P.J. (2007) Antidepressants for neuropathic pain. *Cochrane Database Syst Rev*:CD005454. [PubMed] [Reference list]. In: *Fitridge R, Thompson M, editors (2011). Mechanisms of Vascular Disease: A Reference Book for Vascular Specialists [Internet].* Adelaide (AU): University of Adelaide Press. Chapter 22. Schug, S. and Stannard, K.J.D. Treatment of Neuropathic Pain.

Samuel, J. (2023) Universities can cancel your degree for wrongthink – and there's no real right to appeal. The Daily Telegraph, 11 February. P. 19.

Santayana, G. (1905) In: The Life of Reason: 1) Reason in Common Sense, p 284 *Indypublish.com (2008)* Available at: https://santayana.iupui.edu/wp-content/uploads/2019/01/Common-Sense-ebook.pdf (Last accessed 29 April 2022).

Saunders, C. (2000) The evolution of palliative care. *Patient Education and Counselling* 41 (1), August, pp. 7–13.

Savulescu, J. (2006) Conscientious objection in medicine, analysis and comment. Ethics. *BMJ* 332, pp. 294–297.

Scally, G. and Donaldson, L.J. (1998) Clinical governance and the drive for quality improvement in the new NHS in England. *BMJ* 317, pp. 61–65.

Schantz, M. (2007) Compassion: a concept analysis. *Nursing Forum* 42 (2), pp. 48–55.

Schneider, M.P. (2020) Vaccines and Doubly Remote Cooperation in Evil. Public Discourse: *The Journal of the Witherspoon Institute.* Bioethics, Coronavirus, Healthcare, Vaccines, 22 November. Available at: https://www.thepublicdiscourse.com/2020/11/72866/ (Last accessed 15 May 2022).

Scott, J. (1995) Fear and false promises: the challenge of pain in the terminally ill. In: Gentles, I. (ed.) (1995) *Euthanasia and Assisted Suicide: The Current Debate.* Stoddart Books, Toronto. p 96.

Scott, P.A. (2000) Emotion, moral perception and nursing practice. Nursing Philosophy 1, pp. 123–133. In: Herdman, E.A. (2004) Nursing in a post emotional society. *Nursing Philosophy* 5, pp. 95–103.

Scott, B.J., Gentile, M.A., Bennett, S.N., Couture, M. and MacIntyre, N.R. (2013) Apnea testing during brain death assessment: a review of clinical practice and published literature. *Respiratory Care*, March 58 (3), pp. 532–538. Available at: https://doi.org/10.4187/respcare.01962 (Last accessed 29 April 2022).

Scriptorum, G. (pen name) (2019) Book Review: APOLOGIA PRO VITA SUA by John Henry Newman. *Catholic Medical Quarterly.* Available at: http://www.cmq.org.uk/CMQ/2019/Feb/CMQ%20feb%202019_A4%20CMQ%20FINAL.pdf (Last accessed 1 May 2022).

Seale, C. (2009) Continuous deep sedation in medical practice: a descriptive study. Centre for Health Sciences, *Barts and the London School of Medicine and Dentistry, Queen Mary University of London,* London, United Kingdom. Available at: https://pubmed.ncbi.nlm.nih.gov/19854611/ (Last accessed 1 May 2022).

Second Vatican Council (1965) Pastoral Constitution on the Church in the Modern World. Papal Encyclical (promulgated by his holiness Pope Paul VI): Gaudium et Spes (Joy and hope) 27. 7 December. Available at: https://

www.vatican.va/archive/hist_councils/ii_vatican_council/documents/vat-ii_const_19651207_gaudium-et-spes_en.html (Last accessed 1 May 2022).

Senek, M., Robertson, S., Ryan, T., King, R., Wood, E., Taylor, B. and Tod, A. (2020) Determinants of nurse job dissatisfaction – findings from a cross-sectional survey analysis in the UK. *BMC Nurs* 19 88 (2020) Available at: https://doi.org/10.1186/s12912-020-00481-3 (Last accessed 4 May 2022).

Sevenhuijsen, S. (2000a) Caring in the third way: the relation between obligation, responsibility and care in third way discourse. *Critical Social Policy*. Sage Publications: London. p 12.

Sevenhuijsen, S. (2000b) Caring in the third way: the relation between obligation, responsibility and care in Third Way discourse. *Critical Social Policy*. Sage Publications: London. p 5.

Seymour, J. and Clark, D. (2018) The Liverpool Care Pathway for the Dying Patient: a critical analysis of its rise, demise and legacy in England. *Wellcome Open Res*. Available at: https://pubmed.ncbi.nlm.nih.gov/29881785/ (Last accessed 30 July 2022).

Shakespeare, W. (1592-3) Richard III (V.iv.1.7.)

Shakespeare, W. (1592-3) King Lear (Act II, Scene 4)

Shaw, D. and Morton, A. (2020) Counting the cost of denying assisted dying. *The Journal of Clinical Ethics* 10 March. London, Sage Journals. Available at: https://journals.sagepub.com/doi/abs/10.1177/1477750920907996 (Last accessed 9 April 2022).

Shelley, P. B. (1820) Prometheus Unbound, A Lyrical Drama in Four Acts with Other Poems (1 ed.) London: C and J Ollier. Retrieved 21 May 2015. via Internet Archive. Available at: https://archive.org/details/prometheusunboun00shelrich (Last accessed 9 April 2022).

Sherrington, J. (2021) Don't let 'false compassion' legalise assisted suicide, say bishops of England and Wales. Catholic News Agency. Available at: https://www.catholicnewsagency.com/news/247835/dont-let-false-compassion-legalise-assisted-suicide-say-bishops (Last accessed 11 May 2022).

Shorter, T. (2023) The ruthless tactics of the nursing strike have harmed a valid cause. *Letters to the Editor. The Daily Telegraph*, 2 May.

Sinclair, S., Beamer, K., Hack, T.F. McClement, S., Raffin Bouchal, S., Chochinov, H.M. and Hagen, N.A. (2017) Sympathy, empathy and compassion: A grounded theory study of palliative care patients' understandings, experiences and preferences. Available at: https://pubmed.ncbi.nlm.nih.gov/27535319 Epub (2016) (Last accessed 29 April 2022).

Singh, I. (2018) Debate: The Conscientious Objection (Medical Activities) Bill. *House of Lords*, Available at: https://hansard.parliament.uk/lords/2018-01-26/debates/C4A11F08-ABCF-4EA1-AFB5-18174224A982/ConscientiousObjection(MedicalActivities)Bill(HL) (Last accessed 1 May 2022).

Smith, C.M. (2005) Origin and uses of *primum non nocere* – (above all, do no harm!) *J Clin Pharmacol*, Apr 45 (4), pp. 371–377.

Smith, W. (2017) Euthanasia virus spreads to Australia. *National review. The Corner, politics and policy*. Available at: https://www.nationalreview.com/corner/euthanasia-virus-spreads-australia/ (Last accessed 1 May 2022).

Smith, K. and Godfrey, N. (2002) Being a good nurse and doing the right thing: a qualitative study. *Nursing Ethics* 9 (3), pp. 301–310.

Sodexo (2021) How to improve company culture. Available at: https://uk.sodexo.com/inspired-thinking/insights/improve-company-culture-through-food.html?t=1&utm_source=google&utm_medium=cpc&utm_campaign=UK_CS_GS_PSP_Workplace&utm_content=134746897171&utm_term=improve%20workplace%20culture&gclid=Cj0KCQjw37iTBhCWAR IsACBt1IxAoJgWVUBfMGIv-6mhHKY4XJoEyEjCwHIzcmSIlA7xu8o-ADLeONQaAuxBEALw_wcB (Last accessed 1 May 2022).

Solzhenitsyn, A.I. (1973) *The Gulag Archipelago.* 1st ed. Harper and Row: New York.

Society for the Protection of Unborn Children. (2021) Nobody should have to pass a test to deserve to exist. 'Preborn babies don't have to prove their worth to us': NFL Super Bowl winner Benjamin Watson champions the unborn. Available at: https://www.spuc.org.uk/Article/385009/Preborn-babies-dont-have-to-prove-their-worth-to-us-NFL-Super-Bowl-winner-Benjamin-Watson-champions-the-unborn (Last accessed 1 May 2022).

Somerville, M. (2021) We need to offer alternatives to legalising euthanasia. Mercatornet, Euthanasia. 29 October. Available at: https://mercatornet.com/we-need-to-offer-alternatives-to-legalising-euthanasia/75541/ (Last accessed 1 May 2022).

Somerville, E. (2023) University cancels Lent because 'it's too Christian'. The Daily Telegraph, 30 January. P. 9.

Spiegelhalter D. and Best N. (2004) Shipman's statistical legacy. Significance. *Royal Statistical Society: Data, Evidence, Decisions.* 1: pp. 10–12. Available at: https://rss.onlinelibrary.wiley.com/doi/abs/10.1111/j.1740-9713.2004.00002.x (Last accessed 13 May 2022).

Spooner, A. (2001) Mini Oxford School Thesaurus (Dictionary)

Sprinks, J. (2012) Trust says shorter shifts will give nurses more time at the bedside. Nursing Standard 27 (7), p 8.

Stack, M. (2022) It is not the healthy who need a doctor but the sick (Mark 2:17). Further reflections by a retired hospital chaplain©. P. 16. With permission from the author. Lent. UK. IBSN 978- 1-5272-354-9

Stanford Encyclopaedia of Philosophy (2018a) Aristotle's Ethics *First published Tue May 1 2001. Substantive revision Fri Jun 15, 2018.* pp. 20–22.

Stanford University Encyclopaedia of Philosophy (2018b) Voluntary Euthanasia. *Plato.stanford.edu. Metaphysics Research Lab.* USA. Available at: https://plato.stanford.edu/contents.html (Last accessed 1 May 2019).

St John Henry Newman (1875) *On occasion of Mr Gladstone's recent expostulation.* Chapter 5, p 75. The Catholic Publication Society. London.

St John of the Cross (2009) Dichos 64. Catechism of the Catholic Church. Section 12. 1022. http://www.catholic-catechism.com/ccc_1022.htm (Last accessed 2 August 2022).

Sundin-Huard, D. and Fahy, K. (1999) Moral distress, advocacy, and burnout: theorizing the relationships. *International Journal of Nursing Practice.* 5(1) pp. 8–13.

Sutherland, M. (2021) Euthanasia: you can put lipstick on a pig, but a pig it remains. Contemporary euthanasia is an updated version of early 20th century eugenics. Mercatornet 22 September. Available at: https://mercatornet.com/euthanasia-you-can-put-lipstick-on-a-pig-but-a-pig-it-remains/74831/ (Last accessed 9 April 2022).

Symons, X. (2019) Is the campaign for euthanasia a product of neoliberalism? Bio Edge, bioethics news from around the world. 30 March. Available at: https://bioedge.org/uncategorized/is-the-campaign-for-euthanasia-a-byproduct-of-neoliberalism/ (Last accessed 9 April 2022).

Symons, X. (2021) Are people with advanced dementia still persons? Dementia can yield a richer understanding of what it means to be a person. Mercatornet: Bioethics. 21 October. Available at: https://www.google.com/search?q=Dementia+can+yield+a+richer+understanding+of+what+it+means+to+be+a+person.+Mercatornet%3A+Bioethics.&rlz=1C1CHBF_en-GBGB900GB900&oq=Dementia+can+yield+a+richer+understanding+of+what+it+means+to+be+a+person.+Mercatornet%3A+Bioethics.&aqs=chrome.69i57.5672j0j4&sourceid=chrome&ie=UTF-8 (Last accessed 9 April 2022).

Tabouada, P. (2008) Ordinary and Extraordinary Means of the Preservation of Life: The Teaching of Moral Tradition. *Catholic Culture*. A Conference dictated during the International Scientific Congress: "Accanto al malato inguaribile e al morente: aspetti scientifici ed etici". XIV General Assembly, Pontifical Academy for Life (Roma, 25-27 Febrero 2008). Available at: https://www.catholicculture.org/culture/library/view.cfm?recnum=8772 (Last accessed 13 December 2022).

Tallo, D. (2016) The principles and practice of palliative care in the year of mercy. Summary: Catholic Medical Association. Annual Conference. *Catholic Medical Quarterly* 66 (4).

Tasioulos, J. (2017) Are human rights anything more than legal conventions? Available at: https://aeon.co/ideas/are-human-rights-anything-more-than-legal-conventions (Last accessed 2 May 2022).

Taylor, C. and White, S. (2000) *Practising reflexivity in health and welfare: making knowledge.* Open University Press: Buckingham, UK.

TCW defending freedom (2021) Scientists warn of 'premature and reckless' vaccine rollout. Available at: https://www.conservativewoman.co.uk/scientists-warn-of-premature-and-reckless-vaccine-rollout/ (Last accessed 8 April 2022)

The Daily Telegraph (2023) More people should go private, not fewer. Thursday, 12 January.

The Guardian (2012) NHS accused of deaths of disabled patients: Mencap inquiry finds institutional discrimination against people with learning disabilities led to at least 74 deaths. Available at: https://www.theguardian.com/society/2012/jan/02/nhs-accused-disabled-patient-deaths (Last accessed 29 April 2022).

The Imaginative Conservative (2011) Aleksandr Solzhenitsyn on the Spiritual Life of a Nation. Available at: https://theimaginativeconservative.org/2011/03/aleksandr-solzhenitsyn-spiritual-life.html (Last accessed 6 July 2022).

The Week Staff (2020) What are the pros and cons of 'opt out' organ donation? All adults in England are automatically organ donors from today. Available at: https://www.theweek.co.uk/35635/automatic-organ-donation-the-pros-and-cons (Last accessed 1 May 2022).

Thomas, G. (2016) a brief history of Nursing in the UK. Available at: https://memoriesofnursing.uk/wp-content/uploads/A-Brief-History-of-Nursing-in-the-UK.pdf (Last accessed 30 April 2022).

Thomas, K. (2007) Briefing Paper on the Gold Standards Framework in Care Homes (GSFCH) Programme. 12 March. Gold Standards Framework National Team, Birmingham. In: *Hansford, P., Meehan, H. (2007) Gold Standards Framework: improving community care. Clinical Practice Development. End of Life Care* 1 (3) Available at: https://www.goldstandards framework.org.uk/cd-content/uploads/files/Library%2C%20Tools%20%26%20resources/Gold%20Standards%20Framework%20-%20improving%20community%20care.pdf. (Last accessed 28 April 2022).

Thomas, W.I. and Thomas, T.S. (1928) The child in America: Behavior problems and programs. Knopf: New York. pp. 571–572.

Thorns, A. and Sykes, N. (2000) Opioid use in last week of life and implications for end of life decision making. *The Lancet* 356 29 July. pp. 398–399.

Tomaschewski-Barlem, J.G., Lerch Lunardi, V., Davos Barlem, E.L., Ramos, A.M., Belletti Figueira, A. and Cerutti Fornari, N. (2015) Nursing beliefs and actions in exercising patient advocacy in a hospital context. *Rev Esc Enferm* USP 49 (5), pp. 811–818.

Tourani. S., Khosravizadeh, O., Omrani, A. and Sokhanvar, M. (2016) The relationship between organisational justice and turnover intention of hospital nurses in Iran. *Materia Sociomedica* 28 (3), pp. 205–209. Available at: https://www.researchgate.net/publication/303798475_The_Relationship_between_Organizational_Justice_and_Turnover_intention_of_Hospital_Nurses_in_Iran/link/57552ff308ae17e65eccd3c1/download (Last accessed 28 April 2022).

Treloar, A. (2018) Care of dying children and adults. Ethics, principles and issues for law reform. *Catholic Medical Quarterly* 68 (3), pp. 13–17. Available at: http://cmq.org.uk/CMQ/2018/Aug/CMQ%20AUG%202018%20FINAL.pdf (Last accessed 3 May 2022).

Treloar, A. (2020a) Catholics call for a national inquiry into UK nursing home deaths. Available at: https://www.catholicnewsagency.com/news/44616/catholics-call-for-public-inquiry-into-uk-nursing-home-deaths (Last accessed 28 April 2022).

Treloar, A. (2020b) The beginning of the end for catholic emancipation? *Editorial, Catholic Medical Quarterly* 70 (1) Available at: http://www.cmq.

org.uk/CMQ/2020/Feb/beginning_of_the_end_of_catholic.html (Last accessed 24 April 2022).

Trufin, F. (2021) In: *Devos, T. (ed.), Euthanasia: Searching for the full story. Experiences and insights of Belgian Doctors and Nurses.* New York City. Springer. Available at: https://library.oapen.org/bitstream/id/7114f6e0-c25e-4a23-9b31-42694608b619/9783030567958.pdf (Last accessed 3 May 2022).

Turner, J. (2019) Physician, heal thyself and why doctors won't. *The Physician Philosopher* 17 September. Available at: https://thephysicianphilosopher.com/physician-heal-thyself/ (Last accessed 3 May 2022).

Twomey, D.V. (2019) Newman on conscience. Opinions, Letters. *The Irish Times* 21 October. Available at: https://www.irishtimes.com/opinion/letters/newman-on-conscience-1.4056789 (Last accessed 3 May 2022).

Tylee, A. and Gandhi, P. (2005) The importance of somatic symptoms in depression in primary care. *Prim Care Companion J Clin Psychiatry* 2005 7 (4), pp. 167–176. Available at: https://www.ncbi.nlm.nih.gov/pmc/articles/PMC1192435/ (Last accessed 2 May 2022).

UKCC (2000) Project 2000 A new preparation for practice. Available at: https://discovered.ed.ac.uk/discovery/fulldisplay?vid=44UOE_INST:44UOE_VU2&tab=Everything&docid=alma993446453502466&query=sub,exact,Nurses%20--%20Supply%20and%20demand%20--%20Great%20Britain&context=L&lang=en (Last accessed 5 May 2022).

UK cancer incidence data (2020)

England – Office of National Statistics (ONS) available at: www.ons.gov.uk

Scotland – Information Services Division ISD Available at: https://beta.isdscotland.org

Wales – Wales Cancer Intelligence and Surveillance Unit (WCISU) Available at: http://www.wcisu.wales.nhs.uk

Northern Ireland – Queens University Belfast, Northern Ireland Cancer Registry In: Urology News. (2020) October.

UK Association of Catholic Nurses and UK Catholic Medical Association (2022). Protocol for Care of the Dying Patient. A reference document for specific guidance on required details of holistic, palliative care. Catholic Medical Quarterly, Available at http://www.cmq.org.uk/CMQ/2022/May/Protocol-for-care-of-dying-2022.pdf (Last accessed 11 July 2022).

UN (1989) Convention on the Rights of the Child. (Entry into force 2 September 1990) *Office of the High Commissioner for Human Rights (OHCHR)* Available at: https://www.ohchr.org/en/instruments-mechanisms/instruments/convention-rights-child (Last accessed 3 May 2022).

UN (2015) Universal Declaration of Human Rights. Available at: https://www.un.org/en/udhrbook/pdf/udhr_booklet_en_web.pdf (Last accessed 14 May 2022).

UN Charter (2016) Chapter IX: International Economic and Social Co-operation. Article 55. *Office of the High Commissioner for Human Rights (OHCHR)*. Available at: https://legal.un.org/repertory/art55.shtml (Last accessed 26 July 2022).

Uniform Determination of Death Act (UDDA) (1981) *National Conference of Commissioners on Uniform State Laws*. Available at: https://www.uniformlaws.org/HigherLogic/System/DownloadDocumentFile.ashx?DocumentFileKey=4d19d096-be64-3c0f-ae71-a514b64c06a6&forceDialog=0 (Last accessed 3 May 2022).

University of Leicester (2016) Research: NHS policies failing to stop bullying by managers and staff sickness. Available at: https://le.ac.uk/news/2016/january/study-suggests-nhs-policies-are-failing-to-stop-bullying-by-managers-and-staff-sickness (Last accessed 3 May 2022).

Urology News (2020) UK cancer incidence data. COVID-19 cuts prostate cancer referrals in half. Available at: https://www.urologynews.uk.com/features/features/post/covid-19-cuts-prostate-cancer-referrals-in-half (Last accessed 3 May 2022).

Valko, N. (2007) Whatever happened to common sense at the end of life? *Bioethics Watch, Voices Online Edition*, Women for Faith and Family 22 (3) Available at: http://archive.wf-f.org/07-3-Valko_EndOfLifeIssues.html (Last accessed 11 May 2022).

Valko, N. (2012) Letter from Dr. Truog on why he doesn't have an organ donor card – *Letters to the Editor* – WSJ.com.

Valko, N. (2017) The changing rules on organ donation. A nurse's perspective on life, healthcare and ethics. Available at: https://nancyvalko.com/2017/10/26/the-changing-rules-for-organ-donation/ (Last accessed 8 April 2022).

Van der Arend, A.J.G. and Van den Hurk, C.H.M. (1995) Morele problemen de verplegingen verzorging. Maastricht: Rijsuniverseteit Limburg/Landelijk Centrum Verpleging & Verzoging. In: Georges J .and Grypdonck M. (2002) Moral problems experienced by nurses when caring for terminally ill people: a literature review. *Nursing Ethics 9 (2), March, pp. 155–178*. Abstract available at: https://pubmed.ncbi.nlm.nih.gov/11944206/ (Last accessed 11 May 2022).

Van de Velde, M. and De Buck, F. (2012) Fetal and maternal analgesia/anesthesia for fetal procedures. *Fetal Diagn Ther 31* (4), pp. 201–209. Epub 2012. 25 Apr. Available at: https://pubmed.ncbi.nlm.nih.gov/22538233/ (Last accessed 1 May 2022).

Varden, E. (2018) The Shattering of Loneliness: On Christian Remembrance. Bloomsbury Publishing: London.

Vernon, P. (2021) 10 Black Britons everyone should know about. *The Big Issue*, Issue 1484.

Watt H. (2016) The Ethics of Pregnancy: Exploring Moral Choices in Childbearing. New York: Routledge.

Watt, H (2022) Conscientious objection. Talk given online: Catholics in Health and Social Care: Ethics and Practice. 14 May. *St Mary's University, Twickenham, the Anscombe Bioethics Centre and the Bios Centre*.

Watt, H. (2022) Rapid response to: Overturning Roe v Wade has had an immediate chilling effect on reproductive healthcare. Available at: https://www.bmj.com/content/377/bmj.o1622/rr (Last accessed 26 July 2022).

Weaver K. (2007) Ethical sensitivity: state of knowledge and needs for further research. Research Article. *Nursing Ethics* 14 (2) 1 March. London. Sage Publications. Available at: https://journals.sagepub.com/doi/10.1177/0969733007073694 (Last accessed 4 May 2022).

Webb, C. (2017) St Christophers Hospice – Pharmacy presentation. Common Symptoms in the dying person: individualised methods of relief. *Nursing conference: Patient Advocacy,* 8 May. Held at the RCN.

Wee, M. (2019) The Tafida Raqeeb case and the trouble with 'best interests. Editorial: *Catholic Medical Quarterly* 69 (4), p 5.

Weinstock D. (2014) Conscientious refusal and health professionals: does religion make a difference? *Bioethics*; 28 (1): pp. 8–15.

Wenrich, D.M., Randall, J., Shannon, S.E., Carline, J.D., Donna, M., Ambrozy, D.M. and Ramsey, P.G. (2001) Communicating With Dying Patients Within the Spectrum of Medical Care from Terminal Diagnosis to Death. *JAMA Internal Medic*ine. Original Investigation. Available at: https://jamanetwork.com/journals/jamainternalmedicine/fullarticle/647723 (Last accessed 4 May 2022).

West, M. and Coia, D. (2019) Caring for doctors, caring for patient. How to transform UK healthcare environments to support doctors and medical students to care for patients. *General Medical Council,* London GMC. Available at: https://www.gmc-uk.org/-/media/documents/caring-for-doctors-caring-for-patients_pdf-80706341.pdf (Last accessed 1 May 2022).

White, F. (2019) US doctors vote to oppose assisted suicide. *Bio Edge*. Bioethics news from around the world. Available at: https://bioedge.org/end of life-issues/us-doctors-vote-to-oppose-assisted-suicide/ (Last accessed 1 May 2022).

WHO (2011) Palliative care for older people: better practices. Edited by Hall, S., Petkova, H., Tsouros, A.D., Costantini, M. and Higginson, I. Available at: https://www.euro.who.int/en/publications/abstracts/palliative-care-for-older-people-better-practices. (Last accessed 9 July 2021).

WHO (2017) Facilitating evidence-based practice in nursing and midwifery in the WHO European Region. Available at: https://www.euro.who.int/en/health-topics/Health-systems/nursing-and-midwifery/publications/2017/facilitating-evidence-basedpractice-in-nursing-and-midwifery-in-the-who-european-region-2017 (Last accessed 30 April 2022).

Whyte, L. and Gajos, M. (1996) A study of nurses' knowledge of the (UKCC) code of conduct. *Nursing Standard* 47 (1), pp. 35–39.

Wilkinson, J. (1987) Moral distress in nursing practice: experience and effect. *Nursing Forum, an independent voice for nursing. Nurs Forum.* 1987–1988; 23(1), 16–29. Wiley Online Library.

Wilmot, S. (2001) Nurses and whistleblowing: the ethical issues. *J American Nursing. Leading Global Nursing Research* 32 (5) 25 December. Abstract available at: https://pubmed.ncbi.nlm.nih.gov/11114987/ (Last accessed 11 May 2022).

Wilmot, S., Legg, l., Barratt, J. (2002) Ethical issues in the feeding of patients suffering from dementia: a focus group study of hospital staff responses to conflicting principles. Available at: https://journals.sagepub.com/doi/10.1191/0969733002ne554oa (Last accessed 1 May 2022).

Williams, A. (2022) Archie Battersbee: 'Why we supported his family's legal battle'. 22 July. *Christian Concern*. https://christianconcern.com/comment/archie-battersbee-he-deserves-a-fighting-chance/ (Last accessed 2 August 2023).

Winston, R. (2021) Assisted Dying Bill [HL] (Meacher Bill.) (Vol 815) Debated on 22 October. Hansard UK Parliament. Available at: https://hansard.parliament.uk/lords/2021-10-22/debates/11143CAF-BC66-4C60-B782-38B5D9F42810/AssistedDyingBill(HL) (Last accessed 11 May 2022).

Wolf, Z. and Zuzelo, P. (2006) 'Never again' stories of nurses: dilemmas in nursing practice. *Qualitative Health Research* 1 November 16 (9), pp. 1191–1206.

Wood, E., King, R., Senek, M., Robertson, S., Taylor, B., Tod, A. and Ryan, A. (2020) UK Advanced Practice Nurses experiences of the COVID-19 pandemic: a mixed-methods cross-sectional study. Available at: https://pubmed.ncbi.nlm.nih.gov/33727270/ (Last accessed 30 April 2022).

WMA (2021) *The International Code of Medical Ethics*. A proposed revision of the international code governing the duties of physicians. Available at: https://www.wma.net/news-post/physicians-code-of-ethics-updated/ (Last accessed 30 April 2022).

WMA (2023) International Code of Medical Ethics, 14 April. *World Medical Association*. Available at: https://www.wma.net/policies-post/wma-international-code-of-medical-ethics/#:~:text=In%20providing%20medical%20care%2C%20the,the%20patient's%20values%20and%20preferences. (Last accessed 13 May 2023).

Wuest, J. (1997) Illuminating environmental influences on women's caring. *Journal of Advanced Nursing* 26, pp. 49–58.

Wurster, M. (2018) What does the Bible teach about euthanasia and physician assisted suicide? *Ethics and Religious Liberty Commission*. Available at: https://erlc.com/resource-library/articles/what-does-the-bible-teach-about-euthanasia-and-physician-assisted-suicide/ (Last accessed 30 April 2022).

Wyatt, J. (2021) What's wrong with the Assisted Dying Bill? End of life in depth series. *Christian Action, Research and Education* (CARE) Available at: https://care.org.uk/cause/assisted-suicide/whats-wrong-with-the-assisted-dying-bill (Last accessed 16 April 2022).

Xianyu, Y. and Lambert, V. (2006) Investigation of the relationships among workplace stressors, ways of coping and the mental health of Chinese head nurses. *Nursing and Health Science* 8, pp. 147–155.

Yanke, G., Rady, M.Y., Verheiljde, J and McGregor J. (2020) Apnea Testing is Medical Treatment Requiring Informed Consent. *The American Journal of Bioethics*. *JAMA Network JAMA neurology*. Published online: 22 May 2020. 20:6, 22–24, DOI: 10.1080/15265161.2020.1754509. Available at: https://jamanetwork.com/journals/jamaneurology/fullarticle/781174 (Last accessed 17 November 2022).).

Yeadon, J. (2021) Ex-Pfizer science chief: you are being lied to about Covid, TCW defending freedom. (Formerly *The Conservative Woman*). Available at: https://www.conservativewoman.co.uk (Last accessed 8 April 2022).

About the Author

The wonderful parable of the Good Samaritan encourages nurses to firmly commit to the sometimes-challenging role of the patient advocate.

Nurse-patient advocacy requires respect and support from the profession as an inevitable right of all those, whether Christian or not, who are committed to ethical patient care. Our aggressively secular age can often pose a risk to patient advocacy and true care.

A long-held interest in nursing ethics, holistic patient care and patient advocacy has been developed over years in nursing, together with an interest in medical anthropology and medico-legal issues.

A nursing career, covering elderly care, oncology, palliative care, and nurse education, all experienced in both NHS and private healthcare settings, developed an interest in nurse-patient advocacy. Research undertaken during MSc studies, investigated this important role.

Due to worrying healthcare developments such as the LCP, a need was identified for the creation of a national nursing network for education and support for those nurses opposed to euthanasia, who wished to promote life, and advocate for compassionate and positive care for the true benefit of their patients.

Responsibility for acting as the patient advocate, or Good Samaritan, in all care settings, must be considered as a privileged role for nurses at all levels of the profession.

"This detailed work has been written for the nursing profession. As such, it offers a great deal of wisdom about the background to the profession as it is now and, in particular, its Christian inspiration and commitment. It also highlights the moral dilemmas faced by professionals in this area and suggests compassionate but principled responses to these. It alerts, both professionals and others, to developments that may work against the welfare of patients and the cornerstone principles of doing good and not harm in the practice of medicine. The traditional commitment here of respect for the person and the valuing of life at all its stages is congruent with the teaching of the Catholic Church and Catholics and other Christians should uphold it in every way that they can.

There is an emphasis on the wholeness of approach in both the curative and the caring aspects of the profession. The nurse, especially, must be seen to be one who values patients as persons, who keeps their best interests in mind and who intercedes for them both with the divine and with authority in the medical world.

Teresa has not been afraid to tackle the most difficult issues in her extensive work and always with her loyalty to the best in the nursing tradition and to authentic Christian teaching.

Those not in her profession, such as clergy, moral theologians, seminary teachers etc, will also benefit from the thoroughness of this book which will become a compendium not only of good nursing practice but also of serious moral issues to be addressed in the world of medicine. For this service, we should all be grateful to her".

Msgr Dr Michael Nazir-Ali.
OXTRAD: Oxford Centre for Training,
Research, Advocacy & Dialogue.

"Teresa Lynch is a founder member of UK pro-life nurses who are opposed to Euthanasia. A Christian nurse, she has a great knowledge of nursing and the professional expectations of both Christian and non-Christian nurses, regarding the sanctity of human life, especially relating to assisted suicide and euthanasia.

I was very pleased to see her interesting book with the inspiring title of: *The Good Samaritan Nurse in a secular age.* This is a needed book for every nurse especially those affected by the culture of death and by the rising and engulfing ideas of secularism.

I believe that many nurses today are becoming more influenced by the culture of death in our society, especially in helping the "doctors" who kill our innocent, unborn babies through abortion.

By looking at the contents of the book, varieties of relevant issues may affect all of us today in our society, especially our nurses and their patients. Assisted suicide is such a current focus of debate, together with the many vital and interesting topics, included in this book, of which all health professionals must be aware.

No doubt, by producing a great book which is very much needed today to address all relevant ethical medical issues, it will be a light to all our nurses in any care setting in order to know about the missing Samaritan.

Nurses and doctors are well placed to provide true care, concern, and compassion for each patient as a unique individual, needing holistic care. I believe Teresa Lynch is a role model by impressing on all health professionals, the vital need for acting as a Good Samaritan. She achieves by this book, her other aim as a role model, to educate nurses and other health professionals in any care setting today about the need to adopt the great qualities and characters of the true Samaritan which are explained well in the book.

I believe this book will appeal also to our Muslim nurses and they can learn a lot from reading it. Many doctors too, will benefit from reading this guidebook on many medical ethical issues. Finally, I sincerely feel that after knowing about this book, I am tempted myself to produce a similar book but for doctors".

Dr A. Majid Katme (MBBCh, DPM).
Retired Psychiatrist, Ex-President of the
Islamic Medical Association UK/UN
Leader of the Pro-life, Pro-family Muslim Campaign.

Milton Keynes UK
Ingram Content Group UK Ltd.
UKHW022314050524
442189UK00008B/130